YOU: ON A DIET

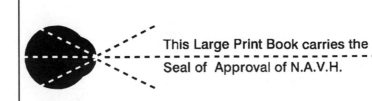

This Large Print Book carries the
Seal of Approval of N.A.V.H.

YOU: ON A DIET

THE OWNER'S MANUAL FOR WAIST MANAGEMENT

MICHAEL F. ROIZEN, MD, AND MEHMET C. OZ, MD

With Ted Spiker, Lisa Oz, and Craig Wynett
Illustrations by Gary Hallgren

THORNDIKE PRESS
An imprint of Thomson Gale, a part of The Thomson Corporation

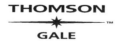

THOMSON
GALE

Detroit • New York • San Francisco • New Haven, Conn. • Waterville, Maine • London

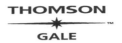

LIBRARY OF CONGRESS CATALOGING-IN-PUBLICATION DATA

You on a diet : the owner's manual for waist management / by Michael F. Roizen . . . [et al.] ; Illustrations by Gary Hallgren. — Large print ed.
    p. cm.
    Includes index.
    ISBN-13: 978-0-7862-9433-6 (hardcover : alk. paper)
    ISBN-10: 0-7862-9433-7 (hardcover : alk. paper)
    1. Low-fat diet. 2. Low-fat diet — Recipes. 3. Weight loss. I. Roizen, Michael F.
RM237.5.R65 2006b
613.2'5—dc22

2006102008

Published in 2007 by arrangement with Free Press, a division of Simon & Schuster, Inc.

Printed in the United States of America on permanent paper
10 9 8 7 6 5 4 3 2 1

Disclaimer

This publication contains the opinions and ideas of its authors. It is intended to provide helpful and informative material on the subjects addressed in the publication. It is sold with the understanding that the authors and publisher are not engaged in rendering medical, health, or any other kind of personal professional services in the book. The reader should consult his or her medical, health, or other competent professional before adopting any of the suggestions in this book or drawing inferences from it.

The authors and publisher specifically disclaim all responsibility for any liability, loss, or risk, personal or otherwise, which is incurred as a consequence, directly or indirectly, of the use and application of any of the contents of this book.

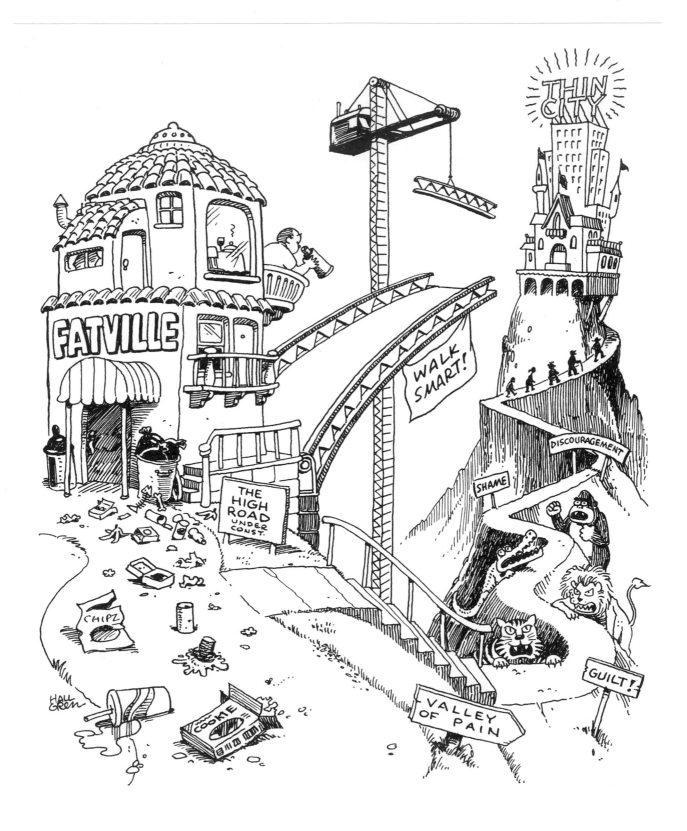

To the millions who have dieted hard,
so they can learn to diet smart

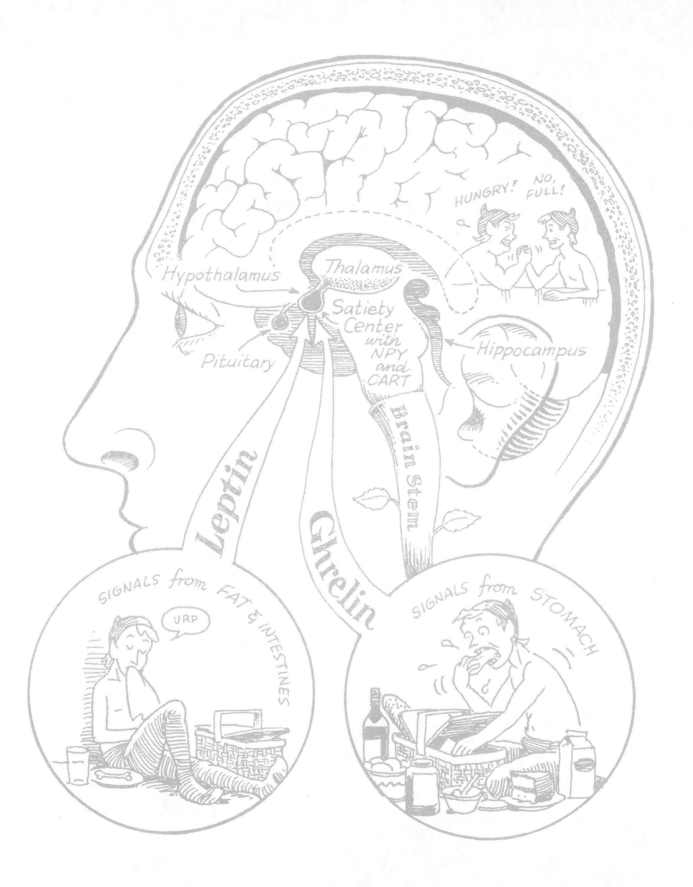

Contents

Part 1: What a Waist!

INTRODUCTION: YOU: ON A DIET 15
Work Smarter, Not Harder

Chapter 1:   The Ideal Body 41
What Your Body Is Supposed to Look Like

Part 2: The Biology of Fat

Chapter 2:   Can't Get No Satisfaction 55
The Science of Appetite

Chapter 3:   Eater's Digest 73
How Food Travels through Your Body

Chapter 4:   Gut Check 97
The Dangerous Battles of Inflammation in Your Belly

Chapter 5:   Taking a Fat Chance 133
How Fat Ruins Your Health

Chapter 6:   Metabolic Motors   165
             Your Body's Hormonal Fat Burners

Chapter 7:   Make the Move   177
             How You Can Burn Fat Faster

Part 3: The Science of the Mind

Chapter 8:   The Chemistry of Emotions   199
             The Connections between Feelings and Food

Chapter 9:   Shame on Who?   209
             The Psychology of the Failed Diet

Part 4: The YOU Diet and Activity Plan

Chapter 10: Make a YOU-Turn   241
             *How to Change What You Thought You Knew about
             Dieting — and Change Your Life for Good*

Chapter 11: The YOU Activity Plan   255
             Physical Strategies for Waist Management

Chapter 12: The YOU Diet.   285
             The Waist-Management Eating Plan

Appendices: The Medical Options

Appendix A: This Is Your Fat on Drugs   377
             The Medical Jump Start to Waist Management

Appendix B: Skinny Skin Skin 391
        When Plastic Surgery Is an Option

Appendix C: The Extreme Team 407
        What to Do if Your Weight Is Out of Control

ACKNOWLEDGMENTS 423
INDEX 429

11

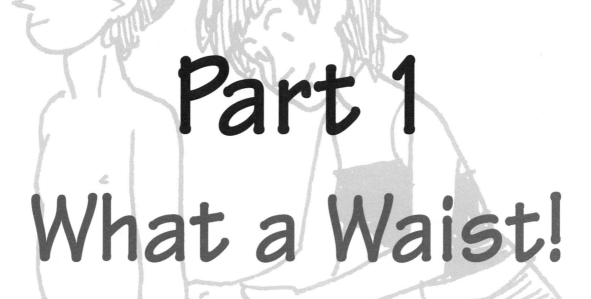

Part 1
What a Waist!

How Your Body Is Supposed to Look — and Work

Introduction
YOU: On a Diet
Work Smarter, Not Harder

Most diets promise commonsense solutions to tight-pants problems: Eat less, and you'll weigh less. Keep your mouth closed, and you'll keep the pounds off. Sweat like a sauna-dwelling sumo wrestler, and you'll wind up skinnier than a sheet of paper. Straightforward enough. But if it really worked that way, our bodies wouldn't be large enough to be spotted by Google Earth. If it really worked that way, then most diets wouldn't fail. If it really worked that way, then we all must be a bunch of rebellious hellions with mayo-covered lips and belt-busting bellies who don't feel like following a few simple instructions.

Or it could be that most diets have it all wrong.

We believe it's the latter.

You know why? Because most diets instruct you to take on the corn chips, meatball specials, and dessert trays with brute force. It's you versus food in a lifetime heavyweight fight. But in that scenario, the fight is always fixed — and not in your favor. That's because the battle against extra pounds isn't won with force, with sweat, with *trying* to diet. It's won with elegance, with smarts, and with healthy choices that become as automatic as a Simon Cowell barb.

When it comes to dieting, trying to whip fat with our weapon of willpower is the food equivalent to holding your breath under water. You can do it for a while, but no matter how psyched up you get, at some point your body — your biology — forces you to the surface gasping for air. And with most diets, your body forces you to gasp (or gulp) for food. No matter how hard you try not to eat, some hidden force deep inside is always prying your mouth back open, making it impossible for willpower to win. Instead of sparring with your waistline, it's time you made your body an ally in the fight against fat.

Our process is to look at our overweight bodies the way scientists would: Identify the underlying biology of the problem, then find the cures. Why? Because we're lucky enough to be in the right place at the right time — a time when the scientific world has just now started to unlock the biological mysteries that have caused us to store fat and gain weight. For the first time in our history, the scientific community is uncovering the medical evidence about food, appetite, and satiety that will allow you to tackle weight problems with the real weapon against fat: knowledge. By making this knowledge simple and accessible, we're going to give you tools and actions to crack the code of true and lifelong waist management. In fact, our plan will help you avoid the dangerous yo-yo cycle of weight gain and weight loss. We're going to help you reprogram your body so that you can keep off the weight you lose forever.

Through the years, many of us have been led to believe that our weight problem is about two things: calorie counting and mental toughness. While some of us may say that the weight problem is too much of the twelve-cheese lasagna, the real problem is that most of us have as much of a clue about how our bodies work as we have about how our cars do. Sure, we know the major parts and generally what they're supposed to do. The real danger of thinking we have most of the answers is that we stop asking the questions. If we look under our hood, do we really understand the systems that make our bodies accelerate to a life of fat and the ones that slam the brake on the dangerous cookie-and-cake collisions that take place every day? Probably not, and that's what we're here to help you learn.

Above all, we're going to teach you that when it comes to dieting, you need to work smart, not hard.

Following our plan, you can expect to drop up to two inches from your waist (or a dress size) within two weeks and see results steadily after that. While the end goal is what many of us look for, we believe that the path you choose to get there is what really dictates whether you make it or not. Our path looks like this:

Part 1: What a Waist! Starting here, we'll talk about our major principles for how the body is designed to work and how our program is geared toward those functions. And we'll also give you the biological ideals of the human body — how our bodies originally looked and functioned. We'll also give you some self-assessment tools for figuring out your own body's ideals. Once you know where you're going, you'll have a better idea of how to get there.

Part 2: The Biology of Fat. Here you'll follow morsels of food from the pantry to the porcelain bowl and everywhere in between. We'll start by exploring the physiology of appetite, and then we'll dive into the science of fat — how we store it, how we burn it, how we fight it. You'll learn what a truly amazing system your body is when you steer it in the right direction through wise nutritional and activity choices.

Part 3: The Science of the Mind. When it comes to overeating, most of us put more emphasis on what we're noshing than on what we're thinking. But you can't discuss weight issues without exploring the scientific and chemical (and even spiritual) reasons why your brain hormones and your emotions drive you to the eight-enchilada special. More important, we'll show you the strategies for making your emotions and the chemicals that drive them work for, not against, your waistline.

Part 4: The YOU Diet and Activity Plan. After you read and learn about the intricacies of your body, you'll find the eating and activity plan that will teach your body to eat and work smart. Your body will become your gym as you gain sleek strength in your body's foundation muscles — all without using weights. And you'll learn to make the right decisions in the supermarket aisle and at the fast-food window. The fourteen-day plan outlines recipes, exercises, and actions you can take to live leaner and healthier.

(In our appendices, we'll explore the medical options for dealing with weight issues — for times when you may plateau, and for those people whose weight problems have led to major medical problems.)

Now, with all the diet information that's circulating today, sometimes it's hard to know what's right, and sometimes it's hard to remember what to do even if it is. That's why we feel that while the program is important, how you learn it — how you ingrain it as part of your lifestyle — is just as vital. As we travel through the four parts of the book, you'll notice various ways you'll learn about your body and how to change it. These are the five main elements we'll use along the way:

YOU-reka Imp

YOU-reka Moments! Like Einstein suddenly realizing that $E = mc^2$ you'll develop deep insights that challenge your preconceptions about diets, about fat, and about your body. In the margin, you'll see our **YOU-reka** imp — the signal that we're about to come upon a moment of enlightenment by busting a myth or explaining something to you about diets that may seem 180 degrees from what you believe is true.

YOUR Body: In parts 2 and 3, as we explore the biology of your body, we'll start each chapter by giving quick biology lessons about what really happens inside your body. We ask that you put on your metaphorical scrubs and gloves as you whiz through your arteries, travel through your intestines, and hang out in your stomach. We'll get up close to your fat so we can see how your body handles it and how it manipulates your body. We believe that by learning about how the inside of your body works, you'll develop the smarts you need to change how the outside looks.

YOU Tests. Through interactive quizzes and measurements, you'll establish baselines for such vital statistics as your ideal body size and your eating personality. And you'll also be able to test for the secret things that could be contributing to a weight problem (get a load of our tongue test on page 95). You can start in a few pages by taking the Fat Facts Test on page 31.

YOU Tips: After we explore the biology of your body to show you what bad things can happen if you make the wrong choice or have cross-wired genetics, we'll immediately give you actions that can help turn your body around. At the end of each chapter, we'll outline intelligent strategies — big and small — for living, eating, and moving in a more healthful way.

The YOU Diet and Activity Plan: In Part 4 (on page 239) we'll detail the specific and simple strategies, recipes, and exercises that will lead you to the body you want — for the rest of your life. The fourteen-day YOU Diet (it's actually so easy that we crafted a seven-day plan that you do twice) and the no-weights-required YOU Workout provide all the tools and instructions you'll need. Best of all, they don't take a lot of time, and they're so easy that you can incorporate them into your life today.

So where do we start? With our first **YOU-reka!** moment: Your body naturally wants to take you to your optimum weight, as long as you don't get in its way.

That's right. For almost everyone, no matter what your genetics, the systems, organs, and processes of your body all want you to function at an ideal weight and size. With the following few principles that we'll develop throughout the book, we're going to teach you how you can make that happen without having to bludgeon yourself in frustration with a butter knife. These are our major principles of achieving your very best and very healthiest body.

YOU Will *Choose* Elegance over Force

Most dieters try to defeat their Oreo/Cheeze Doodle/custard pie infatuations with will, with deprivation, with sweat, with a "my-brain-is-stronger-than-your-crust" attitude. But trying to beat your body with mind power alone may be more painful than passing a melon-size kidney stone. Instead, you have to learn about the systems and actions that influence hunger, satiety, fat storing, and fat burning to fine-tune your corporeal vehicle so it runs on autopilot and takes you to your ultimate destination: a healthy, ideal body. (For those who want to skip ahead, you've probably already peeked at Part 4; however, getting to know the nuances of your body is what will help you achieve and maintain a truly healthy-size body.)

YOU Will Learn How Your Body Thinks

True body improvement is about science. It's about making the leap from witchcraft to hard data, from alchemy to chemistry, from speculation about what works for your body to explanations of how your body actually works. The only way you'll understand the way calories and fat travel from that 2,000-calorie onion loaf to the back of your arm is by bringing alive the physiology of hormones, blood, organs, and muscles — by explaining the processes of digestion, starvation, fat storage, and muscle movements.

FACTOID

When you lose weight without exercise, you lose both muscle and fat, but when you gain weight without exercise, you gain only fat. It's much easier to gain fat weight than it is to gain muscle weight, which is one of the reasons why yo-yo dieting fails so miserably: When you continually gain and lose and gain and lose, you end up gaining proportionally even more fat, because of the muscle loss that takes place every time you lose.

When you understand the magic of physiology and the fun of biology, you'll know what actions to take — and why you're taking them — to reboot your body back to where it wants to be. Just as when you're trying to help a tantruming toddler or kick-start a frozen computer, you can't fix it unless you know what's wrong. Know the *why,* and it's much easier to handle the *how* — when you need to. Let's face it, we're not going to be sitting next to you at 10:30 p.m. when you're pilfering a Pop-Tart. So you need to be equipped with knowledge of how your body works and reacts to that Pop-Tart so that you can defend against the little sugar-coated bugger.

YOU Will Challenge Your Beliefs about Diets

Throughout our lives, we've been conditioned to believe that if one thing is good for us, then more of it must be better. If you eliminate 100 calories from your daily diet, then eliminating 400 must qualify you for size 2. If you walk to lose weight, then running a marathon must nuke the fat right off your body. Well, neither idea is true. Worse, not only aren't they true, but many of the diet myths perpetuated today actually *hurt* our bodies. Food deprivation, for example, drops your metabolism and makes your body want to *store* fat. Many of the rules, ideas, and principles you may believe about dieting — that you assume work when dieting — simply aren't true and can very well contribute to weight issues because they keep the vicious cycle of fat loss and fat gain revolving faster than Lance Armstrong's front wheel.

In a way, we live on the two extremes of a pendulum. Either we swing all the way in one direction (strict, tedious dieting with a draconian low

> **FACTOID**
>
> In men, the supplement L-carnitine — at a dose of 3 grams a day — helps muscles use carbohydrates, but it is also good for blood vessel function in both men and women.

daily calorie intake), or we swing all the way in the other direction (popping cream-cheese-smothered bagels like grapes). We have to stop swinging so much and start living in the middle of that pendulum by striking a balance and avoiding the periods of extreme "ons" and "offs."

One of the reasons why most so-called diets fail is because of a psychological and behavioral flaw that many dieters have. We desperately want to believe the simple, comforting promises that diets make — that doing A always gets us B. Because once we see that A (eating wheat germ 24-7) doesn't always equal B (the cover of *Vogue*), then we get frustrated and angry, and give in to the gods of cream-filled baked goods.

Unfortunately, your body and your fat do not have a linear, two-step relationship. Instead, think of your body as an orchestra. All of its systems, organs, muscles, cells, fluids, hormones, and chemicals play different instruments, make different sounds (your intestines have dibs on first-chair tuba), and produce different results depending on how you use them. They work independently, but only when they're played together can you appreciate the magnificent symphony of your own biology. As the conductor of your biological orchestra, you control how the instruments interact and what the final result will be.

YOU Will Make Dieting Automatic

While we want you to "not think" about eating good foods, we also know that "not thinking" may be how you got into this pants-stretching mess in the first place. When you don't think about the consequences of ordering football-size calzones, you wind up with such pleasantries as high LDL (lousy type of) cholesterol, low HDL (healthy type of) cholesterol, inflammation in your arteries, and a higher risk of aging arteries that cause memory loss, heart disease, even wrinkles, as well as a steady stream of coupon offers from the large men's department. We want your body to guide you to the *right* choices — without thinking about them — so that they'll lead to the results you want. It will take some effort at the start to retrain your habits, palate, and muscles, but this program will serve as a lifelong eating, activity, and behavior plan that will become as routine as going to the bathroom before bed.

Unless you're the rare kind of person who responds to dietary drill sergeants, you won't find long-term solutions using traditional weight-loss methods: willpower, deprivation, fads, phases, or deadbolting the lid of the butter pecan. Instead, using this plan, you will train yourself to *never* think about how much you're eating, *never* think about getting on a diet or worry about coming off one, and *never* have to figure out formulas, zones, or, for the love of (fill in the deity of your choice), place a chicken breast on a food scale.

YOU Will Focus on Waist Management

Our society seems almost as obsessed with pounds as it is with celebrity breakups, but it's time to shift your thinking: Studies have shown that waist circumference, not overall weight, is the most important indicator of mortality related to being overweight. Of course you'll lose pounds on this plan, but we want you

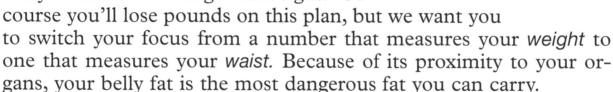

to switch your focus from a number that measures your *weight* to one that measures your *waist*. Because of its proximity to your organs, your belly fat is the most dangerous fat you can carry.

In addition to helping you shrink your waist through diet, we'll also teach you the exercises that will help you achieve and maintain a healthy waist size. Now, we don't want you to think that exercise must involve sweating like a waterfall and panting like an obscene caller, because it doesn't. But you do need to start thinking about your body as a dartboard: it's all about what's in the center. You'll be focusing on the physical activities that will help control your waist size — specifically walking and foundation-muscle training of your entire body (without growing igloo-size muscles). We'll teach you simple moves that will develop all of your foundation muscles, and we'll teach you how to tighten your belly, improve your posture, and develop the muscles that will make you fit into your clothes better. That translates into a shapelier waist, which, studies show, makes you more attractive to others.

But let's not overlook the management part of the waist management equation. We all know how good managers work: they plan ahead and create systems that play to people's strengths, they set realistic goals, they measure progress, and they don't force their employees down roads that are designed to give them a pack-your-

crease. For men, the ideal is 35 inches, and the dangers to your health increase once you hit 40 inches.

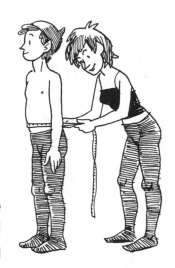

While we're going to emphasize waist over weight in this book, we also know that many of you won't be able to resist the siren of the scale. When it comes to actual weight, you do need to stop thinking about one specific number. ("I want to get down to one hundred thirty.") All of us have an ideal playing weight — not a weight for running marathons or making All Pro linebacker or posing for an airbrushed-anyway centerfold. This ideal playing weight is a *range* in which you live lean and healthy, and one in which you significantly reduce the risks of aging diseases associated with being overweight (more on all of this in Part 2).

things meeting with HR. You need to train yourself to be a good waist manager by following a plan that's designed to help you become the CEO of your body.

You Will *Focus* on YOU, but Not *Rely* on YOU

It doesn't matter whether you look at presidents (Lincoln or Taft), musicians (Usher or Heavy D), or tennis players (Sharapova or Serena), it's clear that we all have different builds, just as we all have different genetics, metabolic rates, and chemical interactions. Still, there are some fundamental biological facts that are true whether

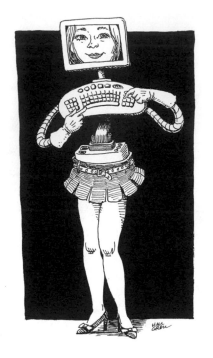

you're built like a branch or a stump. As a species, we're programmed to gain and preserve the right amount of weight. That's simply what our bodies are designed to do (more on that coming up). The trick is to figure out your factory settings. Then, we'll give you the all-important lock-setting tools that will help you to reboot those factory settings so that your body maintains its ideal size and shape.

While this is a very individual challenge, it doesn't have to be a lonely one. Life is a team game; you've got sports teams and surgical teams, restaurant staffs and office staffs, hip-hop clubs and calculator clubs. And of course you have the ultimate team: your family. The most successful teams all work the same way: Everybody plays a different role and contributes in his or her own way. You may have a Shaq, Kobe, or LeBron on your team, but the team can't win the title unless everybody, not just the stars, works for the team goal.

Somehow, though, when it comes to weight control, you believe that you're solely responsible for dropping your excess pounds and changing your habits. To make it worse, when you're gaining weight, even the fans are chipping in on your side; the world around us wants us to gain weight in the form of big portions, drive-throughs, and family dinners that could feed a small municipality. Then when you're trying to lose weight, it's as if everyone's against you; they bring junk food into the home, suggest that everyone goes out for ice cream, and feast on pork fat while you're trying to gnaw on cauliflower.

You have to stop thinking that this game is you versus a stadium full of rib-loving opponents. Sure, you need to be the quarterback of your waist control team, but you won't achieve success without a team that can block for you, high-five you when you're doing well, and give you an encouraging smack on the butt when you're not. Your starting lineup should include your doctor, maybe a nutritionist, maybe a personal trainer, and certainly scads and scads of fans like your family and friends (online or in person) who can push you, support you, and yank the bowl of candy corn away from you. But you shouldn't be the only one relying on other people; you should use this opportunity to find a support partner who needs you as much as you need her. After all, the best kinds of satisfaction shouldn't come from the sixth spoonful of cake batter, but from sharing knowledge and support, and helping others lose inches.

YOU Will *Stop* Blaming Yourself

The classic psychology of fat is this: If you're thin, then you believe that fat people must be doing something wrong to make them fat. But if you're fat, then you blame the environment, or your genetics, or anything else. Well, we're going to try to eliminate that blame and use medical insights to explain the epic saga of weight-related problems. We want to move dieting past a guilt-driven and blame-ridden system, and make it a science-based system.

Of course, not everyone can look like a Cameron Diaz or a Brad Pitt. To get an idea of what your healthy weight, waist, and shape should be, you'll need to take into account such things as bone

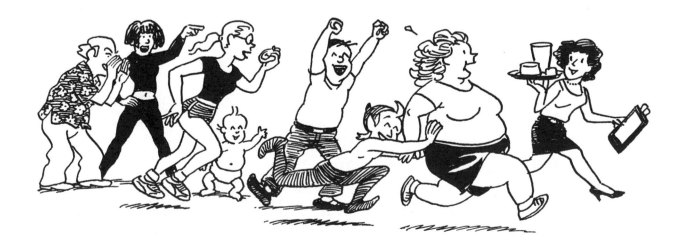

structure, muscle mass, genetics, and risk factors associated with your weight. Here's a fact that goes virtually unmentioned: There are clinically obese people who live with no risk of health problems, and there are CD-thin people whose risk of dying prematurely is more than a chuteless skydiver's. Our goal is to get you to the point where you strip away inches, you strip away the risks of being overweight, and you strip away the guilt associated with the process of always trying to do so.

YOU Will Never Be Hungry

We know exactly how you've felt when you've dieted in the past. Hungry. Famished. Three seconds away from steamrolling through a triple-dip cone with sprinkles. That recipe for dieting is one you can tear up. In fact, the only place hunger ever got you was a pair of pants that could double as curtains. To eat and work smart, your goal is *never* to be hungry and *never* to be in a state of dietary angst, where your only salvation is the 99¢ menu at the drive-through window. By keeping your hunger (and internal chemicals) in check, you'll avoid the impetuous behaviors that send fat on an express ride to your belly.

YOU Will Make Mistakes

Look, we don't care how motivated you are, how willing you are, how inspired you are by Eva Longoria's body. Someday, and someday soon, a volleyball-size muffin is going to get the best of you and nudge, bribe, or cajole its way into your stomach. That's OK. Hear that? That's *OK*. You're going to have moments when your eyes, body, and curious fingers won't be able to turn radar lock off of the queso dip. You have to get past the concept that diets have *side effects* — that is, unexpected negative consequences. Instead, realize that eating plans have *effects* — offshoot actions, behaviors, and emotions that are simply part of everyday living. One of those effects is that you will occasionally eat things that are nutritional cigarettes;

while one may not hurt you, it can get you addicted to some bad behaviors. Because of that, waist management is about developing contingency plans — plans that allow you to make mistakes and then get back on the right road. We're going to teach you how to make a YOU-Turn when you do make mistakes with Twinkies or Tootsie Rolls or any bad-for-your-waist foods. That way, your dietary fender benders won't turn into 100-car Autobahn pileups.

YOU Will *Be* Flexible — and Have Fun

Most of us want our diets to be a little like having the remote control; we want the power to make lots of choices, depending on everything from our mood to the time of day. It's clear from research that the most successful eating plans are low-maintenance: You can follow them with your family, and you won't feel overwhelmed by cravings. If you can do that, you'll get results. But try to stay on a diet where you feel more isolated than a Yankees fan at Fenway Park, then chances are that the result will feel like the box-office numbers of a B-level horror flick — a miserable failure.

Eating right shouldn't be about feeling bad. It should be about feeling strong, increasing energy, living better, feeling healthier, and having more fun than a front-row rock fan. It should be about eating without thinking and without obsessing about every forkful. Of course, we all have reasons for overeating or eating the wrong kinds of food (stress, boredom, comfort, five-cent wing specials). But our goal isn't just for you to make by-the-book food substitutions or come to grips with your Devil Dog demons. You should be grinning — not grimacing, grunting, and growling — as the inches melt away from your waist, and laughing as your lipid profile improves. You'll understand how, after we show you how the mind-stomach connection works by explaining how brain and belly chemicals control what the mind thinks, how the fork acts in your bodily orchestra, and how this relationship can become a cacophony in the wrong hands.

So now that we're about to begin, you're probably asking, What are we going to do, and how are we going to do it? Well, we're going to give you everything you need to make a body change — through a series of elegant and effective changes based on hard science — that will stick with you for your life. Simply, this book will serve as your lifelong waist management, body-changing plan.

Best of all, when you put it all together and integrate automatic actions into your life, you'll live by the principles you'll need to stay fit and healthy, so that you can achieve and maintain exactly what you're striving for:

Your ideal body.

The Fat Facts Test

What Do You Really Know about Fat, Diets, and Other Weight-loss Solutions?

To help you determine your level of dietary knowledge, take this Fat Facts Test. In less time than it takes to listen to an *American Idol* off-key clunker, you may just learn more about your body and belly than you've ever known before.

1. **What is the first historical event that we can point to as contributing to the rise in excess pounds?**
   a. The development of agriculture.
   b. The development of whipped cream in coffee.
   c. The development of more office jobs.
   d. The development of fast food.

2. **What is the reason most diets fail?**
   a. They're designed so that they're impossible to stick to long-term.
   b. They're so complicated that you need a math degree to follow them.
   c. There are only so many carrot sticks and celery stalks a person can take.
   d. Mozzarella sticks. Mmm!

3. **Which of the following strategies is most recommended for people trying to lose weight?**
    a. Weighing yourself once a week.
    b. Eating two to three small meals a day.
    c. Eating nuts every day.
    d. Ex-Lax smoothies for everyone!

4. **What's the most important number for determining whether an increased waist size is putting you at risk for health problems?**
    a. Bra size.
    b. Blood pressure.
    c. Cholesterol.
    d. Heart rate.

5. **What is ghrelin?**
    a. The name of a *Harry Potter* character.
    b. A hormone that makes you want to eat more.
    c. The name of fat cells in your belly.
    d. The chemical in your brain that makes you feel good.

6. **What is leptin?**
    a. The name of the dude on the Lucky Charms cereal box.
    b. The muscle-building protein that helps burn fat.
    c. The nutrient in fruit that works in conjunction with fiber.
    d. A chemical from fat that tells your brain you are full.

7. **Which spice has been shown to be helpful for controlling weight?**
    a. Cinnamon.
    b. Thyme.
    c. Oregano.
    d. The one married to David Beckham; Posh, is it?

8. **Complete this sentence with the most accurate response. Fructose _____ .**
   a. Is responsible for decreasing the number of calories in many foods.
   b. Tricks your mind so you stay hungry longer.
   c. Is responsible for increasing the amount of bad-for-you trans fat in foods.
   d. Sure makes my Trix taste darn good.

9. **What does your body most want to do in periods of extreme stress?**
   a. Stay away from food.
   b. Gorge on food.
   c. Seek crunchy foods.
   d. Crumple up into a pile of jelly and retreat to a warm bath.

10. **Which choice is most recommended to cut your appetite?**
    a. Whole-grain foods.
    b. Whole aisles of fruit.
    c. Whole lot of a diet soda.
    d. Whole boxes of Girl Scout cookies.

11. **Of the following choices, which is least dangerous to a long-term waist management strategy?**
    a. A 1,000-calorie-a-day diet.
    b. Higher than usual colonics ro remove all fat.
    c. Training for a marathon.
    d. Playing video games.

12. **Which organ is most responsible for metabolism?**
    a. Heart.
    b. Stomach.
    c. Liver.
    d. Kidneys.

13. Which condition is responsible for weight gain in about 10 to 20 percent of younger women?
a. Vulvodynia.
b. Hyperthyroidism.
c. Polycystic Ovary Syndrome (PCOS).
d. I've had six kids, so cut me a break, would ya?

14. Calorie for calorie, what fills you up for the longest amount of time?
a. Fat.
b. Fiber.
c. Fructose.
d. French fries.

15. At least how much must you walk daily for optimum waist control?
a. Thirty minutes.
b. Two hours.
c. Any time you can spare.
d. Any, as long as it's not traveling to and from the fridge.

16. What is the main purpose of liposuction?
a. To help people lose weight.
b. To target problem body parts.
c. To keep some Hollywood docs in business.
d. To ensure another season of successful reality TV.

17. What is your omentum?
a. A badly misspelled word.
b. The part of your brain that's stimulated to store fat.
c. A chemical that controls hunger.
d. A fat-storing tissue.

18. Health-wise, what is the optimal waist size for a woman?
   a. As little as possible.
   b. 32 1/2 inches.
   c. Under 35 inches.
   d. Whatever slides into that little black dress, honey.

19. Which part of your body that plays a role in weight gain works most like your brain?
   a. Your stomach.
   b. Your heart.
   c. Your small intestine.
   d. Your unmentionables.

20. What is CCK?
   a. The former Soviet Union.
   b. A hormone that regulates insulin levels by changing your blood sugar level.
   c. Colonic Creations by Katherine.
   d. Cholecystokinin, a chemical that tells your brain to stop eating the waffle.

21. Of the following items, what contributes most to weight gain?
   a. Periods of low levels of willpower.
   b. Short periods of high-intensity stress.
   c. Long periods of low-intensity stress.
   d. Periods of high-intensity dessert trays.

22. What is a duodenal switch?
   a. An effective surgical technique for losing weight.
   b. An intestinal transplant.
   c. The hot new band from Seattle.
   d. A program for cleansing your colon of toxins.

23. Which of the following can be an effective medical option for weight loss?
a. Aspirin.
b. Beta-blockers.
c. Statins.
d. Antidepressants.

24. Which activity is most helpful for waist control?
a. Crunches.
b. Cardiovascular training like running.
c. Resistance training like weight lifting.
d. Naked salsa dancing every other Tuesday.

25. What's the worst side effect of losing weight?
a. Increased risk of chocolate withdrawal.
b. Increased risk of muscular and joint aches.
c. Increased risk of yo-yo dieting.
d. Increased risk of astronomical tailor bill.

Answers

1. a. The development of agriculture meant that we could now have foods we wanted, not needed. And that's what provided the foundation for indulgence.

2. a. Most diets don't reprogram you to think and eat automatically, so that eventually you'll go *off* the diet just as surely as you went *on* it.

3. c. Eating a handful of nuts has been shown to help you stay full, while skipping meals can be detrimental because your body will go into a fat-storing, starvation mode when it doesn't have enough calories.

4. b. Of these risks, blood pressure is the greatest indicator of health risks associated with being overweight.

5. b. Ghrelin makes you want to eat more.

6. d. Leptin keeps you full.

7. a. Cinnamon increases insulin sensitivity, which helps enhance the satiety center in your brain (and also reduces blood sugar levels as well as cholesterol levels).

8. b. Fructose, as in high-fructose corn syrup, doesn't appear to turn off your hunger chemicals, so you do not feel full; thus you eat more.

9. a. Extreme stress (as in the case of a car accident, or even exercise) turns off your hunger. Chronic stress (like a long line of looming deadlines or family problems) can make you crave feel-good carbohydrates.

10. a. Whole-grain foods are loaded with filling fiber.

11. d. Playing video games works because it keeps your hands busy, so you can't eat. (Training for a marathon is actually destructive to your body because of the risk to your joints, and for most people, 1,000 calories is a dangerously low daily caloric intake. Do we really need to explain colonics?)

12. c. Your liver is responsible for most metabolic functions.

13. c. PCOS is responsible for weight gain in at least 10 percent of women under age fifty. It's now clinically called androgen excess; androgen refers to the male hormone.

14. b. Fiber fills you. A cup of oatmeal in the morning has been shown to prevent you from afternoon gorging.

15. a. Walk at least thirty minutes — at once or in intervals—every day.

16. b. Liposuction should be used to sculpt problem areas, not to remove a lot of fat.

17. d. Located next to your stomach, your omentum is fat that can cause damage to surrounding organs.

18. b. While 32 1/2 inches or less is ideal, 37 inches is when women start seeing a greatly increased risk of weight-related disorders.

19. c. Your small intestine — with 100 million neurons — has anatomy similar to your brain.

20. d. CCK is a chemical that directly and indirectly sends a message to your brain from your guts that you're full.

21. c. Chronic stress makes your body store more fat.

22. a. A duodenal switch is one of several surgical options for people with morbid obesity.

23. d. Bupropion, an antidepressant, has been shown to help control cravings and lead to about a 7 percent weight loss. Other antidepressants, such as tricyclic antidepressants or selective serotonin reuptake inhibitors (SSRIs), can often be associated with weight gain.

24. c. Adding a little muscle through resistance training helps your body burn more fat throughout the day.

25. c. Yo-yo dieting not only has physiological effects, because you end up gaining more weight after you've lost it, but it also has psychological effects.

Scoring

You get one point for each correct answer.

20 and above: Congratulations, doc. You're an anatomical expert.

11–19: You're average, but then again, the average person is over-weight, so maybe this isn't so good. Maybe you'd better read on.

10 and below: Don't worry, you're about to enroll in the ultimate course in the biology, history, and anatomy of fat — which is the best way to change your body.

Chapter 1
The Ideal Body

What Your Body Is Supposed to Look Like

Diet Myths

- Your body doesn't need any fat.
- Fast food is responsible for most of our fat problems.
- Dieting has to be hard.

The most common question heard among overweight people isn't "Can I have more sour cream?" It's "Why can't I lose weight?" While you may think you know the answer (severe pancake addiction), the real reason is biological:

We're actually hardwired to store some fat.

Our bodies have more systems that allow us to gain weight than to lose it. Historically, as we'll see in a moment, that served us well. Today, though, we've poisoned the systems that help us lose weight and empowered the ones that allow us to gain it — botching up our anatomy and turning our bodies into fat-storing machines. One of your goals will be to reprogram your body so that your internal systems can work the way they did when the greatest enemy we faced was a charging wildebeest, not a cheese-drowned pork roll.

Our ancestors survived by gaining and storing weight to survive periodic famines. That has left our bodies prone to storing fat and gaining weight, tendencies that willpower alone can rarely overcome. To see how our bodies have morphed from rock-hard to sponge-soft, let's look inside the bodies of early man and woman. They looked like stereotypical superheroes: strong, lean, muscular, able to jump snorting mammals in a single bound.

As we evolved, we created systems and behaviors to survive when droughts and poor eyesight made picking and hunting less than successful. We learned to thrive, and we learned to eat. In early times, our diets consisted of fruits, nuts, vegetables, tubers, and wild meat — foods that were, for the most part, low in calories. That's not to say our ancestors didn't enjoy their foods. They consumed their sugars through fruit, and they even splurged when they came across the Paleolithic Cinnabon — a honeycomb. The difference between their splurges and ours? They came across the sweet treats only rarely; it's not as if they popped in for a 900-calorie sugar bomb every time they went shopping for a new buffalo hide. Add that to the fact that their definition of "searching for food" included walking, stalking, and chasing, not sliding the milk carton out of the way to find the pudding pack. It was a lot of work to get food, so they naturally burned many of the calories they consumed through the physical activity of hunting and gathering.

Because salt and sugar were scarce, our ancestors mostly feasted on grains, vegetables, and meats — for good reason. The meat provided the protein, vitamins, minerals, and fatty acids that helped them grow taller and develop larger brains, while the other foods gave them nutrients such as glucose, a simple sugar found in fruit and the complex carbohydrates of plants, that they needed to grow and develop, and for energy to move. And, of course, food was always fresh, as there was no canning or refrigeration to store up food for Super Bowl parties, or to sneak in an 11 p.m. bowl of sugar-coated oats.

FACTOID

The difference between obese people and thin people isn't the number of fat cells, it's the size of these cells. You don't make more fat cells the fatter you get; you have the same number of fat cells you had as an adolescent. The only difference is that the fat globules within each cell increase as you store more fat. By the way, muscles work the same way: you don't make more muscle cells; the muscle cells get larger.

Another difference was that the meat our ancestors ate wasn't like the meat we know today. Theirs was low in fat and high in protein; ours often comes in the form of corn-fed cows pumped up to make fattier, tastier cuts. Even today's buffalo burger is corn-fed. Truly wild game has about 4 percent fat, while now most commercially

The Heavyweight Fight: Genetics Versus Environment

It's easy to argue that lifestyle choices and lack of willpower are responsible for weight problems (it's the argument that lean people tend to make). But it doesn't explain the 95 percent failure rate after two years of people who have lost fifty pounds or more; they had plenty of willpower to lose but regained the weight nonetheless. Researchers argue that obesity is more genetically linked than any other trait except height — and at least 50 percent of obesity cases clearly have genetic components. Our take: The waist control game requires two players — environment and genetics. Even if your genes have made you predestined for a life of taking up two seats, that doesn't mean you should abdicate control over your body. When you make the right behavioral and biological changes that we outline, you'll be able to stay healthy and avoid the bad side effects of excess weight, like diabetes, high blood pressure (hypertension), and arterial inflammation. While 10 percent of the obese population has genetic challenges that may make a supermodel contract impossible, the bigger risk with these genes is not in the

available beef has nine times that amount. (The theory behind protein-heavy diets like Atkins is that protein reduces overall food intake and could reduce calories as well. The flaw is that eating proteins dripping in saturated fat, like bacon, isn't exactly the same as eating the leaner, healthier forms of protein like chicken and fish.)

The result: Your tribal forefathers and foremothers could eat anytime they could harvest or catch something, and still not put on excess weight.

The lesson: Our ancestors never thought about a diet in the way we do — and their bodies had the approximate density of granite. Us? We obsess about diet more than red-carpet reporters obsess about designer dresses, and our bodies have the consistency of yogurt.

weight itself but in the predispositions for risks associated with obesity. For example, one genetic problem associated with being overweight is called leptin deficiency (leptin is a hormone associated with satiety, which we'll discuss in the next chapter). Folks who either don't produce leptin or block its signals usually become morbidly obese, and the problem is surely genetic.

While some people have these abnormalities, they tend to be the minority of the population. If you need to worry about losing twenty-five, thirty-five, even fifty pounds, your problem is not likely to be genetic. Only when your excess weight exceeds one hundred pounds would most doctors consider testing for genetic abnormalities. Still, the example of leptin is only the tip of the scientific iceberg as far as genetics and obesity are concerned. As the fight against obesity continues, we'll see more and more drug companies target genetic reasons for weight gain — that is, drugs that attack the genetic biochemical problems that may be contributing to your weight problem. That said, the onus of waist management still falls on you, to improve your environment and your behaviors so that your genetics can work for you, not against you.

Still, we can't blame the advent of fast food and waffle cones for all of our weight issues. The downfall started in the pre-G.A. (pre–Golden Arches) era — over 10,000 years or so ago, when agriculture first appeared. Agriculture allowed us to make more advances than a seventeen-year-old **Myth Buster** boy in a movie theater, but we paid a price for them. Besides sparing the lives of countless mammoths, the rise of agriculture ensured that we'd always have a steady supply of food — an advantage during times of famine, a disadvantage at the $6.99 Mama's Kitchen Eat-Everything Buffet. With a constant source of food, people became less nomadic, and communities grew closer together. While the average life span increased (thanks to the elimination of the extreme sport of tiger chasing, with, perhaps, some help from sanitation and immunization), agriculture also brought its share of downsides: more bacterial infections, shorter stature, and rotting teeth that comes from eating refined sugar and less nutritious farm-raised food (overused soil depletes food of its nutrients). Our ancestors' diets shifted from vegetables and meat to grains from the farms, essentially hindering them from getting the diverse mix of protein and micronutrients needed for brain development.

FACTOID

During the Muslim holiday of Ramadan, people eat only after sunset, so they consume all their calories at night. Should they lose weight? Anecdotal evidence, gathered by doctors watching residents working all-night shifts, indicates that people who eat all their 2,000 daily calories in one meal gain more weight than those who space those calories over three meals. Why? Because the one-timers are kicking in their starvation mode, making their bodies want to store fat rather than burn it.

The advent of agriculture essentially started the socio-logical shift that altered the way we lived — and the way we eat — up until this day. We could now produce food, so we could now produce what we wanted, not necessarily what we needed. Instead of making foods that could both complement our bodies and appeal to our taste buds, we started making ones that were kinder to our tongues and pocketbooks than they were to our waists.

We're not in the business of trying to make you live like cavemen, or help you score a blue-jeans billboard, or help you become thin enough to escape between two jail bars. What we should acknowledge is that we live in a world with free will, with temptations, and with more eating options than the Mall of America. Biologically, our bodies want us to eat right. But in today's society (cavemen didn't have bad bosses or deadlines for annual reports), our biological drive to be the right weight and to eat right can be overcome by stress or temptation. And that has shifted many dietary decisions from biological necessities to psychological reactions. What we're going to do is teach you how to reprogram your body to work the way it's supposed to work — so that you eat to satisfy and to fuel rather than to console or excite. Controlling your fat isn't about being banished with a life sentence of broccoli florets. It's about teaching your body a little bit about the way our ancestors ate. Naturally and automatically.

YOU TIPS!

Automate Your Eating. If your waist management plan is going to work — as in, really work, for your whole life — then eating right has to become as automatic as it was for our ancestors. That's not as insurmountable as it seems. Just look at one study from the *Journal of the American Medical Association.* Two groups were assigned two different diets. **Myth Buster** One went on a diet rich with good-for-you foods like whole grains, fruits, vegetables, nuts, and olive oil, foods found in the typical Mediterranean diet. The other group was not given any specific direction in terms of foods to eat but was instructed to consume specific percentages of fat, carbohydrates, and protein daily. In short, they had to think a lot about preparing foods and dividing amounts, while the first group only had general guidelines about foods to eat.

The groups weren't given guidelines about how much to eat; they let their hunger levels dictate their hunger patterns. And when they did that, what happened? Without trying, the first group ate fewer calories, lost inches, and dropped pounds.

YOU-reka! The point: The people in the good-foods group ate the foods that naturally kept them satiated so their bodies could seek their playing weights.

- The "good-for-YOU-foods group" ate significantly more fiber than the control group (32 grams versus 17 grams).
- The "good-for-YOU-foods group" ate higher amounts of good-for-you omega-3 fats in the form of olives, fish, and nuts (especially walnuts). Those fats help increase the level of chemicals that make you feel satiated.
- The "good-for-YOU-foods group" more than doubled their consumption of fruits and vegetables.

The "good-for-YOU-foods-group" ate the foods we recommend in the YOU Diet, didn't obsess about calories, and enabled their bodies to do what they're supposed to do: regulate the chemicals that are responsible for hunger and for satiety (more on this in Chapter 2).

Don't Undereat. When our ancestors couldn't find food and went for long periods of time without it, their bodies acted like a life preserver, storing fat in anticipation of the inevitable periods of famine. The same system works today. **YOU-reka!** When you try to "diet" by going for long periods of time without eating or by eating way too few calories, your brain senses the starvation and sends an SOS signal through your body to store fat because famine is on its way. That's why people who go on extreme fasts and extremely low-calorie diets don't lose the expected weight. They store fat as a natural protective mechanism. To lose weight, you have to keep your body from switching into starvation mode. The only way to do it: Eat often, in the form of frequent, healthy meals, and snacks.

Plan Your Meals. Start every day knowing when and what you're going to eat. That way, you'll avert the 180-degree shift between starving and gorging that occurs when you skip meals. Our fourteen-day diet (in Chapter 12) will show you how to plan your meals so that you feed your body regularly to avoid extreme periods of overeating and undereating that can lead to a gain in weight and inches.

YOU Test

Remember Your Ancestry

Some people say their family has big bones or big cells. Some say their family has big appetites. Some say their family just has big beer coolers. If you gained weight as an adult, you can get a relatively accurate picture of what your ideal size should be by thinking about what you looked like when you were eighteen (for women) or twenty-one (for men); a time when you were at your metabolically most efficient and when you weren't stapled to an office chair for sixty hours a week. Most people gain their weight between the ages of twenty-one and sixty, so by looking at your size at eighteen or twenty-one, you'll have a good, though not quite scientific, idea of your factory settings. It's not perfect, but it's a thumbnail sketch of where you want to be. You can record your waist size (or closest guess) from when you were eighteen, but, more important, think about your shape. Ask your parents about their body sizes — or find pictures of them — when they were eighteen, to help give you a good idea of what you're supposed to look like.

YOU Test

Stand in Front of the Mirror. Naked.
Without Sucking in Your Belly.

For some of you, this assignment may feel natural, but for most, the exercise is as uncomfortable as a coach-class airline seat. We're having you do this not to benefit the neighborhood peepers, but for two other reasons. First, we want you to realize that we're emphasizing healthy weight. Not fashion-magazine weight, not featherweight, but *healthy* weight. And we think that means you have to start getting comfortable with the fact that every woman isn't as light as a kite, and every man won't have the body of Matthew McCanoughey. Where you want to be may not be *exactly* where your body wants you to be. We're not saying you need to accept a belly that looks like four gallons of melted ice cream, but we want you to get closer to your ideal health — and that means physically and emotionally.

   Second, we want you to look at your body. Now draw an outline of your body shape (both from the side and front views). Ask a partner or close friend to look at the shape you drew and tell you — honestly — if that's approximately what your body looks like. (Your clothes can be back on at this point.) This is just a quality-control check to make sure you have an accurate self body image. (Those with eating disorders have very distorted body images, making it an obstacle for getting back to a healthy weight.) This might be the first time you've ever had to articulate things about what your body looks like — and that's good.

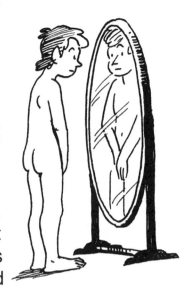

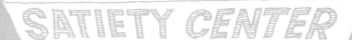

Part 2
The Biology of Fat

Food, from Start to Finish — Why Our Bodies Want It, How We Store It, and How We Burn It

Chapter 2
Can't Get No Satisfaction

The Science of Appetite

Diet Myths

- Hunger is primarily dictated by what's happening in your stomach.

- The biggest battle in dieting involves willpower.

- As long as a food is low-fat, it's not going to make you fat.

As much as an iPod bud in the ear, fat has become a regular part of our landscape. We see it *everywhere.* We see it tethered to a hunk of prime rib. We see it masquerading as a Nutter Butter. We see it crammed into evening gowns or cascading over belt buckles. We've seen paparazzi-haunted celebrities gain it and lose it, lose it and gain it. And, if we can bear a confidence-crushing six seconds of nudity in front of a mirror, most of us have seen our own share of flesh that droops, sags, or jiggles. So, reason would tell you that we should know as much about fat as we know about Angelina Jolie's private life. But we don't.

Sure, we know what it looks like, what it feels like, and that it can be as bad for our health as a steak knife lodged in our hand. But few of us really know how fat works biologically — how the Twinkie morphs from a wonderfully yellow spongy cake to the flab that conjoins our inner thighs, or how our skinny-as-a-straw friend can wolf down a meat-lover's supreme while we feel bloated if we as much as sniff four carrots.

Starting in this chapter and continuing throughout the rest of part 2, we'll show you the way that food travels — from the time your body wants you to eat it, to the time it exercises squatter's rights on your hips, to the time you fry it into oblivion. The best place to start? With your appetite. Appetite really comes in two forms: physiological signals that make you hungry and emotional coaxes that lure you to food.

In this chapter, we'll explore those physiological signals, because understanding and controlling your hunger and satiety signals will help you adopt a healthy eating plan. (We'll explore the psychological and emotional aspects in part 3.) Once you know that those mechanisms have much more powerful control over how you eat than do your taste buds, then you can make the behavioral, attitudinal, and biological adjustments you need to live at your healthy weight.

Above all, there's one sign that will clue you in to whether you've become an effective processor of food. It's the sign that you, not a bag of gummy bears, are in control of your weight. It's the sign that

Fat's Bad Rap

Sure, nobody likes body fat, especially when it beats you through the door by five or six seconds. But despite potentially serious consequences, fat, by nature, is good. (That's not a typo.) Besides helping Santa hopefuls land December jobs, it also helps your cells function and provides insulation. Most of your fat is stored in a reservoir throughout your body. You have drums and drums of it, sitting passively, just waiting to be burned. But you have another kind of fat, too. It's called brown fat and is usually found on the back of your neck and around your arteries (and has absolutely nothing to do with how much chocolate you eat). This increases in outdoor workers during cold spells to protect them from the weather; it insulates our vital organs. Though you have a fairly small percentage of brown fat as an adult, about one-third of fat in babies is brown fat, and it's used primarily to keep them warm. What makes brown fat different? **YOU-reka!** Brown fat is *alive.* It has nerve fibers, like any organ, and it also has leptin receptors. When the level of this hormone goes up, it turns on energy consumption in the brown fat and burns it. This is important because it shows that the right leptin levels can signal you to immediately get rid of this fat. And it's also symbolic of the inherent goodness of body fat — when it's found in the right amounts.

you, without having to work at it, have been promoted to captain of your waist management vessel. And it's the sign that you've ultimately reprogrammed your biology so that your body uses food as a medicine to make you stay healthier so that you live long enough to see how *Lost* ends.

That sign? Satisfaction.

As you change from *always* thinking about diet to *never* thinking about it, you will be reprogramming your body so that it's not your eyes, tongue, or overzealous utensils that will guide you.

YOU-reka! Instead, it will be the chemicals in your brain and body.

By tuning in to your body's signals, you'll allow your anatomy to work the way it's supposed to: so that you'll never be famished, you'll never pop a button at the table, and you'll never bounce between hunger extremes. Instead, you'll get a little hungry, you'll eat, you'll stop. Satisfied.

The Anatomy of Appetite

You'd think that the first place we'd start to talk about how appetite influences fat would be the spot that's covered by an XXXXL shirt. But to understand appetite, you have to navigate farther north — to the place that may hold the least fat. In your brain, you'll find the hypothalamus, a key command center for your body. Among the biological functions it controls are your temperature, your metabolism, and your sex drive. Located in the center of your brain, the hypothalamus (see Figure 2.1) also coordinates your behaviors that involve appetite — not just for food but also for thirst and even for sex. So while it may appear that call-to-duty signals come from your stomach growling or your loins tingling like a static shock, it's actually your brain that's sending out the signals that you crave either a quiche or a quickie. (At least one person we know helped curb an eating problem by having regular, monogamous, healthy sex. When the appetite function for sex was satisfied, the appetite function for food was diverted.)

Hidden in your hypothalamus, you have a satiety center

Myth Buster

> ## FACTOID
>
> As you get older, you have fewer leptin receptors in your hypothalamus — meaning that you have fewer satiety signals, which makes you more prone to gaining weight.

Figure 2.1 **Food Fight** In your hypothalamus, you have hunger and satiety chemicals. The hormone leptin goes to the satiety center to make you feel full and satisfied, while the signal from the hormone ghrelin makes you want to eat, gorge, and slobber over your every feast.

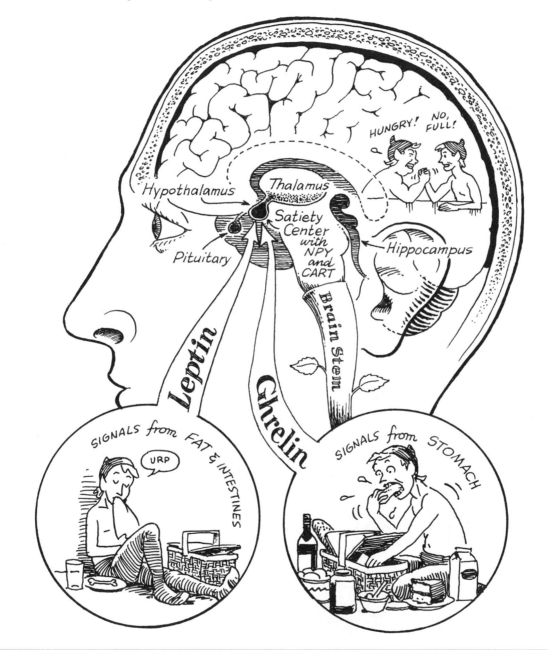

Figure 2.2 **Chemical Reaction** If we look closely at the hypothalamus, we see that a small nucleus at the bottom houses NPY and CART, which fight the yin-yang battle to control the brain biochemistry of hunger. Each chemical readily travels to other nuclei in the hypothalamus. NPY causes our temperature to drop and our metabolism to decrease as we feel hungry. CART stimulates the opposite influence. The nearby mammillary body (literally shaped like a nipple) is part of our limbic system, where we store memories and emotions — just the right combination to create a craving for a favorite food. The thalamus is the body's relay station and rapidly transmits orders throughout the brain based on the desires of the eating center.

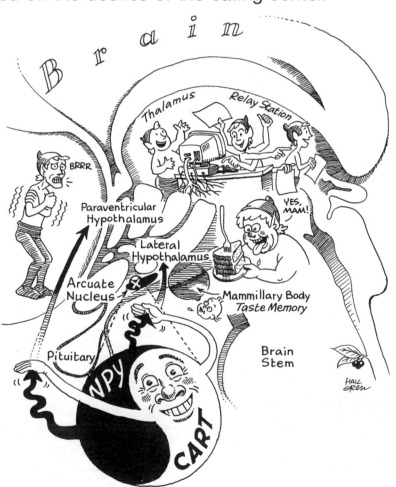

that regulates your appetite. It is controlled by two counterbalancing chemicals that are located side by side (see Figure 2.2).

- The satiety chemicals led by CART (the *C* stands for cocaine and the *A* for amphetamine, since these drugs put this chemical into overdrive). CART stimulates the surrounding hypothalamus to increase metabolism, reduce appetite, and increase insulin to deliver energy to muscle cells rather than be stored as fat.
- The eating chemicals driven by NPY (a protein called neuropeptide Y). NPY has the opposite effect on the hypothalamus; it decreases metabolism and increases appetite.

Think of these two command chemicals as any game or sport that involves offense and defense, like soccer, checkers, or even dating. The offense is always trying to make advances, trying to score points, and trying to attack, while the defense protects its territory.

Your eating chemicals play offense. They want as many points as possible, so they fire off those signals for your body to score: eat, eat, eat, calories, calories, calories, chimichanga, chimichanga, chimichanga. The biological message: Prevent starvation by eating. Meanwhile, your satiety chemicals play defense, like a goalkeeper, the back row of checkers, or a protective parent. They send the messages to your brain that you're full, to shield you from steadily pumping bacon-wrapped scallops down your gullet. How do we know these centers work this way? For one, by looking at extremes and seeing what happens when the feeding system is turned completely on or off. When we study animal models, we see that if a rat's eating center is destroyed, for instance, it forever forgets to eat. The resulting severe anorexia starves the body of all energy and nutrients so that it withers away to the approximate width of an envelope. In rats whose eating center is overstimulated, though, food is always on the radar screen. And those rats eat themselves to death — literally — by increasing their fat-induced diseases like diabetes, hypertension, and arthritis.

FACTOID

CART (cocaine-amphetamine-regulatory transcript, for those scoring at home) is the reason why cocaine addicts don't gain weight. Cocaine and amphetamine stimulate this chemical, giving you a double brain bat to help you control appetite and increase metabolism. It's unclear whether CART will be the basis for effective weight-loss treatments, but researchers are studying the neurological effects these drugs have on appetite to see if they could lead to long-term pharmaceutical solutions to weight loss (without, of course, the dangerous side effects of illicit drugs). Marijuana, by the way, has its own receptors that overwhelm leptin, which is one *big* reason why pot smokers get the munchies. It's also an area that's a promising new approach to weight-loss drugs. By figuring out how the drug turns off the gene that produces leptin, we'll be able to figure out how to flick it on — to keep leptin (and thus satiety levels) high. The prototype drug has done great in trials and symbolizes a new generation of smart weight-loss medications that work hormonally.

In a perfect system, your offense and defense complement each other; you get the foods you need and stop when you've had enough. Unfortunately for everyone except elastic-waistband manufacturers, a lot of things can mess up those systems (many of which we'll discuss in a moment). But these obstacles aren't insurmountable. You can take comfort (and find motivation) in the fact that your body wants you to reach your goals. Your body doesn't want to be bigger than it should be. Your body doesn't want lots of excess fat. Take the case of rats made obese by force-feeding. When they're allowed to eat freely, they go back to their control weight. *They eat what they should eat, without thinking.* Same goes for starving rats. When allowed to eat again, they don't gorge. They naturally go back to their control weight. And we know from years and years of research that what rats do is a pretty fair indication of what humans will do under the same circumstances. (Humans, of course, will do what rats do when they're motivated only by biology. A rat isn't upset by stress at home or work, which is why controlling the emotional aspect of eating plays such a big role in effective waist management, as we'll discuss in Part 3.)

YOU-reka! If you can allow your body and brain to subconsciously do the work of controlling your eating, you'll naturally gravitate toward your ideal playing weight. You do it by developing a well-trained defense that naturally balances the offense. When you do, you'll win the diet game every time, whether you have willpower or not.

Though it may not always be the case in football or Scrabble, when you pit offense against defense in your body, the offense in your body typically attacks more aggressively. It's simply easier to scoop up bean dip than it is to leave it for others.

The Hunger On and Off Switches

Duct tape over your mouth isn't how your body regulates food intake. Your body does it naturally through the communication of substances controlled by your brain. Although there are many hunger- and obesity-related hormones waiting to be discovered, there's enough evidence to suggest that two hormones have as much influence for dictating our hunger and satiety levels as a head coach does on offense and defense — hour to hour and year to year.

Lovin' Leptin: The Hormone of Satisfaction

In sumo champions, a little extra fat can produce good results. But we also think that fat has an unfair knock against it. Fat is treated a little like an accused suspect; it sometimes gets a bum rap. Fat produces a chemical signal in your blood that tells you to stop eating. Left to its own devices, fat is self-regulating; the problem occurs when we override our internal monitoring system and continue to stuff ourselves long after we're no longer hungry. Your body knows when it's had enough, and it prevents you from wanting any more food on top of that. How does fat curb appetite? Through one of the most important chemicals in the weight-reduction process: leptin, a protein secreted by stored fat. In fact, if leptin is working the way it should, it gives you a double whammy in the fight against fat. The stimulation of leptin (the word comes from the Greek word for "thin") shuts off your hunger *and* stimulates you to burn more calories — by stimulating CART.

But our bodies aren't always perfect, and leptin doesn't always work the way it's supposed to. In some research, when leptin was given to mice, their appetites decreased, as expected. When it was given to people, they initially got thin, but then something strange happened: They overcame the surge of leptin and stopped losing weight. This indicates that our bodies have the ability to override leptin's message that our tank is full. How? When leptin tells your defense — the satiety chemicals — to kick in and protect you against stray bonbons, the pleasure center in your brain says, "Uh, yeah, three more this-a-way." That surge from the pleasure center, which we'll discuss in more detail in part 3, can overrule leptin's messages that you're full. That's called leptin resistance (there's another form of leptin resistance as well, which happens when cells stop accepting leptin's messages). Most obese people, by the way, have high leptin levels; it's just that their bodies have the second form of leptin resistance — they don't receive and respond to leptin signals.

That doesn't mean leptin is always on the losing end of this chemical battle. **YOU-reka!** The challenge is to let leptin do its job so that the brain demands less food. One way to do it: Walk thirty minutes a day and build a little muscle (that's part of our activity plan in part 4). When you lose some weight, your cells become more sensitive and responsive to leptin.

Ghrelin Is the Gremlin: The Hormone of Hunger

Your stomach and intestines do more than hold food and produce Richter-worthy belches. When your stomach's empty, they release a feisty little chemical called ghrelin. When your stomach's growling, it's this gremlin of a hormone that's controlling your body's offense; it sends desperate messages that you need more points, you need to score, you need to FedEx the chili dogs to the GI tract immediately. Ghrelin makes you want to eat — by stimulating NPY. **YOU-reka!** To make things worse, when you diet through deprivation, the increased ghrelin secretion sends even more signals to eat, overriding your willpower and causing chemical reactions that give you little choice but to line your tongue with bits of beef jerky.

Ghrelin also promotes eating by increasing the secretion of growth hormone (*ghre* is the Indo-European root word for "growth"). So

FACTOID

Scientists found how ghrelin works accidentally: in gastric bypass surgery, doctors cut out the part of the stomach that secretes ghrelin. They soon realized that it wasn't just the smaller stomach but the reduced ghrelin production that helped surgery patients eat less food. The eat-everything signal was shut off, clearing the way for the satiety center to take care of its business.

when you increase ghrelin levels, you stimulate that growth hormone to kick in, and growth hormone builds you not only up but out as well.

Your stomach secretes ghrelin in pulses every half hour, sending subtle chemical impulses to your brain — almost like subliminal biological messages (carrot cake, carrot cake, carrot cake). When you're really hungry or dieting, those messages come fast — every twenty minutes or so — and they're also amplified. So you get more signals and stronger signals that your body wants food. After long periods, your body can't ignore those messages. That's why sugar cookies usually trump willpower, and that's why deprivation dieting can never work: **YOU-reka!** It's impossible to fight the biology of your body. The chemical vicious cycle stops when you eat; when your stomach fills is when you reduce your ghrelin levels, thus reducing your appetite. So if you think your job is to resist biology, you're going to lose that battle time after time. But if you can reprogram your body so that you keep those ghrelin gremlins from making too much noise, then you've got a chance to keep your tank feeling like it's always topped off.

Food Fight: The Ghrelin Versus Leptin Grudge Match

So now let's get back to that offense and defense. The natural state is for you to have a give-and-take relationship between your eating and satiety chemicals — between your ghrelin and leptin levels — to influence NPY and CART, respectively. It's the relationship between the impulse that says, "I'll take a large pepperoni with extra cheese," and the one that says, "No more passengers, this belly is full."

This battle over eating isn't between your willpower and the Belgian waffles; it's between your brain chemicals. The NPY is the villain — encouraging you to buffets, driving you to the pantry, pointing its chemical finger to the convenience foods, while CART is your dietary guardian angel, which encourages a cascade of allies to keep you full

Myth Buster

and satisfied and in no way interested in creamed anything. Think of the two substances — NPY and CART — competing for the same parking space, the one that will ultimately determine whether or not you eat (see Figure 2.3). They both arrive at the same time and want that space. Either more NPY or more CART sneaks into the spot, thus sending the all-important go or stop signal to your brain to influence the hormones that make you feel full or hungry.

Here's how they all work together: Ghrelin works in the short term, sending out those hunger signals twice an hour. Leptin, on the other hand, works in the long term, so if you can get your leptin levels high, you'll have a greater ability to keep your hunger and appetite in check. Isn't that great? Leptin can outrank ghrelin — to keep you from feeling like feasting on anything short of fingernails every few minutes. If you focus on ways to influence your leptin levels, and, more important, leptin effects (through leptin sensitivity), your brain (through CART) will help control your hunger.

Sometimes, it may seem like we don't have much control over the chemical reactions taking place within our arteries or inside our brains. But just as you can control things like cholesterol and blood pressure by changing the foods you eat or altering your behaviors, you can also control the satiety center of your brain. How? Through your choice of foods.

At least as far as your body is concerned, foods are drugs; they're foreign substances that come in and switch around all those natural chemical processes going about their business within your body. When your body receives foods, different chemical reactions take place, and messages get sent throughout your system — turning on some things, turning off others. While your body internally gives orders, you set the tone and direction of those orders through the food you're feeding it. Eat the right foods (like nuts), and your hormones will keep you feeling satisfied. But eat the wrong foods (like simple sugars), and you'll cause your body to go haywire hormonally, and that ends up with one result: the next notch in your belt.

A major gang leader against your body is fructose, found in high-

Figure 2.3 **In a Jam** The satiety center is waiting to be turned off by NPY or stimulated by CART. Whichever fills up the receptor docks first is what controls whether you want to eat more or not. In turn, these two proteins are influenced by lack of water, sleep, and even sex. They're also influenced by ghrelin coming from your stomach, which stimulates NPY so you get hungry, and leptin from your fat, which is further stimulated by a chemical called CCK, released from your intestines after a meal.

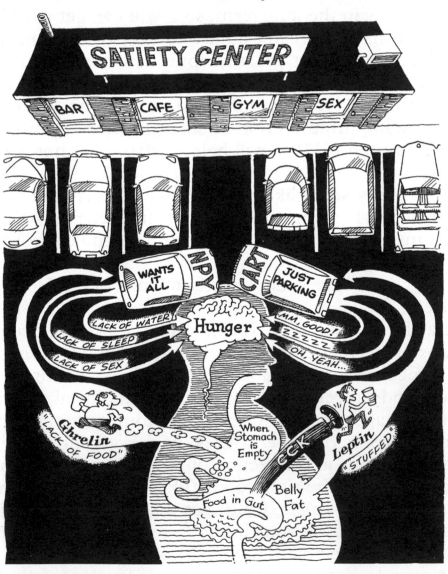

fructose corn syrup (HFCS), a sweetener in many processed foods. Here's how it works: **YOU-reka!** When you eat calories from healthy sources, they turn off your desire to eat by inhibiting production of NPY or by producing more CART. But fructose in the HFCS, which sweetens our soft drinks and salad dressings, isn't seen by your brain as a regular food.

Because your brain doesn't see any of the fructose in the thousands of HFCS-containing foods as excess calories or as NPY suppressants, your body wants you to keep eating (which means that even low-fat foods can have extremely bad consequences, calorie- and appetite-wise). Americans have gone from eating no pounds of this stuff per person in 1960 to eating more than sixty-three pounds of it every year (that's 128,000 calories). That's a contributor to weight gain, since the fructose in HFCS doesn't turn off your hunger signals. Foods with fructose — which may in fact be labeled as low-fat — make you both hungry and unable to shut off your appetite. They are also rich sources of calories: the perfect storm of weight gain. So you constantly get the signal that you're hungry, even after you've jammed your gut with two baskets of calorie-laden, fructose-loaded biscuits.

Myth Buster

YOU TIPS!

Get Over Sticker Shock. You should read food labels as actively as you read the stock ticker or the horoscopes. Don't eat foods that have any of the following listed as one of the first five ingredients:

- Simple sugars
- Enriched, bleached, or refined flour (this means it's stripped of its nutrients)
- HFCS (high-fructose corn syrup — a four-letter word).

Putting them into your body is like dunking your cell phone in a glass of water. It'll cause your system to short out your hormones and send your body confusing messages about eating. Today's yearly per capita consumption of sugar is 150 pounds, compared to 7.5 pounds consumed on average in the year 1700. That's twenty times as much! When typical slightly overweight people eat sugar, they on average store 5 percent as ready energy to use later, metabolize 60 percent, and store a whopping 35 percent as fat that can be converted to energy later.

Any guess as to where 50 percent of the sugar we consume comes from? HFCS in fat-free foods like salad dressings and regular soft drinks.

Choose Unsaturated over Saturated. Meals high in saturated fat (that's one of the aging fats) produce lower levels of leptin than low-fat meals with the exact same calories. That indicates you can increase your satiety and decrease hunger levels by avoiding saturated fats found in such sources as high-fat meats (like sausage), baked goods, and whole-milk dairy products.

Don't Confuse Thirst with Hunger. The reason some people eat is because their satiety centers are begging for attention. But sometimes, those appetite centers want things to quench thirst, not to fill the stomach. Thirst could be caused by hormones in the gut, or it could be a chemical response to eating; eating food increases the thickness of your blood, and your body senses the need to dilute it. A great way to counteract your hormonal reaction to food is to make sure that your response to thirst activation doesn't contain unnecessary, empty calories — like the ones in soft drinks or alcohol. Your thirst center doesn't care whether it's getting zero-calorie water or a mega-calorie frap. **YOU-reka!** When you feel hungry, drink a glass or two of water first, to see if that's really what your body wants.

Avoid the Alcohol Binge. For weight loss, avoid drinking excessive alcohol — not solely because of its own calories, but also because of the calories it inspires you to consume later. Alcohol lowers your inhibition, so you end up feeling like you can eat anything and everything you see. Limiting yourself to one alcoholic drink a day has a protective effect on your arteries but could still cost you pounds, since it inhibits leptin.

Watch Your Carbs. Eating a super-high-carb diet increases NPY, which makes you hungry, so you should ensure that less than 50 percent of your diet comes from carbohydrates. Make sure that most of your carbs are complex, such as whole grains and vegetables.

Stay — Va-Va-Va-Voom — Satisfied. In any waist management plan, you can stay satisfied. Not in the form of a dripping double cheeseburger but in the form of safe, healthy, monogamous sex. Sex and hunger are regulated through the brain chemical NPY. Some have observed that having healthy sex could help you control your food intake; by satisfying one appetite center, you seem to satisfy the other.

Manage Your Hormonal Surges. There will be times when you can't always control your hormone levels; when ghrelin outslugs your leptin, and you feel hungrier than a lion on a bug-only diet. Develop a list of emergency foods to satisfy you when cravings get the best of you — things like V8 juice, a handful of nuts, pieces of fruit, cut-up vegetables, or even a little guacamole.

Chapter 3
Eater's Digest

How Food Travels through Your Body

Diet Myths

- Fat turns to fat, protein turns to muscle, and carbs turn to energy.

- The fullness of your stomach is what tells you to stop eating.

- Sugar gives you an instant high to help combat hunger.

Once your brain tells you to eat, that's exactly what you do. You eat. Maybe you gorge. Maybe you nibble. And then maybe you forget about that hefty portion of mac 'n' cheese until it winds up on the back of your thighs. But in between mouth and thighs, there's an amazing system of digestion that takes place — a system that determines whether that food gets burned, stored, or expelled faster than a delinquent high schooler.

Figure 3.1 **Gutting It Out** Food pulls over at various spots in the intestinal track, so disease of these areas can cause nutritional deficiencies even if two people are eating the identical foods. Not all of the nutrients that come from food and supplements get absorbed in the same place; they're absorbed throughout your GI tract. Here are the rest stations where nutrients are absorbed:

Stomach: alcohol

Duodenum (first part of the small intestine; takes off from the stomach): calcium, magnesium, iron, fat-soluble vitamins A and D, glucose

Jejunum (middle part of the small intestine): fat, sucrose, lactose, glucose, proteins, amino acids, fat-soluble vitamins A and D, water-soluble vitamins like folic acid

Ileum (last part of the small intestine; leads to large bowel): proteins, amino acids, water-soluble vitamins like folic acid, vitamin B12

Colon (also known as the large bowel): water, potassium, sodium chloride

Now that you know the biochemical reasons why you shuttle food to your mouth, it's time to start exploring the biology of what happens to food once it's in there. In this chapter, we'll discuss what happens in the early part of your digestive system, and in the next chapter, we'll discuss the effects of food as it interacts with the rest of your digestive organs.

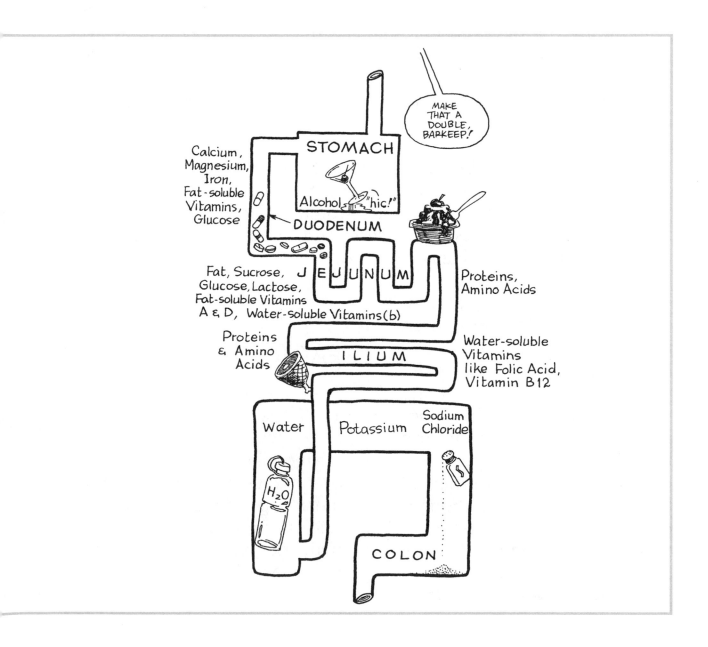

Your Digestive Highway: The On-ramp

On your gastrointestinal interstate, everything enters via your physiological toll booth: your mouth. The nutritious powerhouses slide through the express toll to give you the power, energy, stamina, and strength to live your life. Toxic (though sometimes tasty) foods can enter too, but you'll pay a heavier toll later for the damage they do along the way and after. Throughout its journey, your food and all of its nutrients (and toxins) will pull over at various organs, slow down on winding roads, speed up, merge with other nutrients, and even get pulled over by the bowel brigade for nutritional violations. (See Figure 3.1.)

During every trip, your food hits a symbolic three-pronged fork in the road:

- Either it will be broken down and picked up by your bloodstream and liver to be used as energy.
- Or it will be broken down and stored as fat.
- Or it will be processed as waste and directed to nature's recycling pot: the porcelain junkyard.

Here's how the system starts: Before a morsel even reaches the tollbooth, your body has a radar gun to let you know that food is coming — powered by such physiological cues as sight, smell, and the fact that you've been drooling like an overheated Saint Bernard at the thought of a fried-cheese appetizer special. In response to that sensory information, glands in your mouth start to secrete

FACTOID

The average person has 10,000 taste buds, which are onion-shaped structures. People regenerate new taste buds every three to ten days, but these regenerate at a slower rate as people get older. Elderly people may have only 5,000 taste buds.

enzymes to help break down your food; then your stomach quickly constructs its version of a roadside welcome center by pumping out stomach acid to help prepare your body for the digestion process.

Now, don't underestimate your stamp licker as a player in this digestion process. Back in the day of buffalo-hide cocktail dresses, people relied on their tongues (and their noses) for survival; if it tasted good, then it was safe, and if it tasted like dinosaur dung, then it could be poisonous or toxic.

We do the same things, but in slightly different ways. Since our bodies use our senses to process information, we rely on our tongue for information about food. The information we acquire sends messages to the brain, and then the brain sends messages to our forks: keep eating or stop eating. That message largely comes from our five tastes (sweet, sour, salty, bitter, and unami, which recognizes the inherent deliciousness in foods like juicy filet mignon), but it also comes from what we smell. Some researchers say that three-quarters of how we "taste" certain foods actually comes from how we smell it. What's this have to do with your waist growing? For one, there's the obvious: the more you like a bad-for-you food, the more likely you are to keep eating it. But the genetics of taste and taste buds may play an even more subtle and fascinating role. As you'll see in the box on page 94 ("Are You a Supertaster?"), the physiological makeup of your tongue could make you more or less disposed to eating good or bad foods.

Unlike other animals, we waste very little energy eating because of our highly efficient perfectly opposing molars (see Figure 3.3). The powerful crushing motion helps us extract every possible calorie from the prime rib deluxe.

FACTOID

Maybe the old days were right: It used to be that young docs would criticize older docs for giving B12 shots, calling them nothing more than placebos. But nearly 40 percent of Americans may suffer from a vitamin B12 deficiency.

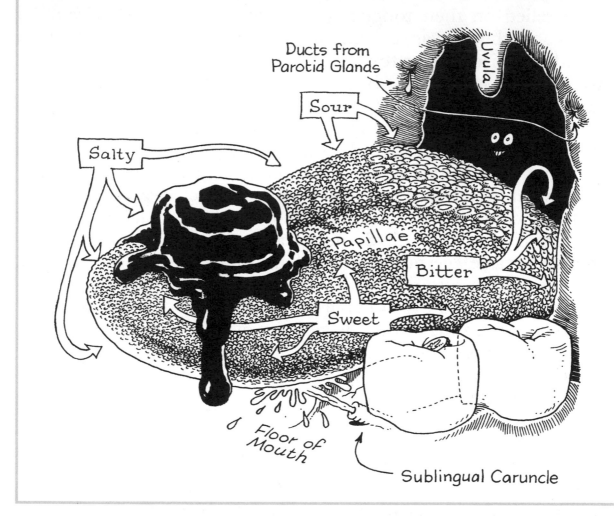

Figure 3.2 **Taste Tester** The most powerful muscle in the body, the tongue, tastes food with papillae that sense the chemicals in foods and tell you whether they're worth your continued attention.

Other animals waste or burn a lot of calories while they eat because their teeth do not efficiently mush the food when they move prey to belly. In humans, once that food actually does breeze past the toll booth, it accelerates onto the on-ramp of the esophagus — that's the tube that links your mouth to the interstate that is your GI system.

After your Double Whopper slides down the on-ramp, it has to

Figure 3.3 **Chewing the Fat** One of the reasons we can gain weight so readily is the efficiency of our teeth, which fit perfectly with one another to ensure that every morsel of food is crushed completely. Salivary glands near the lower teeth and at the back of the mouth secrete enzymes to hasten digestion before swallowing. The sight and smell of food warn these systems of what's to come.

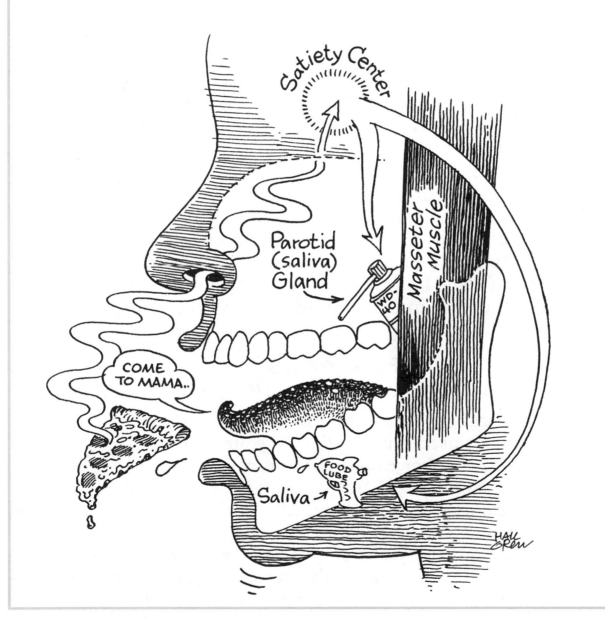

make a tricky merge in the form of a sharp turn to enter the stomach. That angle — the gastroesophageal junction — is what keeps stomach acid from spilling back into your esophagus and making your chest feel like an arson victim. (When you have extra fat in your belly, that angle is pried open, allowing acid to spill upward and cause heartburn. See "The Word on Gerd," page 86.) Once your Whopper chunks have entered your stomach, serious digestion begins. The food is held in your stomach until your body directs it to the small intestine, where most of the nutrients are absorbed and passed along to the rest of your body through your bloodstream (to the liver, which is the next stop for absorbed nutrients), or to the large intestine on the way to evacuation.

FACTOID

Eating nuts does not create the calorie intake that you might expect, because 5 percent to 15 percent of the calories are not absorbed by the intestinal system. That's because the nuts' skin and how well we chew nuts influence digestion. An added bonus: The slow release of calories throughout the intestinal system leads to prolonged satiety.

Food Processor:
How Your Body Breaks Down Nutrients

In terms of weight gain, a calorie is a calorie is a calorie. Calories not used immediately by your body for energy are either eliminated as waste or stored as fat. **YOU-reka!** But that doesn't mean that all calories are treated equally by your body. For example, protein and fiber with high water content have a great effect on satiety, and simple carbohydrates have the least effect on satiety. (Fat, by the way, has an effect on satiety similar to that of protein and fiber, which is why low-fat diets leave

Myth Buster

people hungry all the time.) When it comes to converting calories, your body processes fat most efficiently — meaning that you actually keep more of it, because your body doesn't need to expend as many calories trying to store it. On the flip side, your body works hard to process protein, to make it highly flammable to your body's metabolic furnace.

Contrary to popular belief, not all ingested protein becomes muscle, and not all the fat in your food gets stored on your hips. Everything has the potential to turn into fat if it's not used by your body for energy at the exact time it is absorbed through your intestines. And energy is energy is energy (see Figures 3.4a and 3.4b). Here's how the different nutrients are processed:

Simple sugars (as in a cola): When sugar, which is quickly absorbed and sent to the liver, meets the liver in the digestion process, the liver tells your body to turn that sugar into a fat if it can't be used

Oh, the Gall

Your gallbladder may seem as unnecessary as bad goatees, but one of its functions is to help store bile — that digestive juice that helps your body absorb nutrients. Obese people have a greater than 50 percent chance of developing gallstones. Why? An overworked liver caused by being overweight makes bile, which is more like sludge than liquid, and predisposes them to developing stones. It's also more likely that you'll develop stones when you lose weight fast, like after weight-loss surgery — because the gallbladder doesn't empty enough when it doesn't see any fat. So it's not uncommon for a surgeon to remove the gallbladder during a gastric bypass procedure. The risk factors for developing the painful stones are easy to remember, because they sound like an R & B group. They're the 4 Fs: female, fertile, fat, and forty. (We don't mean this to be a gender issue, but the fact is that women are more likely to have gallstone symptoms than men.)

immediately for energy.

Complex carbohydrates (as in whole-grain foods). They take longer to digest, so there's a slower release of the carbohydrates that have been converted in your bowel to sugar to become sugar in your bloodstream. That means your digestive system is not stressed as much. Still, if your body can't use this slower sugar when it's released, it gets converted to fat.

Protein (as in meat): It gets broken down into small amino acids, which then go to the liver. If the liver can't send them to your muscles (say, if you're not exercising and don't need them for muscle growth or maintenance), then, yep, they get converted to glucose, which then gets converted to fat if you can't use it for energy.

Fat (as in funnel cake): It gets broken into smaller particles of fat and gets absorbed as fat. Good fats (like those found in nuts and fish) decrease your body's inflammatory response, and bad fats increase it. That inflammatory response, which we'll explain in the next chapter, is a contributing factor to obesity and its complications. If you're exercising and have used up all readily available carbohydrates (sugar), your muscles can use fat for energy, which is a great way to erode your love handles.

Your Digestive Highway: The Main Drag

At the bottom of your stomach and top of your intestines, your food hits an important traffic signal: It's the red light that tells your brain you're full and don't need another large order of onion rings (or the cheese sauce for dipping or the beer to wash it down). That red light is delivered by the vagus nerve, which is a large nerve that comes from the brain and stimulates the contraction of the stomach (see Figure 3.5). The vagus nerve is also the main cable controlling the parasympathetic system, which is the relaxation section of your nervous system. **YOU-reka!**

82

Figure 3.4a **Department of Energy** The three major types of energy are contained in carbohydrates, proteins, and fats, which can come from healthy or waist-busting forms. Complex carbs enter the blood slowly, so we do not tax our hormones. Amino acids are converted inefficiently to sugars, and fats cannot be converted at all. Fats come in forms our bodies recognize (like nuts) and naturally less common forms that poison us (like trans fats). Most foods, like meat, are a combination of energy sources; as the food digests (or sometimes rots) in your intestines, nutrients are absorbed in different places. By the way, even though the liver is the symbolic center of the metabolic universe, the intestines, as evidenced by your bathroom time, aren't really a closed loop.

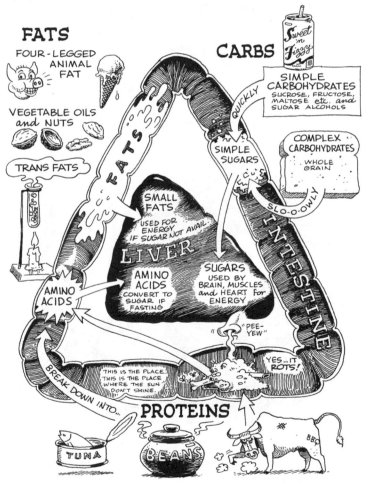

Figure 3.4b **Food Use** Simple sugars from carbohydrates are the most versatile energy source, so they're preferentially used by our organs, especially the finicky brain, which refuses to tolerate any other source. Fats are a backup system to supply muscle with energy; this is why actually using muscles is needed to selectively lose fat, and why exercise works so well. Amino acids from proteins are crucial for building the body, but are used only as a last resource for exercise energy.

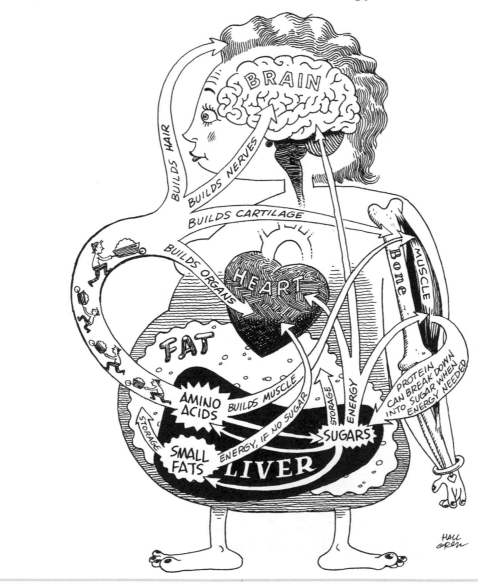

Figure 3.5 **Stop Sign** Food entering the small bowel stimulates release of the substance CCK into the wall of the stomach. That's where the vagus nerve senses that we're full and informs the satiety center in our brains to tell our hand to put down the buttered popcorn.

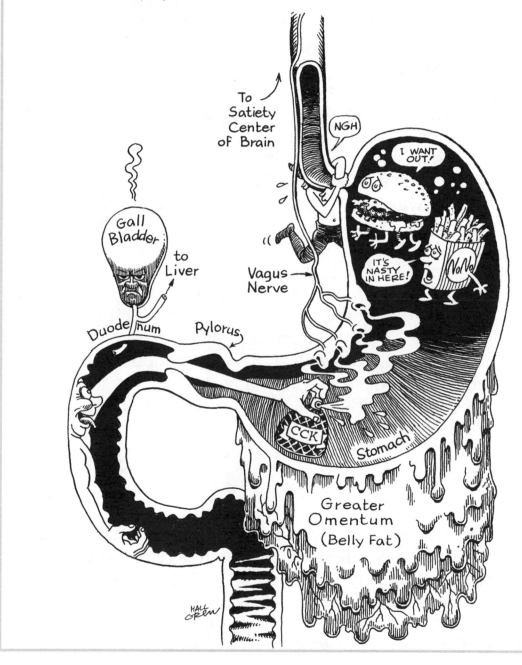

The Word on GERD

Fat doesn't just pose problems for your belly and subway turn-stiles; it also can mess with your throat. About half of obese people have the chest-burning condition called GERD (gastroesophageal reflux disease). The thinking is that extra fat in the belly pushes down on your stomach, thereby opening the angle of the GE junction and pushing it toward the chest. (Remember, it's at an acute angle to keep food from going back up your throat every time you eat.) The pried-open angle makes it easier for acid and food to be pushed back up. Plus, the extra fat in the belly puts pressure on the contents of your bowel. More pressure, more GERD. What's the big deal? Besides the unpleasant sensation of tasting your food on the way *up,* GERD also burns your esophagus — in the same way that the sun burns your skin. After a burn, it takes a couple days to heal, but if the burning happens over and over, it means you're burning the tissues and are more likely to develop cancer there, just like repeated sunburns increase your risk of skin cancer. Taking half a full aspirin or two baby aspirin (you want 162 mg) with a glass of water decreases this risk by about 35 percent. By the way, alcohol, coffee, pepper, acidic foods like tomatoes and OJ, and, to a lesser degree, chocolate increase GERD symptoms. The best way to manage symptoms until you lose weight is to avoid meals within three hours of bedtime and to put blocks under the head posts of your bed so that you sleep at a slight tilt. (Pillows usually don't work, since your head will typically roll off the pillow.)

The key messenger switching the vagus on is a peptide produced in your gastrointestinal track called CCK, which is released when your bowel senses fat. Technically, it stands for cholecystokinin, but for our purposes, let's think of it as the Crucial Craving Killer because its main purpose is to tell your brain via the vagus nerve that your stomach feels fuller than a *Baywatch* bathing suit.

Figure 3.6 **Acid Trip** Fat presses on the gastroesophageal junction and unkinks this connection, which makes acid and reflux move up toward the throat. Pressure on the stomach from intra-abdominal fat increases the backwash.

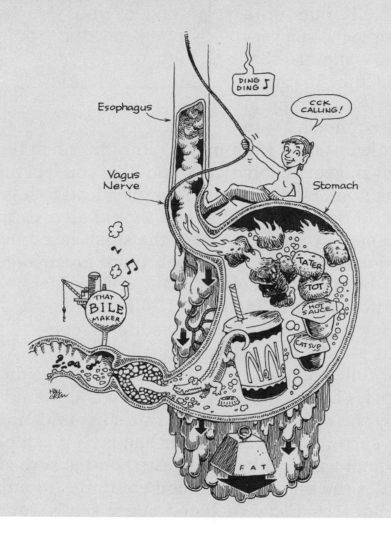

Without having to go through the chemical pathways of your body (your bloodstream), CCK acts as a very direct message and indicator of your fullness. (Remember, leptin is more of a long-term indicator of your satiety; CCK provides a very short-term, intense message.)

After the food spends some time in your stomach, it

Myth Buster

will slowly leave that reservoir and go into the small intestine via the duodenum, the first part of your intestines that comes right after the stomach. That's when CCK puts up a digestive detour sign, in a very clear physical signal that makes you feel full. It causes the pylorus — the opening at the end of the stomach — to

slam shut; that keeps food from moving into the small bowel. That's how your stomach gets full physically and how you feel full mentally. One interesting note: High-saturated-fat diets lead to less CCK sensitivity, so you do not feel as full as you should after eating a steak.

After the stomach, your food enters the small intestine and has a head-on collision with bile. Bile is the thick green digestive fluid that's secreted by the liver, stored in the gallbladder, and released into the small intestine. (CCK also has a third effect: It's what causes the gallbladder to contract.) After fat is broken down into smaller particles

Myth Buster

by substances called lipases, which are released by the pancreas, these tiny particles interact with bile to form a compound that is easily absorbed by the cells of your body. Bile surrounds the fat in our meal like soap surrounds grease on our hands so it can be scrubbed from the intestinal wall and better digested and absorbed.

Once it reaches the bloodstream, food continues to influence how hungry you may feel. Elevated blood sugar sends your brain the message that it's time to take your plate to the sink and hit the couch. When your blood sugar is low, that's what stimulates hunger and causes you to feed like a rat in the Kraft aisle.

Many of us get into trouble when we eat foods with simple sugars (think soft drinks, jelly, cake). Simple sugars create a rebounding effect. You're feeling blah, so you eat a 3 Musketeers. That sugar surge works like an electrical jolt, and you instantly feel more energy. But less than two hours later, that energy surge (in the form of elevated blood sugar levels) plummets, and then you feel blah again. Your conclusion? You must need another Musketeer. That rebound effect (combined with the desire for the taste that's stimulated by the pleasure center in your brain) can put your body in biological turmoil, where you eat to feel better, though what you're eating is actually making you feel sluggish, so you swirl and swirl around, always feeling like you need to eat.

YOU-reka! At the bottom end of your small intestine (before it joins your large intestine), food hits the ileal brake — another signal that you're full. At this juncture there's a traffic signal that slows the passage of the slurry of intestinal contents from the small intestine to the large intestine. It's called the ileocecal valve. The squeezing required to overcome this traffic signal valve is reduced naturally by some foods, since your body feels that you're still digesting and not ready to evacuate those foods yet. Very little absorption of nutrients occurs in the colon, so once the food passes the ileocecal valve, not much more happens except that you reabsorb water while consolidating the waste you've formed. The result: You have a traffic backup in your gut, and if you try to send more cars down the road, the problem's only going to turn into a fuller feeling. It's one of the reasons why fiber kills cravings, because fiber slows down the transit of food from your small intestine to your large intestine, keeping that full feeling. In the next chapter, we'll pick up the rest of the digestive journey in the intestines, where some of the key fat-storing processes take place.

The System of Satisfaction

Though it may seem that we have endless reasons to eat — to celebrate holidays, to beat stress, to pass time between Super Bowl commercials — there's only one real reason why we need food: for energy. That energy allows our organs to function, our muscles to move, and our bodies to keep warm. And to a large extent, our brains help control how we convert food to energy. To help understand the process that your body goes through to use energy, we'll break down the metabolic path into two phases.

Digestive Phase: Your hypothalamus orchestrates this phase of metabolism by receiving signals from throughout your body about whether you're hungry or not, so that your body can use energy to power itself. Here's how: Your body has a short-term reservoir for energy in the form of glycogen, a carbohydrate primarily stored in your liver and muscles. After eating, when you have glucose (sugar) and insulin (the hormone produced in the pancreas to transport glucose), your body uses all of the glucose it needs for immediate fuel but takes the rest and stores it as glycogen. If your blood glucose level falls, your pancreas stops releasing insulin — and then releases another G substance, glucagon, which converts the stored energy (glycogen) to sugar (glucose). So the effect is that when your intestinal gas tank empties of sugar (in other words, when our ancestors were fasting between bison hunts), your body is still able to supply crucial energy to your central nervous system by converting glycogen to glucose.

Fasting Phase: When you're sleeping or go long periods without eating, your body needs to have a supply of energy to keep your organs functioning. Once you use up all of your available glucose during the digestive phase of metabolism (your body stores only about 300 calories in the short-term glycogen reservoir), it taps a long-term reservoir: fatty tissue in the form of triglycerides (molecules that include a carbohydrate-containing glycerol). This keeps you going until you break the fast with breakfast.

Figure 3.7 **First-degree Burning** Feasting allows our livers to store excess sugar as glycogen, so we can access energy without eating for hours. Once glycogen stores are full, we save the excess energy from an ice cream sundae as fat. To break down fat, we first have to use up glycogen, which can take a half hour of exercise. That's when the body automatically begins burning up fat.

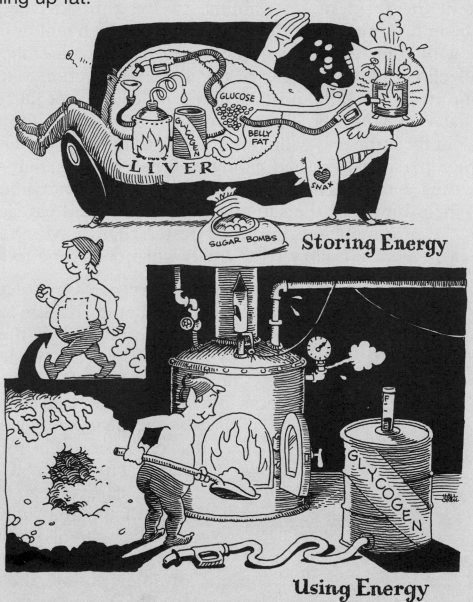

YOU TIPS!

Slow the Process. Especially before your meal. If you have a little of the right kinds of fat just before you eat, you can trick your hormonal system by sending the signal to your brain that you're full. If you eat a little fat twenty minutes before your meal (70 calories or so of fat in the form of six walnuts, twelve almonds, or twenty peanuts), you'll stimulate production of CCK, which will both communicate with your brain and slow your stomach from emptying to keep you feeling full. (CCK release and ghrelin reduction take about twenty minutes to kick in and take about 65 calories of fat to stimulate.) That way, you'll be able to sit down for a meal and eat for pleasure, not for hunger — which is one way to ensure you'll eat less. The average person is finished eating well before his satiety signals kick in, thus counteracting any possibility that his hormones can help him. For the same reason, you should eat slowly. If you down your food faster than a MiniVac, you won't allow your satiety hormones time to kick in.

Set the Early Fiber Alarm. Many of us may associate fiber with better health and increased toilet time, but fiber is the speed bump of your GI interstate. It slows everything way down. Technically, it works by slowing the transit of food across the ileocecal valve, keeping your stomach fuller for longer. The result: a greater feeling of satiety and an increase of appetite-suppressing CCK-like signals. While you should aim for around 30 grams of fiber a day, the key is bulking up in the morning. Studies show that con-

CECUM

suming fiber in the morning (at breakfast) makes you less hungry in late afternoon — a notorious candy-sucking, diet-busting time of day. Great sources of breakfast fiber include oatmeal, cereal, whole grains, and fruit. (You'll note that every breakfast in the YOU Diet — see Part 4 — has a lot of fiber in it, whether it's the cereal or the vegetables in an egg white omelet or the whole wheat bread. And morning snacks, like an apple, also have fiber.)

Besides controlling blood sugar levels and decreasing insulin levels, fiber also reduces calorie intake for up to eighteen hours a day. Start with 1 to 2 grams of dietary fiber before meals and at bedtime and slowly increase to 5 grams. (If you add it all at once, you'll produce more gas than a Saudi oil field.) The supplement konjac root also seems to have a fiber-related effect. One study showed a nearly six-pound weight loss in eight weeks for those who ate 1 gram of it an hour before their meals.

Step Down to the Plate. Monstrous portion sizes are one of our stomach's biggest enemies: Studies show that when you're served bad foods in large containers, you'll eat up to one-third more than if you were served in smaller containers. By getting served in larger popcorn boxes, bigger dishes, and taller cups, we've automatically been tricked into thinking that availability should dictate how much we eat, rather than physical hunger. You don't have to go through drastic changes to make small ones. For starters, change your serving plates to the nine-inch variety to give yourself the visual and psychological clue that you're full when your physical appetite has been sated. That's important, because studies show visual clues help determine how full you are, in that you may not feel satisfied until your plate is clean, no matter how large the plate is. That's also reason never to eat directly out of a box or carton and always to remember that one serving size of a food is often about the size of a fist.

Slow Down. Stomach growling stimulates appetite, but growling doesn't really tell you how hungry you are. It tells you to eat, but not how much to eat. That's why meal size is so important. You're hardwired to eat, but you're not hardwired to eat a lot. Having a big meal quickly won't stop you from wanting to eat a few hours later. So slow down and let your CCK act; it takes about twenty minutes after the nuts to decrease your desire to eat.

Add Pepper. Red pepper, when eaten early in the day, decreases food intake later in the day. Some credit the ingredient capsaicin for being the catalyst for decreasing overall calorie intake and for in-

YOU Test

Are You a Supertaster?

We all know that foods we like may send others seeking gas masks. But your tongue-related genetics may play an even bigger role in waist management. It could mean that you're either not getting the right foods, or more prone to downing an after-dinner pie before the check arrives.

If you're classified as a "supertaster," you tend not to eat fruits and vegetables because they may taste very bitter, thereby putting yourself at a higher risk of certain diseases and colon polyps because you're not getting the nutrients from fruits and vegetables. You should supplement your diet with a multivitamin to ensure you're getting the right nutrients, as well as use fruits and veggies to enliven other things — as in salads and desserts and as moisturizers on breads (tomato sauce works great here). And if you're an "undertaster," you may be more prone to eating (and overeating) sweets because it takes more of a taste to satiate you. By the way, researchers say about 25 percent of us are supertasters and 25 percent are uncreasing metabolism. It also appears to work by inhibiting sensory information from the intestines from reaching the brain, which is particularly effective in reducing appetite in low-fat diets. Capsaicin works by killing — or at least stunning — the messages that you're hungry. So add red peppers to your egg-white omelet.

dertasters, while the rest of us are regular tasters.
Which taster are you?

The Saccharin Test: Mix one pack of saccharin (Sweet'N Low) into two-thirds of a cup of water; that's about the size of the tennis ball. Now taste the water. You'll probably taste a mix of both bitter and sweet, but see which taste is stronger. If sweet is dominant, then it means you're probably an undertaster, and if bitter is dominant, it means you're probably a supertaster. If it's a tie, you are like half the population, so don't sweat it. To be sure, you may have to do the test more than once to tease out differences.

The Blue Tongue Test: Wipe a swab of blue food dye on your tongue and see the small circles of pink-colored tissue that polka-dot the newly painted blue canvas. Those are your papillae. Then put a piece of paper — with a 4-millimeter hole, or the size of a hole punch in three-ring paper — over your tongue. Using a magnifying glass, count the little pink dots you see in the hole. If you have fewer then five dots, it means you're an undertaster, while more than thirty indicate you're probably a supertaster.

Chapter 4
Gut Check

The Dangerous Battles of Inflammation in Your Belly

We all know about the daily skirmishes that play out in the battle against obesity. You versus the ranch dressing, you versus the dessert tray, and in the title fight, your butt versus your college jeans. But it would be a mistake to think that every weight-loss war happens at the table or in the privacy of your own closet. In fact, millions of little firefights break out inside your gut every time you eat or drink — and these are the most influential battles in your personal crusade

How Tolerant Are You?

With more than 100 million neurons in your intestines, gastrointestinal (GI) pain is immediate, but the level of GI discomfort you feel depends on your genetics; specifically on your tolerance of or allergies to certain foods and your genetic disposition for feeling the effects of those GI land mines. While there are certainly pharmaceutical solutions for dealing with the digestive explosions, there are also foods that produce an anti-inflammatory effect and can come in and put out the fire (see YOU Tips). During these inflammatory firefights, your intestines are contracting too much, or are being dilated — a painful process that works through the vagus nerve. Too much stimulation or distension of the bowel is what causes the pain. Some of us are less sensitive to those internal motions, so we may not always be getting the clue from our gut. These are some of the more common GI firestorms involving food intolerance:

■ *Enzyme deficiencies:* When your intestines lack enzymes to metabolize specific foods like milk or grains or beans, the food remains undigested, so you start feeding your intestines' ravenous bacteria. The result: lots of intestinal dilation and more gas than a Hummer fuel tank. The most common of these is lactose intolerance (the lack of GI agreement with dairy products), and a close second is an allergy to the protein gluten from wheat (and rye and barley; nutritional good guys). As an example, when you lack the enzyme lactase, the sugar lactose

against excess weight. Deep inside your éclair-encrusted gut, you have cells and chemicals that react and respond to food in two ways: as an ally or as an enemy.

As we move along in our digestive journey to the second half of our digestive system, we'll explore these battles and how they influence your waistline. Here, your body doesn't just form allies or fight enemies according to how many calories a particular food has, or

in the milk reaching your intestine is not metabolized, so it's presented to your intestinal bacteria, which metabolize the lactose in your intestines, producing a lot of gas.

■ *General GI disorders:* Problems like irritable bowel syndrome, which causes gut-related symptoms like diarrhea and abdominal pain, are caused by sensitive nerves and result in inflammation in the intestinal walls. For example, we usually all pass the same amount of gas a day (about fourteen times, or 1 liter total), but some of us sense discomfort from that gas more than others do.

■ *Psychological responses:* Food aversions can develop if, say, a person had a bad vomit-inducing shrimp dinner one night. The response would be to associate the shrimp dinner with the painful aftereffects and avoid it.

Of course, there are a number of extreme-end GI problems like infections, parasites (worms are the world's most successful weight-loss technique — but we don't recommend the *Fear Factor* diet), and violent and even lethal allergic reactions to food. The point is that we all may have degrees of intolerance in ways we may not even recognize. And we need to start listening to what our small intestine is trying to tell us about what we eat. Once you recognize that the general sense of "feeling off" can be caused by the foods you eat, you can identify — and work to eliminate, reduce, or substitute — the substance that makes your gut twist like an animal balloon.

how greasy it is, or whether its mascot is a red-haired clown. When interrogating nutrients as they pass through your digestive system, your body classifies them by what kind of inflammatory effect they have; the enemies contribute to inflammation, and the allies quiet it.

We're not just talking about the inflammation that happens when your belly balloons to the size of a convention center, or the inflammation that happens to your joints if you have arthritis. We're talking about the chemical reaction of inflammation that happens within your bloodstream and is an underlying cause of weight gain. This process is like the rusting of our bodies. Just like metal rusts when exposed to oxygen, inflammation is caused when oxygen free radicals (no political affiliation) attack innocent bystanders in our bodies.

Inflammation happens on many different levels and through several different mechanisms, many of them having to do with food. Not only can you get inflammation through allergies to food, but you can also get inflammation in the rest of your body — through the way your liver responds to saturated and trans fats, and through the way your body and belly fat respond to such toxins as cigarettes and stress. In turn, these inflammatory responses can cause things like hypertension, high cholesterol, and insulin resistance — and *those* inflammatory responses influence the total-body mother of all inflammation in your arteries, which leads to heart disease. (We'll discuss these at length in the next chapter.)

Here, we'll look at how inflammation happens at the gut level, and then, in the next chapter, how that can lead to inflammation at the total-body level.

Inflamed Gut: The Intestinal Firefights

At the intestinal level, foods can cause inflammation of your intestinal wall through such things as allergies, bacteria, or other toxins. When food incites inflammatory responses in your gut, it's as if a grenade has been launched throughout your digestive system (see Figure 4.1 on page 109). Then in response to this already damaging

100

grenade, your body tosses more grenades to create an apocalyptic digestive War of the Worlds. The effect is that the more inflammation we have in our intestines, the more toxins can enter our bloodstream.

During this firefight along the digestive border, your body perceives a foreign intruder and assigns its special forces — mast cells and macrophages — to eliminate the culprit. These are the cells that start an immune-response process throughout your body by ingesting foreign elements and alerting the rest of your body's protecting cells that intruders have entered the area. Foods that don't agree with your body's sensibilities are seen as foreign invaders, so the macrophages attack these foods and tell everyone that this war is going on. This causes your whole body to start firing away at these foods and at innocent bystanders — and thus causes inflammation in your bloodstream. In that way, eating unhealthy food is really like having a chronic infection that triggers an immune response, which then causes inflammation.

One of your body's goals is to get glucose into your brain cells —

FACTOID

For those of you who've stayed up wondering, here's the reason why your gas may smell and other people's gas may not: Think of your body as a refrigerator. If you let food sit in there, it's going to smell after a while. In your body, sulfur-rich foods like eggs, meat, beer, beans, and cauliflower are decomposed by bacteria to release hydrogen sulfide — a smell strong enough to flatten a bear. Avoiding these foods is the ideal solution, but when stinky gas persists, the best solutions are leafy green vegetables and probiotics (specifically lactobacilli GG or Bifidus Regularis), which work like baking soda in your fridge to reduce odor. Beano can sometimes work with beans, but soaking the beans ahead of time is useful as well.

to feed those brain cells so that they can function. But inflammation in your body prevents sugar from getting to those cells, so you end up wanting more glucose and eating more sugary foods, which then increase inflammation and starts the whole cycle again.

While we should be concerned about decreasing our body fat, we should also concentrate on decreasing our body's inflammatory response so we become more efficient in managing potential complications of our waist size.

There's some genetic component to inflammation (some us have more than others, and smokers tend to have higher levels of inflammation than nonsmokers). Most important, the process of gaining weight is often a process of inflammation. **YOU-reka!** When you decrease your body's inflammatory response, you will decrease your weight and waist as well.

The more inflammation you have, the less efficiently you use your food calories, and the worse you feel. The worse you feel, the more bad foods you eat to try to make yourself feel better. The more bad food you eat, the less well you can respond to the normal stresses of life, and the more inflammation you experience. And the more inflammation you have, the higher your risk of developing:

- diabetes
- high blood pressure
- bad cholesterol numbers

102

■ and all of the other conditions that contribute to your increase in size and your decrease in health

Plain and simple: Inflammation ages your body by making your arteries less elastic and by increasing atherosclerosis (the rusting of blood vessels). Inflammation also makes it more likely that your DNA will be damaged, and a cell will become cancerous. And it increases your risk of infections. If the inflammatory mediators are fighting in the arteries, they can't be defending elsewhere, and this situation increases the risk that your body will turn on itself, causing an autoimmune disease in which you attack your own tissues (for example, some forms of rheumatoid arthritis and thyroid disease).

Inflammation stresses your body.

Inflammation fattens your body.

Myth Buster

Obesity isn't just a disease of doughnuts and baked ziti. Obesity is a disease of inflammation. As we travel through the rest of our digestive journey, we'll be stopping at three

---

FACTOID

We have two main sources that power nature's rear-propulsion system. Gas comes from the air we swallow (20 percent) and the digestion of foods by bacteria in our intestines (80 percent). These bacteria love digesting sugars, fiber, or milk (if you're lactose-deficient). The result is lots of gas made up of carbon dioxide, nitrogen, and methane (which — *duck!* — is flammable). You can reduce swallowing air by avoiding cigarettes, gum, and carbonated beverages, or by eating and drinking more slowly.

---

digestive landmarks to see how foods influence inflammation and how inflammation influences fat:

Your Major Interstate of Food: Your Small Intestine. This approximately twenty-foot-long organ (it's about three times your height) serves as your second brain, deciding which foods agree with your body and which foods cause your body to rebel like sixth graders with a substitute teacher.

Your Parking Lot of Fat: Your Omentum. The omentum, which is located next to your stomach, serves as your primary storage facility of fat, where you park some or (in really bad cases) all the excess foods you eat. Ideally, the garage is empty. But as we gain weight, some of our bellies are housing four stories of Winnebago-worthy fat. Most important, the omentum serves as our body's ultimate stress gauge: **YOU-reka!** As we'll explain in a moment, bigger bellies indicate higher levels of inadequately managed chronic stress — which causes chronic levels of inflammation.

Myth Buster

Abdominal Pain Is a Pain in the Neck

Your abdominal discomfort may be caused not by what's happening inside your belly but by what's happening outside. According to one researcher, there's such a thing as Tight Pants Syndrome, which is abdominal pain lasting two to three hours after a meal. Its cause? Yup: pants that are too tight. (The researcher says there's as much as a three-inch difference between waist size and waistband.) Funny, but the same thing happens with men and shirt size. Two-thirds of men purchase shirts with a neck size that's too small, so they get headaches, changes in vision, and even changes in blood flow to and from the brain.

Your Post Office Processing Facility: Your Liver. Your liver is the second-heaviest organ in your body (the largest, your skin, is actually twice as heavy) and is your body's metabolic machine. Your liver works a lot like an urban postal center, taking in all the incoming mail (in terms of nutrients and toxins), sorting it, detoxifying it, and then shipping it off to different destinations for your body to use as energy.

> **FACTOID**
>
> Fat is like an organ, but the omentum is the supercharged version. Omentum fat has more blood supply than any other kind of fat and is quickest to mobilize itself to feed the liver.

While the three organs all play different roles, the upshot of their relationship is this: The small intestine initially processes your food, and your omentum helps store it. Inflammation occurs in your small intestine and omentum, but the big battle happens in your liver, where the mother of all inflammatory responses takes place. That's the one that makes you store fat — and experience the unhealthy effects of it.

Yes, we know that in-your-gut physiology isn't always pretty, but we want you to keep in mind our main gut goal: By understanding how food travels through this leg of your digestive system, you'll be able to identify the foods

> **FACTOID**
>
> About 10 percent of Americans have fatty livers that are overwhelmed with fat sent from the intestines and omentum for processing. Fatty livers can lead to fibrosis-reduced liver function, and even the serious liver disease cirrhosis over time, although for most folks, you just end up looking like foie gras on the insides.

that will help you reduce harmful and weight-related inflammation. When you do that, you'll have signed a digestive peace treaty that can end the war on your waist.

Gathering Intelligence

They say that a woman thinks with her heart, and a man thinks with his personal periscope, but when it comes to sheer anatomy, the organ closest to your brain isn't the one that flutters over a midnight serenade or the one that tingles over a lingerie catalog. It's the one that coils through your gut like a sleeping python.

From a purely physiological standpoint, your small intestine functions as your second brain. It contains more neurons than any organ but your brain (and as many as your spinal cord), and the physical structure of the small bowel most resembles that of the brain. In addition, after your brain, your small intestine experiences the greatest range of emotions — in this case, your **Myth Buster** feelings manifest themselves in the form of gastrointestinal distress. In your brain, you react to actions: You feel love when your spouse holds your hand, mad when he forgets an anniversary, humiliated when he takes off his shirt at the Bears game and thumps his densely forested chest for a shot at being on SportsCenter. Your small intestine does the same thing. It reacts to foods that enter its pathway, depending on their anti- or pro-inflammatory effect. Your foods dictate whether your small intestine feels mild annoyance (a little bloating), anger (gas), stubbornness (constipation), or all-out temper tantrums (a thar-she-blows case of diarrhea).

Of course, you're the one who decides what foods you'll eat, but your small intestine works like an undercover agent — gathering information about all the nutrients and toxins that enter your body.

Your small intestine feels. Your intestine thinks. And your intestine performs a critical job during digestion: It helps guide you in all of the decisions *you* make about eating, because it tells you which

Why Some People Stall

We'd like to think that our bodies work like cars — press the accelerator to go faster, tap the brakes to slow down. But our body's metabolic switches don't quite work that way: We may not gain or lose weight at the rate in which we expect to. When we have inflammation, our bodies are less efficient, meaning that we burn more calories — as a way to protect you, even as you gain weight. As we lose weight and decrease inflammation, our bodies go back to being efficient, and we may not burn calories at the proportional rate in which we gained them. So when we eat the right foods and more efficiently metabolize them, weight also may stall temporarily — meaning you still may be heavy, but might not have as many health risks associated with the weight.

foods agree with your body and which ones don't. How does it do that? Through the absorption of those foods. Your small intestine has an absorptive surface area that's 1,000 times larger than its start-to-end length because of all of the accordion-like nooks, crannies, and folds within it. Those spaces are where your body actually absorbs nutrients. So your intestinal absorption area isn't just 20 feet long; it's the equivalent of 20,000 feet long. No wonder you absorb so much of what you eat. When you have inflammation in the wall of your small intestine (through a food allergy or intolerance), it dramatically cuts down on that absorptive surface area — from about 2 million square centimeters to 2,000 square centimeters — because of swelling and poisoning of the functional surface cells. And if the intestine can't absorb nutrients, you experience an upset stomach and diarrhea.

While we're all familiar with those overt, emergency intestinal crises, our intestinal emotions also influence us in ways we don't normally associate with food. The reason we may feel groggy or have less energy than a drained nine-volt could be because our intestines are trying to tell us we're choosing the wrong foods. If you pulled out the small intestines of your entire family and laid them on the back deck to compare them (latex gloves, please), you'd see that they all look alike; they're the classic, wormy tubes that wind throughout your gut. In terms of basic physiology, we all have the same intestines, just as we all have the same basic brain structure. But just as all of our brains don't function the same way even though we have the same parts, our intestines don't function the same way either. **YOU-reka!** Our intestines are as different as our smiles, as our laughs,

FACTOID

You may hear that celebrities get colonics because they seem like some sort of miracle weight-loss cure. Here's how they work: You get a tube pushed up into your lower intestines (via your back end). You're infused with a solution, and you roll around to wash out your colon, then the fluid gets sucked out (you're given coffee, to help you go to the bathroom quickly). The purpose is to cleanse out the toxins and "reboot" your intestines. You'll produce a lot of waste after a colonic, but the main waste here is of money. Your colon only absorbs water, so there's no weight-loss benefit from colonics. In fact, you can get the same colon-cleansing and toxin-eliminating effect with a twenty-four-hour fast.

Figure 4.1 **Internal Conflict** Food and toxins continually line the frontier of our intestines. Good foods slip through to provide us nutrition, but combatants stimulate an aggressive response from local immune cells. The resulting inflammation causes swelling, gas, and belly cramps.

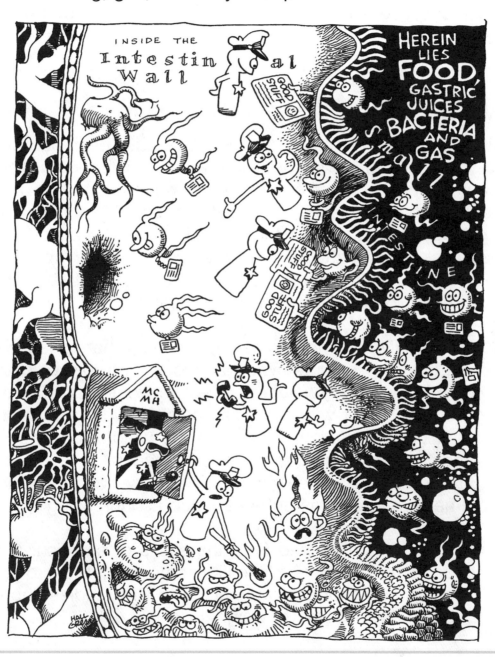

as our political views, as our fetishes. A particular food can make one person feel energized and make another person feel as lethargic as a rag doll.

Anatomically, your intestinal wall is Clint Eastwood tough. With more than a trillion bacteria living in your intestines at any given time (most of them helpful, but at least 500 species of which are potentially lethal), your body protects itself with a fortified infrastruc-

---

FACTOID

While hundreds of herbs and supplements have been purported to help you lose weight, many of them have not been studied well enough to support those claims and are not regulated by the FDA. Safety can be an issue — as was the case with ephedra, which helped people lose weight through adrenalinelike action but put them at risk of heart attacks. Here are some common herbal remedies and why they may not be all they're supposed to be, which is why you shouldn't put your weight-loss faith in any of them:

- Calcium: It's been touted as an ingredient that speeds weight loss. Studies have shown that those with low calcium are more likely to gain weight and be overweight. But the people who lost weight with increased calcium were also on short-term, calorie-restricted diets, so the weight loss was more predictable than an Oscar winner's speech.
- Bitter orange: It's been shown to decrease weight but has the same side effects as ephedra, such as increasing heart rate and blood pressure.
- Chitosan: It's extracted from the shells of shellfish, and the theory is that it works a little like some weight-loss drugs, by blocking fat absorption in your body. But studies show that chitosan doesn't lead to weight loss.

ture to keep the bacteria out of your bloodstream. But your body — though it relies on that Fort Knox–like wall — has to have a way to give clearance to authorized visitors. That is, it needs to allow nutrients to get through the wall to your bloodstream so you can use food as energy to keep your organs functioning, to go to work, to pry the kid's fingers from the panicked frog's leg. (One of the ways this penetration system works is through bile, which tricks the wall's security so fats can get through to the bloodstream.) This selection of what stays in your intestines and what can cross the line is one of the least understood anatomical processes, but it's part of the inflammatory battle that plays out daily in your body. When your intestinal wall is inflamed, some unauthorized visitors get in.

Essentially, alien bacteria are living in your intestines, trying to get into your bloodstream to multiply (which is their goal) and cause havoc, but they're being fought at the intestinal wall by those who guard it. (Your gastrointestinal tract, but especially your intestines, is one of three places where your body interacts with the external world; your skin and lungs being the other two.) In your small intestine, your mast cells and macrophages, which are part of your immune system, serve as the bowel brigade, fighting alien invaders.

When foods enter the small intestine and are transported across the intestinal wall, they're met by this bowel brigade border patrol, which screens the nutrients. The bowel brigade lets the food through because it has an authorized ID card — it's food, and your body wants it. But if it's the wrong kind of food, or if it's got some toxins with it,

FACTOID

About 2.5 percent of us suffer from milk allergies, making it the most prevalent of food allergies. While allergies to dairy products are generally outgrown, peanut allergies are not (and they're the most potentially lethal). By the way, it seems like allergies are more prevalent the earlier in life we're exposed to the foods.

Milking It

If you suffer from a milk allergy, it can make your gut feel like a washing machine in the rinse cycle. Here are some ways you can help manage it:

- Milk's one of the easiest ingredients to substitute in baking and cooking by using an equal amount of either water, fruit juice, or soy or rice milk.
- Watch out for hidden sources of dairy. For example, some brands of canned tuna fish and other nondairy products contain casein, a milk protein. The U.S. Food and Drug Administration (FDA) is currently working on requiring products to eliminate the term nondairy if they contain milk derivatives.
- In restaurants, tell your server about your allergy. Many restaurants put butter (which comes from milk) on steaks and other food after they've been grilled or prepared to add extra flavor, but you can't see it after it melts.
- Some ingredients seem to contain milk products or derivatives but actually don't. These are safe to eat if you have a lactose allergy: cocoa butter, cream of tartar, and calcium lactate.

By the way, there's a higher ethnic predominance of lactose intolerance in those of non-European origin. It's just another example of how genes — not willpower — help dictate what you can and cannot eat.

your bowel brigade responds by calling in more mast cells and setting off time-released bombs throughout your intestines. This is where the inflammation firefight starts. The result? Pain, gas, nausea, or general GI discomfort.

Why is this crucial? Not just because of the initial inflammatory reactions, but for the role it plays in your eating emotions (your small

Figure 4.2 **Belly Up** Not all fat is skin-deep. Deep down under your muscles, the omentum drapes off the stomach like stockings on a hanger. As we store fat, the omentum wraps around to give us the dreaded beer belly.

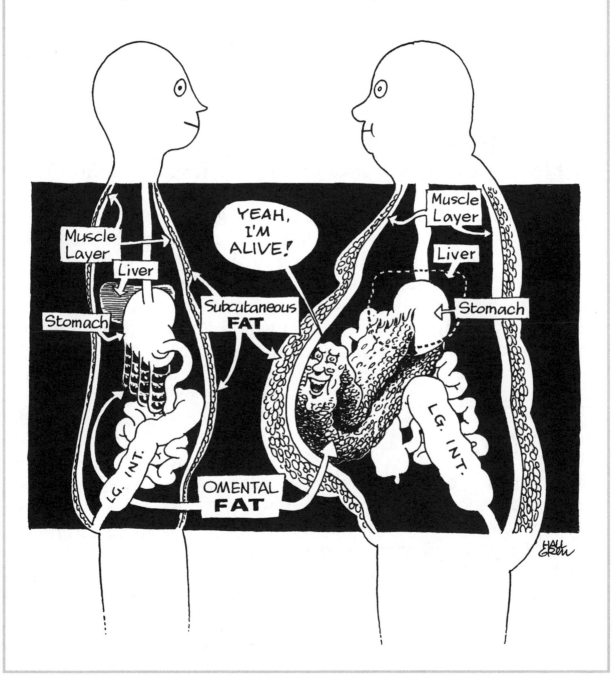

bowel is your second brain, and 95 percent of your body's serotonin, which is a feel-good hormone, is in your gut). How you feel influences how you eat, and how you eat influences how you feel. When you eat food that makes you feel bad, you self-medicate with food that may make you feel good in the short term but will actually contribute to both inflammation and weight gain. Ultimately, when you're caught in a cycle of feeling bad and eating worse, you'll create a chemical stress response in your body — one that's handled by your parking lot of fat.

The Storage of Stress in Your Belly

The best way to tell how stressed you are: Take a look how much belly fat you have. The larger your waist, the higher your stress.

Along the intestinal freeway, the parking garage for fat that is your omentum looks like a stocking draped over a hanger (the stomach is the hanger), but changes depending on how many calories you're storing (see Figure 4.2). In a person with little omentum fat, your stomach looks as if it has nylons hanging off it — thin, permeable, with some webbing. But in a person with a lot of omentum fat, the hanger looks as if snow pants are hanging on it — the fat globules are so fat that there's no netting or webbing whatsoever. (While cells can convert to fat in the liver, getting fatter is more a case of your existing cells growing. When you add body fat, you don't get more fat cells, just more fat in each cell.)

Genetics certainly helps dictate whether you're going to have a full garage (by having lots of belly fat) or an empty one. But your lifestyle — in

FACTOID

Most of our body parts are adaptable enough to use multiple energy sources to survive. Only two organs need sugar directly: the brain and the testes. Evolutionary hints often come in these forms of clues.

terms of stress — often plays a bigger role in deciding whether you'll have large amounts of belly fat or not. Here's how it works:

Historically, mankind has two types of stresses. The first kind is the immediate soil-your-loincloth stress (in other words, the dinner-seeking saber-toothed tiger is closing in fast). In that fight-or-flight scenario, your body produces the neurotransmitter norepi-

nephrine to speed your heart rate, breathing, and 100-yard-dash time to the cave. When that happens, the last thing you're thinking about is grilling up some tubers on the campfire, so your hunger levels are squashed. That's because your body inhibits the peptide NPY during periods of acute stress (it's why exercise cuts appetite, because your body senses that you're in acute stress). So high levels of stress work in favor of your waist: They take away your appetite and speed up your metabolism.

The second kind of stress that early man faced is the chronic struggle brought on by drought and famine. In contrast to the thirty or forty seconds they sweated over tiger fangs, our ancestors worried about survival all the time, and their bodies had to deal with chronic stress. When they faced famine, they sought out as many calories as they could, and their metabolism downshifted to help them conserve energy. While we don't deal with famine, we experience modern-day versions of chronic stress that make us seek out calories and then downshift our metabolism. **YOU-reka!** Our bodies respond by storing the excess energy to call upon during periods where there may not be enough food. Those extra calories are stored in the omentum — our abdominal fat depot — to have on hand in case we are denied food. The

115

liver, which is the relay station for energy circulation in the body, has immediate access to this omental fat, unlike the cellulose cluttering up the back of our thighs.

When people are under stress, their bodies release high amounts of steroids into their bloodstream in the form of the hormone cortisol. In acute cases (the tiger or a car accident), steroids stick around briefly. But when you're under chronic stress (the drought or the nagging task), your body needs to find a way to deal with those high levels of cortisol. So your omentum clears the cortisol steroids; it has receptors that bind to them and can suck them out of the bloodstream. (Unfortunately, this doesn't necessarily reduce the stress level that you feel.) The steroids turbocharge the ability of omentum to store fat, so your belly fat (and subsequent waist size) becomes the best surrogate indicator of how well you are really coping with stress — despite what your brain might be claiming. That uptake of steroids throws your body into metabolic disarray by making your omentum resistant to insulin so that sugar floats around without being absorbed and used appropriately by needy cells. This:

FACTOID

The additive olestra looks like a fat, cooks like a fat, and tastes like a fat, but is not a fat and isn't absorbed as a fat — which is why it's used in some food products to lower their fat and calorie contents. The problem is that olestra gives your stools the consistency of tea and sucks away some of the valuable fat-soluble vitamins, especially carotenoids. So it's smart to eat lots of yellow and green vegetables if you're eating chips made with olestra. By the way, the official name of olestra provides a useful insight into its mechanism of action: "sucrose polyester."

- chronically raises your blood sugar, which damages your tissues;
- supercharges your omentum with inflammatory chemicals that

116

Figure 4.3 **Toxic Dump** All the nutrients we absorb through the intestines pass through the liver via the portal vein. Excess fat and inflammatory chemicals stored in the omentum can dump directly into the liver as well, which can start a cascade of toxic protein release into the body.

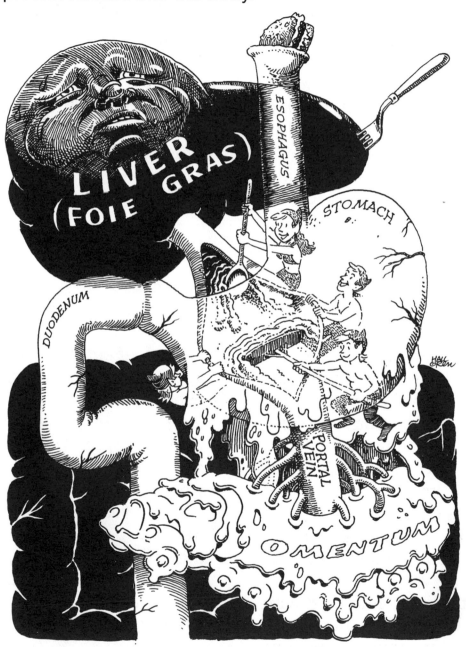

destabilize the delicate equilibrium of your hormones;

■ forces your omentum to pump high-octane fat directly into your liver — causing your liver to make even more inflammatory chemicals.

The Fight Against Inflammation

The liver — the organ that's responsible for your metabolism — receives its blood and nutrients from your gut. What it wants isn't the trans fat from the extra-large fries. It wants the other nutrients: the protein from the meat, the carbohydrates from the bun, the lycopene from the tomato, the calcium from the cheese. The liver is always on the job, processing munchies after midnight, as well as 5 a.m. coffee.

Your liver takes every chemical in your body and processes it by binding it to a protein, transforming it into something the body can use.

So your poor overworked liver also gets the toxic trans fat directly from your intestines and from your omentum via that portal vein that feeds right into it. When your intestines send that convoy of fat pouring down into the vein, the liver sees it as a runaway train and tries to metabolize the foods. But in defending the body, additional inflammatory chemicals are released.

In your liver, nutrients can be met by two substances. In our digestive town along our

FACTOID

Preliminary studies in animals show that the scent of grapefruit oil — yes, just the scent — has an effect of reducing the appetite and body weight. Rats exposed to the scents for fifteen minutes three times a week enjoyed the effect. The cause? It's unclear, but it may work through grapefruit oil's effects on liver enzymes. Grapefruit oil is widely available through aromatherapy stores and websites. As a bonus, try to eat a couple of grapefruit while you're searching.

intestinal highway, let's think of one as the raucous frat house that stimulates inflammation, while the other is a nice, stately nonprofit group that quiets inflammation and performs good deeds throughout your body.

Eating foods that stimulate your liver to release the frat-house substance — which is called nuclear factor kappa B, or NF-kappa B — triggers a chain of events that causes the inflammation in your body and prevents the transport of glucose to your cells (and thus triggers hunger). Glucose (sugar) on the inside of cells stops hunger (in the

Help on the Horizon

"Fat-free" can refer to marathoners and teen pop stars, but when you see it referring to food, you have to be skeptical. That's because either it tastes like a shoe box or it can be loaded with lots of sugar to compensate for fat — making that "fat-free" food more dangerous than a slowpoke in the passing lane. One goal for food manufacturers is to make foods that allow eaters to have the best of both worlds: great-tasting food that doesn't have waist-expanding ingredients. One such substance that may eventually change the way we eat is called Z-trim — it's a natural, zero-calorie fat substitute that's made from the fiber of such ingredients as oats, soy, rice, and barley. While there's no clinical data showing its effectiveness in weight loss, there's some evidence to suggest it can be used to cut the amount of fat usually used in a meal by 25 percent to 50 percent. The resulting food has all the "taste" benefits of fat (better taste, more creaminess, better mouth-feel) without the caloric load. Z-trim, which you can use with your own recipes, might also inhibit the hunger-inducing ghrelin because of its fiber content. The downside seems to be that by adding Z-trim, you also lose the benefit of the healthy oils in the food. Our tasters reported that foods with Z-trim had all the flavor of full-fat food, and that's enough to make us hopeful that nonfat won't always have to mean high-sugar or no taste.

Infected and Inflated

While it's true that everything from your hair to that ankle tattoo technically belongs to you, the truth is that only 10 percent of the cells on and in your body are actually yours. The rest are microbes living on your skin and in your orifices (pleasant visual, eh?), and especially in your gut. Those gut-residing microbes provide the enzymes you need to digest the fiber in fruits and vegetables that would otherwise pass through your system without being absorbed (pleasant visual number two). That's right. Without the bacteria and viruses in your gut, the food-label warning about 100 calories per bite would be a gross exaggeration. Specifically, mice raised without exposure to any germs have 60 percent less body fat than ordinary mice, even though they eat 30 percent more food. More intriguingly, common gut bacteria inhibit proteins that normally prevent the body from depositing fat, so infected mice have more belly fat.

So what do a few blubbery mice have to do with obesity in humans? It turns out that people infected with a specific chicken virus in India carry an extra 33 pounds of fat compared with noninfected humans. More important, they have lower cholesterol and triglyc-

specific satiety center of the brain). But you can also eat foods that stop the inflammation riot or foods that stimulate the release of the do-good substances that have an anti-inflammatory effect (see Figure 4.4). They're called PPARs (it stands for peroxisome proliferator-activated receptors, but we like to think of them as Perfectly Powerful Abdominal Regulators). The reason PPARs are so effective: Once they're activated, they decrease glucose and insulin levels, as well as cholesterol and inflammation. Though we all have different genetic dispositions for levels of PPARs, PPARs aren't self-starters; they need to be activated by foods to work.

Now, if you look at PPAR and NF-kappa B at the cellular level, you can also see how they predispose us to obesity. Every human cell is run by DNA strands that carry blueprints for future growth. When

eride levels — just the opposite of what we expect with weight gain. Why? Perhaps because the germs in the gut also digest cholesterol, so that less of it is absorbed. In an American study, the virus was found in 30 percent of obese subjects compared to only 11 percent of leaner people, and the folks who had the virus weighed significantly more than uninfected people. (And when twins with only one infected sibling are examined, the infected twin has 2 percent more body fat, despite having the same genes.)

Finally, we know that fat cells and our immune cells share lots of similarities. Fat cells can engulf bacteria and can secrete hormones that stimulate the immune system, possibly explaining why obesity causes an inflammatory response and leads to elevated C-reactive protein (a marker of inflammation). So how do you tell if you have a germ civil war inside you that's causing obesity? If your cholesterol and triglyceride levels are low and your C-reactive protein level is elevated, it might be worth testing yourself; Obetech (www.obesity virus.com) makes a kit. This might reduce your guilt level, but since science is still gathering data and a cure is still lacking, you will still need to focus on other approaches. At least for now anyway.

the DNA mutates, it makes our cells less able to reproduce themselves rapidly and accurately, so our bodies age. What makes that DNA break down? Yes, inflammatory responses in your body that cause oxidation (remember that this is your body's rusting process) — namely in the form of increasing NF-kappa B with inadequate PPAR levels to put out the inflammatory fires. How do we stop that mutation, that oxidation, and that inflammation? By eating foods with antioxidant and anti-inflammatory properties — foods that we'll cover in the waist management plan on page 231. These foods are particularly useful for those who are aging and unable either to exercise or to manage stress efficiently.

This is one of the primary battles you want to win — to quiet your inflammation and decrease your fat storage through the regulation

Figure 4.4 **Party's Over** Foods entering the liver can stimulate either proteins (NF-kappa B) that act like drunk frat boys and cause inflammation or soothing receptors (PPAR) that put out the fires. Even if you eat too much, if the PPARs are running the show, the negative effects are far less.

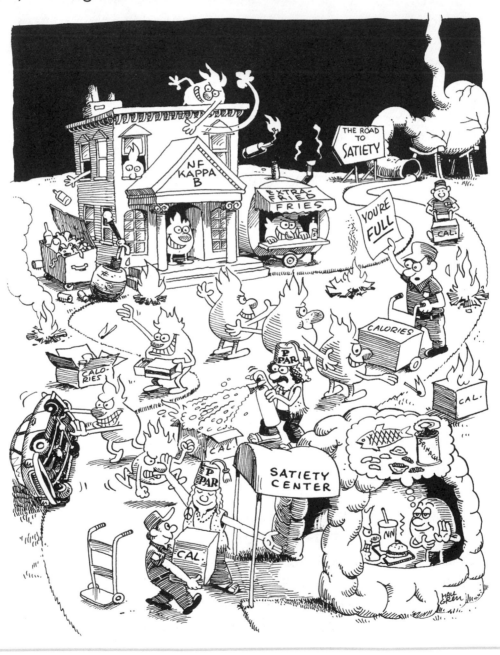

Weird Causes of Obesity

Most people assume that being overweight means one of two things: that you eat too much or move too little. But some research suggests that overeating and inactivity shouldn't be the only things taking the blame for our moon-sized waist circumferences. Studies show that other explanations for obesity include things like — get this — what you stick under your armpits and the age of your mom when she gave birth. Here are some of the more unusual things theorized to be related to obesity:

Deodorants: Some deodorants contain chemicals that can disrupt your normal metabolism, making you more likely to gain weight. While we don't recommend ditching the deodorant and scaring off elevator mates, you should avoid deodorants that contain the ingredient aluminum or sprays with polychlorobiphenols.

The temperature: Air conditioning in the summer and heating in the winter may make you less cranky, but they also may make you fatter. If you're in a cold room, for example, your body has to do more metabolic work to bring your temperature to normal (same for a warm room) — thus increasing your metabolism. You can increase your calorie-burning motors simply by lowering the temperature in your house during the winter or raising it in the summer.

Stopping smoking: We recommend cigarettes about as much as we recommend DIY vasectomies, but nicotine can be a powerful weapon in the fight against fat. See our take on nicotine on page 390.

Your mom: Studies show that the older your mom was when she gave birth, the more likely you are to be fatter. While there's nothing you can do to change your family history, having a mom who was older at the time of your birth means you need to be more vigilant about watching your waist.

Your mate: Studies show that fatter people tend to choose fat mates, and that increases the odds that you'll produce an even fatter child. We're not in the matchmaking business, but it's worth noting that the best place to meet a mate isn't at the burger joint.

of these two chemicals and their allies. To quash those hooligans living in the NF-kappa B house, you need to increase the effects of the noble PPARs throughout your body.

The Stress Response: Putting It All Together

Today, we don't experience droughts or famine, but we do have high levels of chronic stress, whether it comes in the form of workload, relationship troubles, or to-do lists that are longer than Route 66. And our bodies respond the same way as our ancestors' bodies did. But the difference is that we have plenty of food at our disposal. Chronic stress triggers an ancient response of calorie accumulation and fat storage, so we end up continually upgrading the size of our omentum storage unit. Here's where the cycle of fat spins out of control:

- When you have chronic stress, your body increases its production of steroids and insulin, which . . .
- Increases your appetite, which . . .
- Increases the chance you'll engage in hedonistic eating in the form of high-calorie sweets and fats, which . . .
- Makes you store more fat, especially in the omentum, which . . .
- Pumps more fat and inflammatory chemicals into the liver, which . . .
- Creates a resistance to insulin, which . . .
- Makes your pancreas secrete more insulin to compensate, which . . .
- Makes you hungrier than a muzzled wolf, which . . .
- Continues the cycle of eating because you're stressed and being stressed because you're eating.

Interestingly, the more fat you store in your omentum, the more it reduces the effect of stress on your brain — it's your body's way of comforting you, assuring you that you'll be prepared during times of famine. It's why your omentum fat — the fat around your belly —

Figure 4.5 **Stress Mess** The cycle of stress affects weight by increasing hormones above normal levels, resulting in hunger and fat deposition, which causes inflammation, which causes more stress, and off we go.

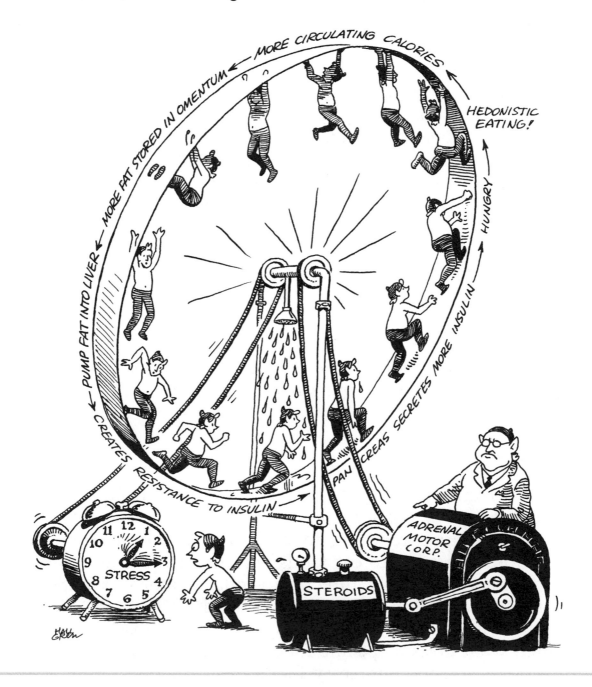

Is There Such a Thing as a Bad Food?

Fast-food franchise owners aren't the only ones who may say that there's no such thing as good or bad food — that it's just the volume of food that you eat. There are plenty of dietitians, nutritionists, doctors, and food growers who believe the same thing. Our research leads us respectfully to disagree. Good, healthy foods satiate you, they decrease inflammation in your body, they decrease the tendency to yo-yo, they're nutrient-dense, and they make you younger. Bad foods make you more hungry, increase inflammation in your body, make you feel sluggish, make it more likely you'll yo-yo, have few nutrients, and make you older. After all, when you eat fries (no matter whether it's two fries or two bags), you're taking in calories that taste good, but have as much nutrient value as plywood. In our words, bad foods add to your waste; good foods make waist management easier because they help keep you satisfied so that you never feel like gorging on nutrient-low and calorie-high foods. We call those good foods the YOU-th-FULL foods.

isn't just an indicator of the size of your waist, it's also your own personal gauge of the size of your stress.

YOU TIPS!

Let Food Fight the Fight. Your best weapon against fat isn't a Tae-Bo video or a self-serve liposuction vacuum. It's food. Good food. Inflammation-reducing food. To reduce obesity-causing inflammation, you need to eat foods with nutrients that can do just that — either by having direct anti-inflammatory or antioxidant properties, or by stimulating the do-good PPARs or inhibiting the party-throwing pledges in the NF-kappa B frat house. Antioxidants are often what gives a specific food its flavor, smell, and color. So eating more anti-inflammatory foods means eating more flavorful and brightly colored foods. (The foods you eat ought to be tasteful; you can magnify a flavor by doubling up on it with two different food sources. For example, add sun-dried tomato bits to tomato sauce, or eat dried apples with applesauce to bring out the flavor.)

Following is a list of nutrients that seem to have antioxidant and/or anti-inflammatory effects, and our recommended doses. While they may not help you lose a ton of weight, they're known or thought to have anti-inflammatory effects, which will help you live healthier no matter what your weight.

Substances known to fight inflammation:

Omega-3 Fatty Acids: Omega-3 fatty acids — found in fish oils — seem to increase the number of PPARs, which will help reduce your inflammation. We recommend you get omega-3s in the form of three four-ounce servings of fish per week or a 2-gram fish oil capsule a day or an ounce of walnuts a day. (Saturated fats, by the way, increase inflammatory properties, and trans fat undermines the effects of omega-3s.)

Green Tea: The thinking is that catechins in green tea inhibit the breakdown of fats and also inhibit production of NF-kappa B. Studies have found that drinking three glasses of green tea a day reduced body weight and waist circumference by 5 percent in three months. It also increased metabolism (all nonherbal teas have substances that increase the metabolic rate).

Substances we think may fight inflammation:

Beer (in moderation, Tiger): The bitter compounds that come from hops derived from beer seem to activate PPARs in animal studies. But you have to get them in the form of only one drink a day. People who drink twenty-one eight-ounce beers, or twenty-one glasses of wine, or twenty-one shots of whiskey a week have a clear correlation predisposing them to belly fat, independent of all other risk factors.

Turmeric: A gingerlike plant that has curcumin as its active ingredient, turmeric seems to activate more PPARs to reduce inflammation. Just add the right dose — a pinch (1/8 of a teaspoon). Add any more and your food will taste like mustard.

Jojoba Beans (They are really seeds): They've been shown to tune up the system in the ways we want, like increasing good cholesterol levels and raising leptin levels to curb hunger. The supplement jojoba extract (the supplement simmondsin is also made from jojoba) seems to work by stimulating CCK. The dose is about 2.5 grams to 5 grams for most people (50 milligrams per kilogram of weight).

The Main Ingredients

Though the effect is not completely proven, there's some evidence that the following substances and ingredients have a meaningful anti-inflammatory effect:

Substance	Found In
Isoflavones	Soybeans, all soy products
Lignans	Flaxseed, flaxseed oil, whole grains such as rye
Polyphenols	Tea, fruits, vegetables
Glucosinolates	Cruciferous vegetables such as broccoli and cauliflower, plus kale
Carnosol	Rosemary
Resveratrol	Red wine, grapes, red or purple grape juice
Cocoa	Dark chocolate
Quercetin	Cabbage, spinach, garlic

Drink Java. Coffee is Americans' largest source of antioxidants (aside from caffeine, which has its own antioxidant properties). It is chock-full (pun intended) of polyphenols and is a great low-calorie fluid when you have cravings. You can drink decaffeinated versions to avoid the side effects. The second-biggest source of antioxidants? Bananas, which have seven times less than coffee.

Go through the Process of Elimination. To change the way you feel, the way you process food, and the way you store fat is to get at the root of the system: You need to figure out what foods may be causing you GI trouble, no matter how subtle your symptoms may be. The best way to do that is through the food-elimination test. What you'll do is completely eliminate certain groups of foods for at least three days in a row. (Sometimes, the elimination of a food takes two or more weeks to show its benefits in how you feel.) During that time, take notes about all the different ways you feel: your energy levels, fatigue, and how often you go to the bathroom. Take notes when you eliminate foods and when you reintroduce them — that way you'll really notice what changes make you feel worse or better.

Here's the order we suggest: wheat products (including rye, barley, and oats), dairy products, refined carbohydrates (especially sugar), saturated and trans fats, and artificial colors (which are tough to get rid of because they're in everything). While the experiment will help you ID your personal digestive destructors, it has an added benefit: Eliminating a group of foods for several days at a time will help train your body to eat smaller portions all the time.

Get Moving after a Big Meal. If you've made a mistake and gorged on a tub's worth of food, make your body work in your favor. Stay awake for a few hours and take a thirty-minute walk to help your body with the breakdown of nutrients and so that it uses the food for energy, rather than storing it as fat. Once the calories are in your stomach, don't try to vomit; vomiting can damage your stomach, burn your esophagus, and even discolor your teeth if you do it enough. Also, don't eat sweets after gorging, because sweets will increase insulin and help deposit excess calories in your belly.

Pick Your Poison. High amounts of sucrose (sugar) cause inflammation; you can reduce the effect by using alternative sweeteners. Besides causing sudden spikes in blood sugar, foods with high sugar content have high calorie content, and if not burned off or used as fuel, those calories will be stored as fat. While some sweeteners are low- or no-calorie, there is a downside: Sweeteners found in diet soft drinks, in diet foods, and on restaurant tables next to the sugar packets go unrecognized by the brain. They're essentially invisible to your brain's satiety centers, so it doesn't count them as real food and still desires to be fulfilled by calories somewhere else. There's no clear-cut proof on the effects of these sweeteners — either on a health level or on a weight-loss level — but we do know one thing: Prehistoric man wasn't putting Splenda in his water. Artificial sweeteners, while lacking calories, may have side effects like intestinal problems and headaches. If you're having a hard time losing weight or don't feel well, these are some of the first things to cut out, even though they can be an alternative to high-calorie sugars. There's no clear-cut data on which sweeteners work most effectively, but here's how we rate them:

Sweetener	The Scoop	Here's the Skinny
Sucralose (Splenda)	Discovered in 1976 but not introduced for widespread use for many years. More than 500 times sweeter than sucrose, stored in body fats, suitable for baking, and does not affect levels of blood sugar.	The research is least complete on this one, but go ahead and keep it in the cupboard. Its widespread use is too new for us to know any of the long-term effects, but it appears the most promising — and it's the best one to use for cooking.
Aspartame (NutraSweet)	Entered the market in 1981. Several studies have found that it has adverse health effects, but those studies were very limited.	It's come under a lot of scrutiny and has basically stood the test of time. But it's the sweetener that hangs around the longest in your body, and it cannot be heated — it turns into formaldehyde (which could help you save on funeral expenses). It's also rumored to limit the brain's ability to use certain vitamins, antioxidants, and the mineral magnesium.

Sweetener	The Scoop	Here's the Skinny
Saccharin	Has been around since the early 1900s, and while some studies found a health risk, those studies have significant limitations.	It appears to be one of the safest sweeteners and the only one with real long-term data, even if some of the data is not positive. (If you consume more than eighty twelve-ounce diet sodas a day, you're at an increased risk of bladder cancer — good luck!)
Agave nectar	It's a hypersweet natural substance.	Try it. While it's very high in calories, you need only a fraction of the amount of sugar needed to gain the same level of sweetness. You can order through vegan essentials.com or blue agavenectar.com.
Stevia	A noncaloric natural herb. Taste isn't ideal, and stevia seems to lower sperm counts in some studies.	For the taste and the potential side effects, no thanks. No diet drink is worth the potential of sterility.

Chapter 5
Taking a Fat Chance

How Fat Ruins Your Health

Diet Myths

- Thin people are automatically healthier than fat people.

- A fat is a fat is a fat. All fat is equally damaging.

- Your ideal blood pressure is anything less than 140/90.

It doesn't matter whether you're just trying to shave a few inches from your waist or trying to morph your slushy belly into an ice-hard one, the fact remains: It's hard to forget about body fat. You see it when you get dressed, get washed, and get jiggy. You feel it when you sit down, when you walk upstairs, when you bend over to lick the last cake crumbs off the plate. And if you're a person who's struggled with weight for a lifetime, you likely stress about fat more than you stress about money, relationships, or anesthesia-free colonoscopies.

Fat is constantly right in our faces. And on our minds. And wrapped around our necks and arms. And hanging from our bellies, raining from our rears, and gyrating during twist contests. But you know what?

Oftentimes, we forget about fat. We eat a lot of food at one meal and go back to do it right again — because we don't see the health risks in the same way we see a slightly larger chin in the mirror. Now that our digestive journey is over, and you've learned how fat is stored, it's time to explore what that excess stored fat can do — to your heart, to your arteries, to your entire body.

Most of us assume that you have to be as skinny as a coaxial cable to be healthy, but the truth is that plenty of so-called thin people are less fit and less healthy than so-called heavy people. **YOU-reka!** That's right: It's actually better to be fat and have few risk factors for bad health than it is to be thin and have a high number of health-related risk factors. Now, that's not to say we're ordering a round of fried pickles for everyone. When all else is equal, carrying extra fat will more likely increase your risk of heart attacks, strokes, and diabetes. But our point is that we want you to stop thinking about pounds and pounds only; we'd rather you start thinking about the numbers that really matter — especially to your husbands, wives, children, parents, and friends. The real story of your body isn't measured by scales or wolf whistles. It's measured by your waist size — and what fat does inside your blood and arteries.

134

What Fat's Got to Do with It

Here's how many of us assess our health: If the pain's not severe enough to call the paramedics, then we tough it out, go on our way, and write off most of our general feel-bad symptoms to fatigue, stress, age, or the jug of vanilla fudge we downed during *CSI*. The problem with that approach? You're probably more in tune with the fall TV schedule than you are with your own body. Of course, if you're overweight, the extra fat is sure to manifest itself in some outward side effects like lack of energy or lack of self-esteem. But many of the risk factors associated with carrying too much fat don't have any outward symptoms at all — meaning that the only way to tell whether being overweight is threatening your life is by taking a microscope underneath the flub and chub and focusing on what's happening at your body's most core levels.

Sure, you know that fat lives on your hips, but it also lives in your blood. If you were to take a vial of blood and let it sit (we don't recommend doing this at home), you'd see a layer of clotty cream that would rise to the top of the vial, sort of like tiramisu. That's fat. How did it get there? (Half credit if your answer was tiramisu.) It's absorbed via your intestines. But the key player is the omentum. And why should we care about that organ that sounds like it's missing the letter *m?* Because the omentum can store fat that is quickly accessible to the liver (meaning it can cause lousy cholesterol and triglyceride levels to rise) and also sucks insulin out of circulation (making your blood sugar rise) — meaning that this cream-converted fat sets up shop in the omentum and puts your organs within very close striking distance of a hammer.

See, fat is like real estate: it's all about location, location, location.

We all have three kinds of fat: fat in our bloodstream (called triglycerides), subcutaneous fat (which lies just underneath the skin's surface), and that omentum fat. (The fourth fat, of course, is the fat in food). As you remember from the last chapter, the omentum is a fatty layer of tissue located inside the belly that hangs *underneath* the muscles in your stomach (it's why some men with beer guts have hard-as-keg bellies — their fat is underneath the muscle).

Because this omentum fat is so close to your solid organs, it's their best energy source. (Why go to the gas station on the other side of town when there's a station at the next corner?) Think of the omentum fat as the obnoxious eighteen-wheeler on a crowded highway — elbowing out the stomach, pushing away other organs, and claiming all the space for itself (see Figure 5.1).

What's most interesting — and encouraging — is that as soon as you make physiological changes to your omentum, your body starts seeing effects. That is, once your body senses it's losing that fat, then your body's blood-related numbers (cholesterol, blood pressure, blood sugar) start traveling in the healthy direction — within days, before you even notice any kind of physical sign of weight loss (especially when you consider that the size of your omentum is impossible to measure without a CT scan).

In addition, the fat released from the omentum travels to your liver rapidly and constantly as opposed to the more patient fat on your thighs. The processed material is then shipped to the arteries, where it is linked to health risks like high LDL (lousy) cholesterol. The other problem with omentum fat is that it secretes very little adiponectin, which is a stress- and inflammation-reducing chemical that's related to the hunger-controlling hormone leptin. When you have less fat, you secrete more adiponectin, which produces a product that reduces inflammation. But more importantly, higher levels of adiponectin are related to lower levels of fat. So the more omentum fat you have, the less fat-regulating adiponectin you'll produce. Those who have low levels of adiponectin have abdominal obesity, high blood pressure, high cholesterol, and other risk factors associ-

Figure 5.1 Belly Bully The omentum greedily bullies surrounding structures out of the way. The squished diaphragm and lungs make breathing difficult, and the squashed kidney and its blood supply secrete hormones to raise the blood pressure in an effort to fight back.

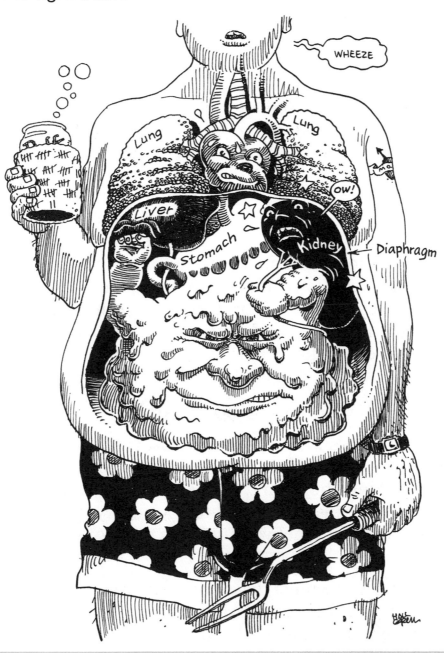

ated with coronary artery disease.

Those are the reasons why the fat in your thighs doesn't matter as much to your health as does omentum fat (even if it matters for your bikini pride), and they help explain why omentum fat (or an "apple" body shape) is more harmful than subcutaneous fat (like thigh fat, which gives you a "pear" shape). Subcutaneous fat isn't supplying a feeding tube to the rest of your vital internal organs, and it's not messing up the levels of substances in your blood that are being supplied to your vital organs.

The closer your waist is to ideal, the healthier your arteries and your immune system will be. The healthier your arterial and immune systems, the longer — and better — you'll live. And the more energy you'll have every day.

Highways to Health

Before you know what's inside your arteries, you need to know how they're structured — so you can see what kind of damage they can sustain and what kind they can't. Made up of three layers, your arteries are the monorails of your body — they transport blood throughout your body and deliver nutrients to all of your organs (see Figure 5.2).

Inner layer: The innermost layer of your arteries (the intima) comes in contact with blood; it's slippery like Teflon so blood can easily flow through. This normally smooth layer helps protect the

138

Figure 5.2 **Moving Through** The artery has three layers — the inner to help blood move through the artery (intima), the outer (adventitia) to protect it from the outside, plus a middle, muscular layer (media). Damage to the inner layer hurts the tile-like layer of cells, injuring the delicate media layer.

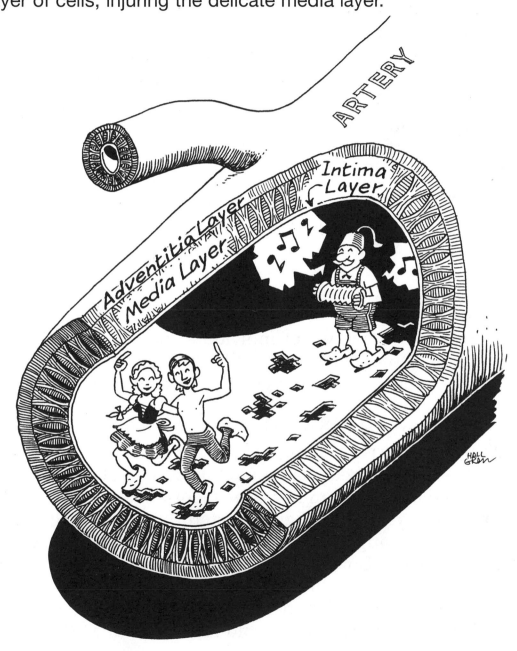

muscular middle layer (the media) and is the layer most susceptible to attacks from outside sources.

Middle layer: The middle layer of your arteries supports the entire arterial structure by working a little like a hand squeezing a hose or a boa constrictor squeezing a neck. When you're depressed or anxious, the layer can constrict, narrowing the amount of space where blood can flow through (the lumen). But it also has an advantage; it can release tension by dilating (the hand releasing the hose) to pull the Teflon layer outward and open up *more* space in the part of the artery where blood flows — say, when you exercise. When that happens, it allows more red cells, oxygen, and other nutrients through. You feel more energy when that layer functions like it did when you were nine years old.

Outer layer: The outer layer (the adventitia) shields the artery from the rest of your body like sausage casing; it holds the artery together from the outside.

Under normal circumstances, the inner layer is lined with delicate cells, and blood runs freely. Think of the structure as a tile wall — it's a smooth wall made up of individual tiles connected together with little gaps throughout. In the tile wall, you have white gooey grout; in the artery, you have tight junctions holding the cells together.

Now, in your arteries, that wall will stay tight unless something comes along and starts chipping away at the junctions between those smooth cells. The most damaging tile buster — high blood pressure — is the arterial sledgehammer. But plenty of other pickaxes can chip away at the arterial lining: cholesterol, nicotine, high levels of blood sugar, stress, anger, and about forty other smaller risk factors, primarily stemming from lifestyle choices you make. The effect? They chip away and cause little nicks in the intima of your arteries, and those injuries trigger the anatomical starter's pistol. As shown in Figure 5.3, the race to destroy — and repair — your arteries is on.

Figure 5.3 **Clog Jam** Low-quality (LDL) cholesterol stimulates white blood cells to attack, and the combatants are soaked up into the artery walls. The resulting toxic terrain creates rough patches, despite the efforts of healthy HDL cholesterol to heal the wound. Ultimately, the irritated areas are sealed off with platelets and blood clots that close off the artery completely and cause a blood-flow traffic jam — a heart attack.

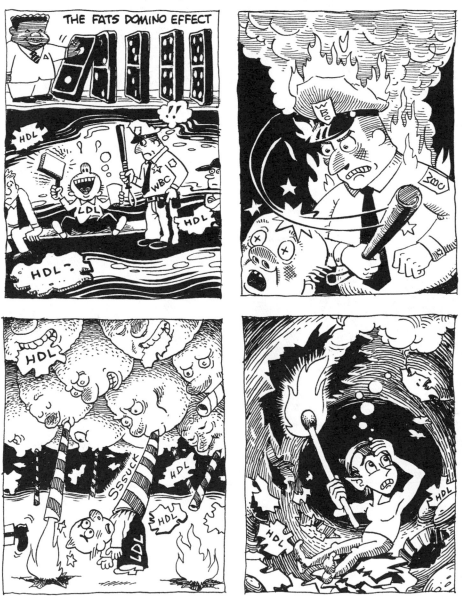

Figure 5.3 **Clog Jam** continued.

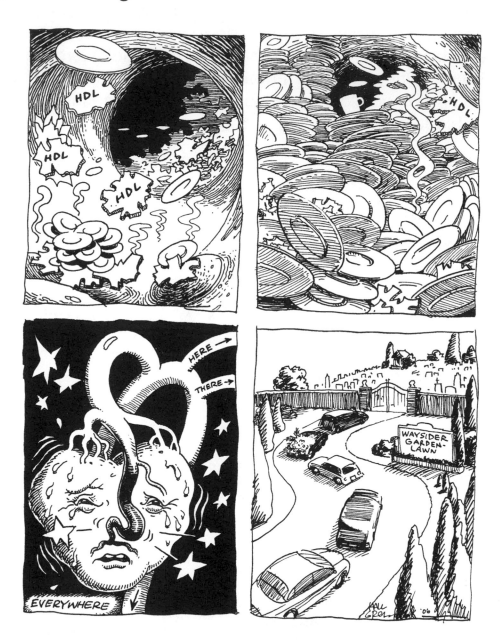

142

Super HDL: The Future of Cholesterol Drugs

In a northern Italian village on Lake Garda, the villagers have low levels of HDL. Science would tell us that, without high levels of the protective cholesterol-carrying protein, they should all be dying of coronary artery disease. But they aren't. It turns out that these villagers have supercharged, Drano-like HDL (called apo-1a-Milano) to clear away the gunk from their arteries and allow blood to flow smoothly. This case study points to the next wave of cholesterol drugs: drugs that enhance HDL action to clear the bad LDL away, rather than those that work by lowering the LDL levels in the first place.

The Effects of Fat

For years, you've been used to looking down at a scale's needle to determine your health. Wrong needle, bucko. What you need: a needle in the hands of someone who can draw your blood. With results from a simple blood test, you'll find out what your current settings are and then be equipped with the data you need to take steps that will reset the settings to the factory originals.

Blood Pressure: These days, blood pressure machines are everywhere — at the pharmacy, in your gym, in mall kiosks. Even in Wal-Mart and McDonald's. That's good. Actually, it's great. (Get your BP, hold the fries.)

That's because you need to track your blood pressure — your most crucial vital sign — even more diligently than Geraldo reacts to the news. High blood pressure still reigns as the leading cause of heart attack, stroke, heart failure, kidney failure, and impotence. While most of your other blood numbers reveal levels of substances inside your blood, your BP gauges how your blood travels through your body. Simply, blood pressure refers to the amount of force exerted by your blood on your arterial walls as it passes through. It's mea-

Figure 5.4 **Pressure Situation** With hypertension, the arteries squeeze down so tightly that the heart struggles to keep the blood moving forward. To compensate, the heart gets too thick, like a muscle-bound weight lifter. It becomes so stiff that it loses flexibility and can't relax. If it can't relax, blood has trouble traveling through the arteries, and the resulting high blood pressure damages the arteries.

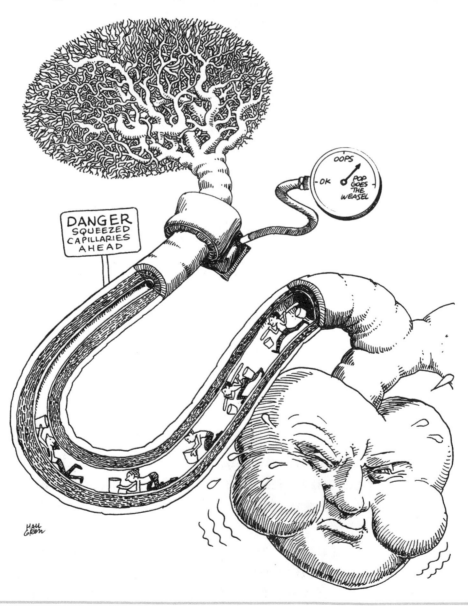

sured through the systolic pressure (the pressure being exerted when the heart contracts; the top number) and the diastolic pressure (the pressure on your arteries when your heart is at rest).

Now, if the force of that pumping is too high, it'll gouge holes in that smooth inner lining of your arteries (see Figure 5.4), causing those nicks in the tile wall that trigger a chain reaction of grouting, then destructive inflammation and clotting (which we'll discuss in detail below). Think of it as the beating of a bongo. If you hit a bongo with your fingers, the drumhead will stay intact. But slug away with two baseball bats, and that bongo head will feel like a roach in an exterminator's crosshairs. Your goal: Treat your arterial walls with a nice steady rhythm — let your blood *tap tap tap* them; not *pound pound pound* them. (Blood pressure fluctuates throughout the day; the goal is to have your total BP picture under control.)

Certainly, many factors can make your blood pressure soar higher than an Albert Pujols home run (stress, high levels of the mineral sodium, lack of the mineral calcium or potassium from not enough fruits and vegetables, lack of physical activity). But it's also clear that being overweight leads directly to high blood pressure. This happens in part when the kidneys, squashed by fat, feign death unless they are fed with a higher blood pressure. (Your kidneys are the organ primarily responsible for regulating blood pressure.)

Luckily, you can reduce your blood pressure quickly and dramatically by addressing your waist issues. Losing 10 percent of the weight you've gained since you were eighteen (that's only four pounds if you've gained forty) can result in a decrease of 7 mmHg (stands for millimeters of mercury to measure the partial pressure of a gas) from your systolic number and 4 mmHG from your diastolic one. The message is clear: Drop your waist and you'll drop your BP.

Cholesterol: Hear the word cholesterol and you're likely to think of eggs, heart attacks, and a mandate from your doctor. But cholesterol is part of your body's arterial repair kit; it's designed to help you, though it doesn't always happen that way.

Let's go back to those nicks in your arterial wall. Whether it's BP,

145

nicotine, or too many cheese curls that damage the wall, your body gets angrier than a cinched-up bull — because it doesn't want the middle lining of the artery exposed to blood. So your body hires a handyman to patch up your nicks with grout, to cover the wounds in the inner lining.

What's that grout? Cholesterol, but not just any ol' cholesterol.

Your handyman — let's call him Lester — carries two things: a bucket of grout and a spatula. The grout can come in the form of lousy cholesterol, which is carried by low-density lipoprotein (LDL). It's big and puffy, and prone to breaking up and scattering bits of cholesterol when it hits the walls of the artery. When your LDL levels are too high to begin with (maybe from your diet or from your heredity), and then you nick the inner lining of one of your arteries, Lester goes crazy and slaps on more and more and more grout. He starts covering up the damage with the bad cholesterol — loads and loads of bad cholesterol.

But look inside Lester's tool belt. He's got a spatula that takes premium-grade grout in the form of cholesterol carried on high-density lipoprotein (it's the healthy HDL cholesterol). Compact and powerful, the spatula works with this slick stuff to take the extra gunk away.

Now, if you have too much of that LDL grout (this can be familial but is primarily a result of eating the wrong kinds of foods — simple sugars and fats — and especially *too much* food) and not enough premium-version HDL grout (from not eating enough of the right kinds of foods and fats, not getting enough physical activity, or not having enough female hormones — yes, even men have them), it can lead to a chain of events that has potentially heart-stopping outcomes. We'll call it fat's domino effect.

146

Domino 1: Having too much bad cholesterol not only means you'll have too much junk (plaque) in your arteries. It also means that LDL cholesterol will get into the middle layer of your artery. That cholesterol in the middle layer acts like a drunk fan with courtside seats, making the environment much more hostile than it's used to being. The presence of LDL cholesterol in that middle layer stimulates the immune system to attract white-cell protectors to try to smooth out and calm down the rotten cholesterol.

Domino 2: Those white blood cells, in turn, spill some of their toxic contents that normally attack infections — and that causes generalized inflammation.

Domino 3: The toxic contents and cholesterol are soaked up by scavenger cells, building up blister-sized spaces in the walls of your arteries. They're called foam cells — and they increase the size of the plaque, or grout, even more to make the artery surface rougher.

Domino 4: Sensing something's wrong, your body responds with more inflammation, creating bulges and potholes in the wall, often in the area of weakness, where the initial nick was and a scar was trying to form over the dangerous plaque. If that plaque ruptures into the middle of your blood vessel, the next domino falls.

Domino 5: These rough patches in the wall then attract sticky blood platelets to form clots in your arteries. Normally, platelets are good (they help form scabs to heal wounds). But when they hit that rough patch in your arterial wall, they grab the lining and form a big clot on top of irritated, inflamed plaque. And this brings in more clotting proteins to the area that act to cement the platelets in place.

Domino 6: All of this gunk piles up faster and faster, and the inside of the arteries becomes so inflamed that the platelets and clots fill the entire artery. **YOU-reka!** This ruptured plaque process take minutes rather than decades, so you can influence its likelihood today by making the right choices about food.

Domino 7: The blood can't get through the artery, and nourishment to the heart is shut off.

Game Over: The chain reaction triggers a heart attack (or, depending where the process happens, causes a stroke, memory loss, impotence, wrinkled skin, or any number of health problems that happen when blood flow malfunctions).

As you can see, it's not the cholesterol by itself that's so bad; it's not having high enough levels of healthy and/or low enough lousy cholesterol to thwart the process before it even begins. And it's not doing things like normalizing your blood pressure and blood sugar to help decrease the chance of developing nicks in the first place.

While genetics dictates some of your cholesterol level, your physical activity levels and poor foods choices — trans and saturated fats, simple sugar, and too many calories — really dictate whether Lester carries the right amount and kind of grout or moves the spatula fast enough to make for a nice, clean wall.

Blood Sugar: Yep, we know how it is. You don't have diabetes, so you're going to blow off thinking about blood sugar faster than a flight attendant blows off a flirty coach passenger. And that would be a mistake. Blood sugar is another substance that can nick your arteries if levels are too high. You may think your level is normal, but most blood sugar levels are recorded when you've fasted. Having "normal" levels for fasting (under 100 milligrams per deciliter, abbreviated 100 mg/dl) and for after meals (under 140 mg/dl) is important. Why? Because there's a good chance that even with normal blood sugar levels, your blood sugar may rise significantly throughout the day as you eat. Studies show that men with a waist of 40 inches or more have twelve times the risk of getting diabetes compared with men with a waist smaller than 35 inches. For women, having a 37-inch waist is that much riskier than having a 32 1/2-incher. (The most sensitive way to diagnose diabetes is to measure the blood sugar fasting, and again two hours after taking 75 grams of sugar — to see how your body can deal with the sugar.)

Many people think that diabetes is a purely genetic disease, and of course, it sure would be nice to blame Aunt Mabel for the medical condition, but it doesn't quite work that way. For type 2 diabetes (type 1 is the juvenile form), your environment (that is, your

148

lifestyle, your behaviors, your macaroons) is a much more dominant trait than genetics.

Yes, type 2 diabetes is a genetic disease. That is, if you are a twin and have an identical twin who gets type 2 diabetes, you have the genetics for it. And it's a tough disease, too: Diabetes ages you one and a half years for every year you live. For example, if you get it at age thirty and live to sixty, you're not really sixty. You have the energy and disability risks of a seventy-five-year-old.

Here's how it works (see Figure 5.5): Insulin in your blood normally takes sugar and puts it into the cells, but in people with type 2 diabetes, the transfer of sugar into your muscle and fat cells is inhibited. While nice in coffee, that sugar in your blood chips away at your arterial wall by weakening the junctions between cells that form the surface lining of your arteries. Ultimately it allows holes to form in these junctions. By causing your insulin levels to go haywire and making proteins in your body less effective, sugar really behaves like nutritional cocaine.

Omentum fat (belly fat) contributes to type 2 diabetes by making it difficult to get glucose inside the cell and let insulin do what it does best: deliver glucose. Simply being overweight, especially having a waist greater than 37 inches (85 centimeters) for women and 40 inches (100 centimeters) for men, makes your body less sensitive to insulin; the insulin receptors on the cells don't allow insulin to transmit the message enabling glucose transport into the cells, leaving the glucose to float around in your blood. That omentum fat is also selfish; it uses up the insulin so it can't do its job (one study shows omentum fat sucks up a quarter of the insulin that passes through the blood supply).

So your blood sugar level remains high because the sugar isn't being admitted to your cells readily and thus isn't broken down properly, meaning that sugar will hang out in your blood like a truant skipping school and causing mischief.

So what? Well, having too much sugar in your blood is like having too much rain in a small pond — the flooding can cause damage for everything around it. Too much blood sugar can:

Figure 5.5 **Carried Away** Resistance to the normal effects of insulin makes cells resistant to taking in glucose (sugar). This forces excess glucose to stay in the blood vessels, where it acts like debris to damage the Teflon-like surface of our inner roads. Cholesterol trucks bounce around and spill junk that ruins our blood highways.

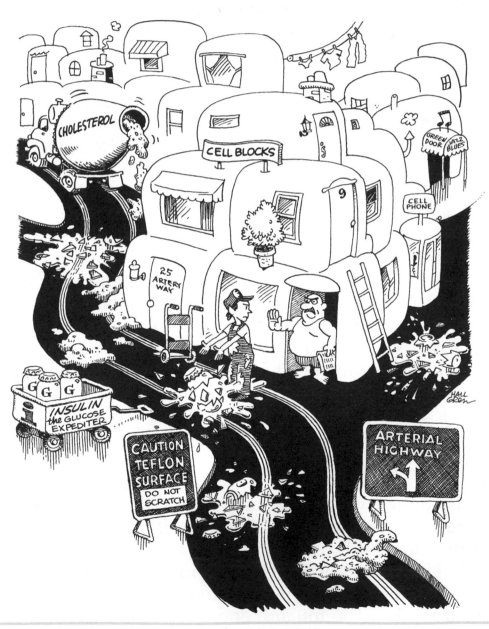

- Weaken the junctions between those smooth endothelial cells lining your arteries, making the Teflon-like lining more vulnerable to nicks.
- Increase the power of the hammer, to cause high blood pressure. (Sugar turns the hammer into a sledgehammer.)
- Cause your white blood cells to stop fighting infections, thus weakening your immune system.
- Trigger a chemical process in your red blood cells, which transport oxygen in your bloodstream, that causes the cells to want to hold onto oxygen more tightly. That keeps oxygen from getting to your tissues. When that happens, the glucose, like a lost puppy, attaches to whatever it can find — most likely, proteins in your blood and tissues. These proteins deposit in tissues, leading to the development of cataracts, joint abnormalities, and lung problems.
- Get into your nerves and cause a reaction that makes your nerves swell, become compressed, and lose their ability to function — usually in the parts of your body farthest from your brain: your hands and feet.
- Flip off a switch in your small blood vessels. Normally your body automatically regulates the flow of nutrients into your small blood vessels. They sort of work on backup (like a generator for when the power goes out), so they can function even when your big vessels might be experiencing problems. But high levels of glucose turn off that automatic regulation — and let a

> **FACTOID**
>
> Talk about being thick-skinned: One early sign of insulin resistance in a few people is the appearance of a brown, thick, velvety patch of skin behind your neck. This condition — called acanthosis nigricans — is an early sign of metabolic syndrome, which is associated with high blood pressure plus elevated levels of blood lipids and blood sugar.

little high blood pressure make more of those nicks and tears in the junctions between cells in your smaller blood vessels. This is like asking someone to use a sledgehammer to do the job of a jeweler's tool; it magnifies that effect and magnifies the size of the nick.

But here's the thing. You can control your genes if you want to. To keep blood sugar levels down, you should avoid foods with simple sugar and lousy aging fats (trans and saturated fats). And about 1,000 calories' worth of activity a week — about thirty minutes of walking a day and twenty minutes of the YOU Workout three days a week — causes your muscles to be so much more sensitive to insulin, which allows sugar to do its duty inside your cells, rather than cause havoc in your bloodstream. A little physical activity goes a long way.

FACTOID

Monosodium glutamate (MSG), the additive found in many Chinese foods, may play a role in messing up the body's metabolic systems. A taste enhancer, MSG is used to overstimulate (some say poison) the glutamine receptors of the brain, so we sense salt and sweets more (but not bitter and sour tastes, interestingly). The downside? That may cause us to eat more and to have higher insulin levels.

Arterial Inflammation: When we think of our arteries and what can damage them, we tend to think of that clog: the hunk of junk that stops the flow of blood like a lemon seed in a straw. If there's a roadblock in the way, then there's no way for traffic to move through. But that's only one mechanism for closing off blood flow. The other occurs through the process of inflammation. Typically, inflammation in our bodies makes us think of things that swell *out* — like a sprained ankle, or swollen gums, or the shiner from the 2 a.m. bar brawl. But

152

when it comes to arterial inflammation, you have to think about swelling *in.* In response to all that clotting action we talked about with LDL cholesterol, inflammation occurs in the middle layer of your arteries. As the middle layer swells, it pushes into the inner layer because the outer sausage layer doesn't give. That pushing into the inner layer reduces the size of the hole that blood can travel through (like drinking with a thinner straw).

One of the ways we determine potential cardiovascular risks is by measuring chemicals in the blood that signal inflammation. C-reactive protein (CRP) is one such chemical; elevated CRP indicates an inflammatory reaction somewhere in your body, from a sinus infection to gum inflammation. If it's high, your risk of heart disease is greater, because any significant inflammation in your body increases inflammation in your blood vessels.

Fat Chance: The Other Major Risks

We're not here to lecture you and pummel you with brochurelike statistics about health risks. But to put fat in perspective, remember that it's an all-body risk factor — with implications everywhere. Even if your numbers in some health categories are as perfect as a Michelle Kwan triple toe loop, you're not risk-free. Being overweight or obese leads to the following:

Higher Risk of Cancer: The inflammation resulting from omentum fat also causes dysfunction in the system that protects you from cancer. In fact, there's a direct correlation between waist size and an increased risk of hormonally sensitive tumors, such as breast cancer in women and prostate cancer in men. Fat contains an enzyme, aromatase, which converts adrenal hormones into a long-acting kind of estrogen, which can cause increased breast cancer risk.

Higher Risk of Sleep Apnea: Fat around your waist correlates with a thick neck, and that can obstruct your breathing (you're at higher risk if your neck size is more than seventeen inches). In its benign form — snoring — you can still move air through your throat,

Figure 5.6 **Bottle Neck** Fat in the throat contributes to sleep apnea. In this condition, the airway is cut off during sleep, and breathing can stop for up to ten seconds at a time throughout the night.

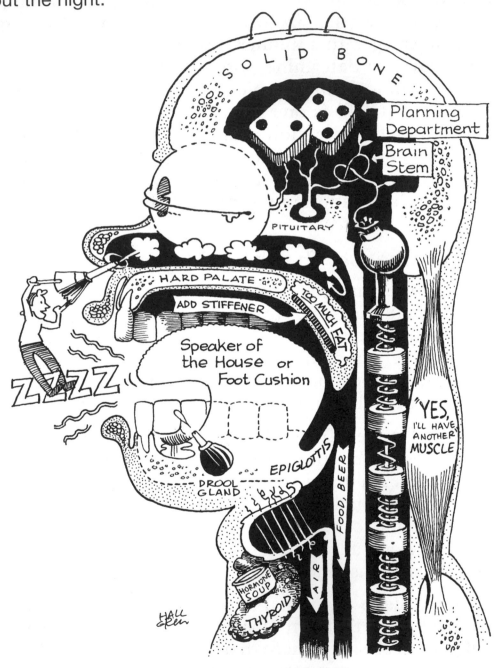

but generate a kazoo sound that violates OSHA requirements and can cause permanent hearing loss and marital strife. In some cases, that obstruction worsens, until eventually no air can pass into the lungs for up to ten seconds at a time (see Figure 5.6). Fortunately, the body instinctively awakens prior to suffocation. As you get older, the tissue in your throat softens, and the area around your tonsils attracts fat. When you're asleep, and your muscles fully relax, the tissue collapses, so there's even less room in the back of your throat.

Sleep apnea makes you miss out on deep, restorative REM sleep. This leads to frequent awakenings at night (though your spouse may know it, you'll probably never feel yourself waking), lack of sleep, and daytime drowsiness. You're more likely to develop nick-causing high blood pressure (caused when your lungs hang onto carbon dioxide when you stop breathing) and, the bitter irony, you're more likely to get fatter because of it. That's because sleep apnea is like a series of rear-end collisions — one accident after another. The lack of sleep makes you tired. You feel like you need more energy. You eat foods that give you quick energy but also have high sugar and fat. You get fatter. You continue to have sleep apnea. And the cycle continues. (As an incentive to embrace a good eating plan, most people will lose fat first in their faces and throats; so with a waist reduction of a few inches you'll probably be able to prevent or reduce these sleep problems by 30 percent early in your program.)

Higher Risk of Joint Problems: While strong, your joints are like parents trying to squash constant whining; they can take only so much before they break down. Your knees are some of the most powerful joints in your body because you use them to both push off and absorb force. But they're also prone to wear and tear if they have to carry a heavier load (that is, more fat in your body) than they're designed to. When you gain ten pounds of body weight, it feels more like a thirty-pound weight to your knees while you're walking. When you walk upstairs, the ten pounds of fat feel like seventy pounds to your knee joint. That extra weight makes you more vulnerable to developing joint-deteriorating conditions like osteoarthritis, which occurs when your joints get nicks in their smooth cartilage from bearing a load they're not designed to carry.

When you reduce your omentum fat and your waist size, you'll automatically reduce your risk in so many areas of your health. Even better, you'll have the potential to see dramatic reductions in risk factors. **YOU-reka!** When overweight people (with an average weight of 225 pounds) lose about 7.5 percent of their body weight (about 17 pounds or four inches of waist size), they improve their HDL and LDL cholesterol levels, BP, and blood sugar numbers by — get this — 20 percent. That's nearly three times the benefit compared with percentage weight loss. Take the following steps to help you get there in terms of both inches and risk factors.

YOU TIPS!

Know Your Fats. Fat in foods, like bosses, comes in two broad categories: those that are good for your well-being and those that want you to suffer. The strongest influence you can have on your levels of cholesterol (not to mention your waist size) is by watching what fats you're eating and what fats you're banishing from your life and your gut. Above all, you want to avoid saturated and trans fats; a serving size should have no more than 4 grams of those two villains combined. They're the foods most associated with long-term weight gain and clogging your arteries. Essentially, bad fats are ones that are solid at room temperature: animal fat, butter, stick margarine, lard. Trans fat contains cross-linked hydrogen bonds, which make it stable for long periods of time at room temperature. Eating trans fat leads to abnormalities in cholesterol (decreasing your good and increasing your bad), as well as increasing inflammation and damaging your arterial cells, which makes you more prone to clotting. (By the way, trans fat was originally designed for candle wax, but the market died with the advent of electricity.) The value of trans fats is that they have a long shelf life; the average food manufacturer would love to make foods with healthy fats if they could have the one-year shelf life that they can get from the unhealthy fats. The good fats, by contrast, are the ones that are liquid at room temperature but get thick when they get cold, like olive oil. They help raise your HDL levels to clear away the guck. Far more important than the calories of fat are what fatty acids can do to your cell functions, and how they influence arterial function and inflammation.

Super (Youthful) Fats: Facilitate Spatula Action	Stupid (Aging) Fats: Cause the Clogs, Clump Up the Spatula
Monounsaturated Fats. They come in two forms: omega-3 fatty acids and *omega-6* fatty acids, in the form of fish (3s) and nut oils (3s and 6s). The omega-3s have been shown to improve arterial and brain function. They're found in olive oil, canola oil, fish oils, flaxseeds, avocados, and nuts (especially walnuts). They've also been shown to reduce blood pressure and lipid levels when used in place of carbohydrates. **Bottom line:** Make about 30 percent to 40 percent of your fats the monounsaturated variety.	**Trans Fat.** This is the fat that contains hydrogenated vegetable oil. It's the worst kind of fat and will stunt weight-loss efforts. Trans-fatty acids are in all kinds of food — especially when long shelf life is important — from buttered popcorn and cookies to chips and margarine. **Bottom line:** Say no. Stay away from them the way you'd avoid highways on the day before Thanksgiving. Clog city.

Super (Youthful) Fats: Facilitate Spatula Action	Stupid (Aging) Fats: Cause the Clogs, Clump UP the Spatula
Polyunsaturated Fats. These are like monounsaturated except that they contain more than one unsaturated bond. They are usually present in vegetable oils and sesame oils. They may improve arterial and brain function, and will help keep up your satiety levels. **Bottom line:** Make 20 percent to 40 percent of your fats polyunsaturated.	**Saturated Fats.** Found in meats and dairy products, these fats will make you gain weight and clog your arteries. **Bottom line:** Limit saturated fat to lean sources like lean cuts of beef and low-fat dairy products. Aim for less than 4 grams of saturated fat per serving. Less than 20 grams, or less than 30 percent of your daily allotment, should be from saturated and/or trans fats combined.

Note: The best oil to have in your home is extra-virgin olive oil or organic (or cold-press) canola oil. For cooking, you can also use sesame or peanut oil. That's because their smoking point — that is, the temperature at which the fat burns — is very high. Cook beyond it, and you'll end up with a burned, charcoal flavor. Once heated, oils can become rancid and also can generate toxic chemicals, so you lose the major benefit of eating these usually healthy foods. Also, it's best to cook the food, rather than the oil. So don't heat the oil directly in the pan; instead, roll your food in the oil first and then heat the food so the oil doesn't become overheated.

Here are smoke points for some commonly used healthy oils:

Unrefined canola oil: 225°
Unrefined sunflower oil: 225°

Extra-virgin olive oil: 320°
Virgin olive oil: 420°
Sesame oil: 410°
Grape-seed oil: 420°
Refined peanut oil: 450°
Semirefined sesame oil: 450°

Clear It All Up. More and more evidence is showing that clog-free living is correlated with raising your amount of HDL to thwart the clot-triggering process. By raising your HDL, you increase the amount of healthy cholesterol that's available to clear away the lousy cholesterol. Things that have been shown to effectively raise HDL include:

- Consuming healthy fats found in olive oil, fish, avocados, and walnuts.
- Walking or doing any physical activity for at least thirty minutes a day — no excuses.
- Taking niacin. Take 100 milligrams four times a day. Regular (and OTC) niacin is much cheaper than prescription niacin, and there seems to be a beneficial effect of extended-release doses. Sometimes higher doses are needed, in which case your doctor needs to peek at your liver function to ensure that you avoid the uncommon toxicity. To reduce flushing (feeling hot and light-headed), take an aspirin a half hour ahead of time and take the niacin as you go to bed. Do not increase the dose above this level without talking to your doctor, and check with your doctor before using niacin at any dose if you have a history of liver problems.
- Taking vitamin B5 (pantothenic acid). We recommend a dose of 300 milligrams a day to decrease LDL and raise HDL with no side effects yet known.
- Having one drink of alcohol every night. You should not be drinking just to get your HDL up, but if you do drink alcohol, stick to one drink, and you may see some small beneficial effects.

159

- Substituting protein or monounsaturated fat in place of carbs. Recent research suggests that this can help reduce BP and modify lipid levels.

Just Say Yes to This Drug. If there were one magic pill for fighting fat and saving lives, the pharmaceutical industry would send everyone from scale makers to diet-book authors into bankruptcy. There's no pill that will do it all. (At least not yet. More on drug solutions in the appendix.) But that doesn't mean you can't use drugs to improve your health and reduce your cardiovascular risk factors. Our recommendation — and the closest thing to a pill with mystical powers — comes in the form of two baby aspirin (162 milligrams total) a day. You need two rather than one, since many folks are resistant to the lower dose. (There is no measurable increased risk of stomach problems in studies with this small increase in doses from 81 milligrams to 162 milligrams, and the reduction in heart attacks or ischemic strokes goes from around 13 percent to around 36 percent.) Aspirin makes platelets less sticky and decreases inflammation that occurs to narrow the space where blood flows through your arteries. And it's been shown to reduce arterial aging and immune system aging, and that means decreasing your risk of everything from heart attack, strokes, and impotence to colon, rectal, and esophageal cancers, and maybe even breast and prostate cancers. To reduce the gastric side effects, drink a half glass of warm water before and after taking the pill. (See your doc if you have any history of serious bleeding, are taking blood thinners, or do extreme sports.)

Have Regular Readings. Not just with your book club or by an astrologer. These regular readings are about tracking your health numbers. Instead of measuring your success through the scale, the real measurement — and test — of your success is seeing whether you've reduced your cardiovascular risk, as evidenced in the following test readings:

Blood Pressure: Optimum level is 115/76. Blood pressure readings can be variable, so have your BP taken in the morning, during the day, and at night, as part of your normal activities (except for thirty minutes after exercise, when it will naturally be higher). Take the average of three readings to come up with your base number. After that, take readings every month to help you monitor your progress. (If BP is high, then you can track it daily.)

Lipid Profile Blood Test: Have one now to establish your baseline measurement, then have your blood analyzed every other year so that you and your doctor can watch changes and make appropriate adjustments to your eating and/or drug plan.

HDL (healthy) cholesterol: You're at a low risk if your HDL is greater than 40 mg/dl. But like basketball players, the higher the better. In fact, if your HDL is over 100 mg/dl, the chances of heaving a heart attack or stroke related to lack of blood flow are smaller than the chance that a Hollywood celeb could walk through Boise unnoticed. (Except in some extremely rare cases where HDL malfunctions inside the body, there has never been a heart attack or stroke due to lack of blood flow reported in the entire medical literature in a person with a functional HDL over 100).

LDL (lousy) cholesterol: You're at a low risk if your LDL is less than 100 mg/dl. By the way, research shows that for all women, and for men over sixty-five years old, the LDL number isn't nearly as important as the HDL. So women and men over sixty-five don't need to obsess too much over LDL levels unless their HDL levels are too low.

Fasting blood sugar: Below 100 mg/dl.
C-reactive protein: Below 1 mg/dl.

Get a Lift. Muscle isn't just for football players, bouncers, and souped-up cars. Everyone benefits from adding some muscle to his or her body; in fact, adding some muscle will help lower your levels of blood sugar. The more muscle you have, the more you increase insulin receptivity — that is, the process by which insulin transports glucose into your cells. If you gain muscle and lose weight, you change the chemistry of your cell membranes so that you absorb more glucose throughout your body rather than having it stay in your blood. You add muscle by doing strength exercises (more coming up in the YOU Workout).

Stop Freebasing Sugar. One thing that causes blood sugar to spike is, uh, sugar. That is, straight, pure sugar — not eaten with any other substances like fat or protein around it. Though we recommend eating as few simple sugars as possible, if you do eat them, you should always be sure not to eat that candy bar or cookie dough by itself. Have a handful of nuts or some olive oil with bread first; that slows your stomach from emptying and will keep sugar levels from creating a pyrotechnical effect in your blood.

Go Chrome. Chromium, a mineral found in a variety of foods (especially mushrooms), seems to help control blood sugar. Taking 200 micrograms a day of the supplement chromium picolinate can help aid the uptake of insulin, to help your cells use blood sugar for fuel. Though the studies aren't definitive at this point, we recommend the supplement for waist — and blood sugar — control. Chromium increases your cells' sensitivity to insulin and is depleted by refined sugars, white flour, and lack of exercise. One study showed users lost four pounds over ten weeks compared with no pounds in a control group. You should take it with magnesium, which reduces low-grade inflammation that can be associated with insulin resistance. A dose of 600 micrograms of chromium has been shown to be effective for those with type 2 diabetes, but for others, stick to the recommended dose of 200 micrograms. Just because a little is good doesn't mean that taking a lot more is better. Taking too much chromium can hurt your kidneys.

Become Sensitive. Here's a tantalizing observation: Cinnamon (with an *m*, not a *b*) seems to have an insulinlike effect, enhancing the satiety center in your brain while also reducing blood sugar and cholesterol levels. Just a half teaspoon a day can have some effect. Sprinkle it in cereal or on toast, or add it to a smoothie.

Get in the Zone. Studies show that meditation has a statistically significant reduction of risk factors for coronary heart disease, such as blood pressure and insulin resistance. Find a quiet room, take a few minutes, close your eyes, and focus on one healthy word or phrase, like "om" (or "omega-3 fatty acids").

YOU Test

Hey There, Good Looking, Can I Get Your Number?

In most cases, like a bike fall or a noodle-size hangnail, seeing your blood is not a good thing. But for our purposes, you need to look deep inside your blood to get an assessment of the effect of the extra weight you're carrying. That's where you'll find all the numbers that indicate the risks that may be associated with carrying extra weight. If you don't know these numbers, see your doctor for your latest blood results or request a blood test from your primary-care physician.

Blood Pressure: _____
(Measures the force of blood being pumped through your arteries. Ideal is 115/76)

HDL Cholesterol: _____
(Measures the amount of good clog-clearing cholesterol in your blood. Greater than 40 mg/dl is acceptable. And you've hit the lottery if you're above 60 mg/dl.)

LDL Cholesterol: _____
(Measures the amount of bad clog-forming cholesterol in your blood. Ideal is less than 100 mg/dl if you have any risk factors of heart disease, or 130 gm/dl if you are otherwise healthy as a horse and your ancestors never suffered heart disease.)

C-Reactive Protein: _____
(Measures levels of inflammation in blood vessels, a marker for many types of diseases. Ideal in most labs is less than 1 mg/dl.)

Chapter 6
Metabolic Motors

Your Body's Hormonal Fat Burners

Diet Myths

- It's your habits that are entirely to blame for fatness.

- Your body burns most of its calories through activity.

- You can't adjust your "slow metabolism."

Bad genes aren't something that you wore in high school. They're what can make you have a propensity for heart disease, baldness, mental problems, and putting on weight. Though diet and physical activity play the lead roles in losing fat and maintaining a healthy weight, your genes are part of the supporting cast. It is possible to eat like a guppy but grow bigger than a beluga. Simply, some people can have a bad genetic response to a good diet (that is, they put on weight), while other people (the scoundrels!) can have a good genetic response to a bad diet.

Myth Buster How do we know there's a genetic component to obesity? For one, studies of twins raised apart from each other show it. Two people with the same genes raised in different lifestyles and on different diets show about 30 percent of the same propensities for gaining weight. But genes don't just dictate how you metabolize fat — that is, whether you come from a "big-boned" family or one that could fit through slats in air vents. Genes help dictate many things regarding why you put on fat — like cravings for certain foods or the way you cope when you're stressed. And family ties also govern whether or not the homemade sauce has butter or olive oil.

Nevertheless, what we're trying to do is shrink the size of your jeans by shrinking the effect of your genes. While you have genetic influences that steer you toward a particular body type and behaviors, those dispositions and unhealthy decisions can be neutralized and minimized by eating the right foods, rebooting your body, and, in effect, changing which of your genes are turned on and which are turned off. That's right; your choices turn on or turn off specific genes you have. For example, the flavonoids (antioxidants) in grape skins turn off the gene that makes an inflammatory protein that ages your arteries.

Now that we've discussed why you eat, how your food moves, and the effects of storing excess fat, you need to know how your body burns fat. In this chapter, we'll discuss the body's natural ways of doing so — ways determined by your genes — and in the next chapter we'll discuss ways you can add horsepower to your natural fat-burning engines.

Of course, the place to start is with your metabolism, your body's thermostat — the rate at which you burn off extra fat (metabolism literally means "change").

Most of the 1 million calories you consume every year are burned without your ever thinking anything of it. It takes energy for you to breathe and sleep, and for all of your organs to function.

Myth Buster

The energy you consume and store is used primarily to power your anatomical systems and structures. **YOU-reka!** Only 15 percent to 30 percent of your calories are burned through intentional physical activity such as exercise, walking, or doing the wumba wumba on your anniversary. So while you may think that spinning class or Bikram yoga is the primary pathway to frying fat, physical activity is only a fraction of it. You burn most of your calories by keeping your heart pumping, your brain remembering your spouse's birthday, and your liver disposing of last night's vodka concoction.

Now, that doesn't mean there aren't many outside influences that slow down and speed up your burn rate. Any movement speeds metabolism, including fidgeting (called nonexercise activity thermogenesis in scientific lingo, or NEAT for short). Every increase in body temperature of one degree increases your metabolic rate by 14 percent (eating protein appears to do the same thing naturally, by the way). When you sleep, your metabolic rate decreases by 10 percent. **YOU-reka!** When you starve yourself for more than twelve hours, your metabolic rate actually goes down by 40 percent. When you skip meals, your body senses a dietary disaster and quickly goes into storage mode rather than burning mode. That's the primary reason why deprivation diets don't work. Your body panics about going into a famine, so it slows metabolism into emergency-storing mode rather than a steady state of burning. Breakfast eaters are on average thinner than those who skip breakfast because they keep their metabolism genes turned on; this means that calories are more likely to be burned off before they can turn into fat.

In our battle to reduce our waistlines, we have several fearsome adversaries. And some of the greatest foes we will meet on the battlefield are our hormones. Sure, we all know that raging hormones can make a teenage boy become sex obsessed or give a menopausal woman hot flashes so bad she feels as though she's in Death Valley in August. But you may not know that your hormones have a lot to do with whether or not you're going to look good in a Speedo.

Is Something Secretly Making You Fat?

Before you hit yourself over the head with a stick of salami for lacking the willpower to resist aforementioned salami, or if you can't figure out why you eat less than all your friends but still gain weight, consider that your hormones may be influencing your body more than you think. Glands, which make up your *endocrine system* and produce your hormones, are responsible for the genetic conditions that could be influencing your metabolism and your weight. The primary metabolic glands are:

Thyroid gland: Thyroid hormone influences how quickly or slowly you burn energy. Too much hormone forces the body to waste energy too quickly (in extreme cases, it actually causes your heart muscle to become hypermetabolic and weaken). But if you don't produce enough, you develop a condition called hypothyroidism, in which your metabolic rate turtles way down. The best way to check levels of thyroid hormone? A simple blood test. You have elevated thyroid-stimulating hormone (TSH) if it's above 5 IU/liter. This

168

Figure 6.1 **Gland Inquisition** Too much stress overstimulates the adrenal gland, which releases too much cortisol (the stress hormone), testosterone, and estrogen. This witch's brew encourages us to eat more and rapidly stores those calories in your belly fat.

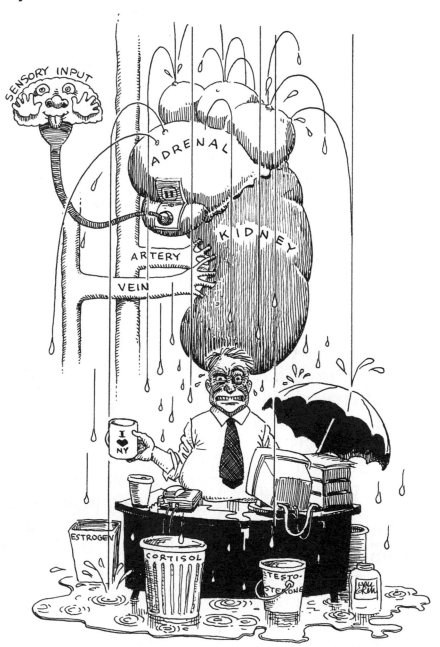

means your body is desperately trying to build up your body's circulating free thyroid hormone levels but is failing. TSH is released from your pituitary gland and tells your thyroid to produce two hormones that help control metabolism. Though decreased thyroid levels are rarely the sole cause of being overweight, abnormal levels may indicate that you should see your doctor or an endocrinologist about whether you need to supplement your thyroid function in the form of a thyroid pill to boost your metabolism. (Symptoms of hyperthyroidism include anxiety, heart palpitations, sleeplessness, and fast-growing hair and nails. For hypothyroidism, you may be lethargic, gain weight, have a reduced appetite, or have brittle nails.)

Adrenal glands: Adrenal glands sit like a dunce's cap on the kidneys, but they are controlled by corticotrophin-releasing hormone (CRH), which is made by the hypothalamus. This valuable relationship enables the adrenal to be very responsive to sensory input from the world around us, like a charging woolly mammoth. When chronically stressed, your adrenal glands produce cortisol, and cortisol inhibits CRH — which is too bad, because CRH will decrease your desire to eat. High cortisol levels reduce insulin sensitivity, so diabetes becomes more common and adversely influences fat and protein metabolism. The kidney responds to high cortisol levels by retaining salt and water

FACTOID

The average woman gains twenty-four pounds between the ages of twenty-five and sixty-five. Considering that the total food intake of women over forty is more than forty thousand pounds of food, the difference between food intake and food expenditure that produces such a weight gain is .06 percent — or just 8 calories a day. And if you want to lose weight, the whole fight comes down to measly 100 calories a day — that's ten permanent pounds and roughly three inches off your waist every year.

so that blood pressure increases. At the same time, other hormones created by the adrenal gland, including testosterone and its derivative estrogen, increase; this can lead to obesity-linked diseases like uterine fibroids and breast cancer. To measure cortisol levels, you need a blood test or a twenty-four-hour urine collection. Above 100 milligrams in twenty-four hours generally indicates a high level of cortisol. (Note: In some people, the cutoff number varies, depending on the lab.) By the way, this is also the reason why people on steroidal medications (for asthma, for instance) seem to gain weight; cortisol is a form of steroids. (These are not the same steroids that some athletes are abusing. Those *anabolic* steroids are related to testosterone.)

Pancreas: A normally functioning pancreas secretes insulin, the substance that helps glucose travel from the blood into muscle to produce energy and fat for storage. Insulin actually works a lot like leptin; it has a mechanism that tells you to eat less. But when insulin resistance occurs in cells, it negates the appetite-control effect. Especially in early diabetes, you can naturally avoid high blood sugar with your food choices. But when you eat high-sugar foods without adequate insulin secretion to overcome insulin resistance (type 2 diabetes), you have less feedback of being full and less appetite reduction than appropriate, so the vicious hunger cycle continues.

Hormones in Action

Now, your goal shouldn't be to burn all of your fat (though you may often consider it to be so). The average person has about 2,500 calories of carbohydrate reserves — stored mostly in liver and muscle — to use for all kinds of functions that need energy, especially immediate energy, like when you're trying to catch a bus or escape a charging rhino. An average person has about 112,000 calories stored in fat (that is, if you are at your ideal weight, you typically have about fourteen pounds of fat). The message: Your body fat isn't the enemy, unless you're carrying more than you need. We need fat to function; it's an energy bank account that we can withdraw from. (Remember how food is processed. See figures in Chapter 3.)

The trick, of course, is to make sure we don't let our banks open up branches in every single part of our bodies.

In all, you have nine known hormones that tell you to eat more and fourteen that tell you to stop eating. Hormones, like your own anatomical sports agent, are on your side. They're looking out for your health. But that doesn't mean you can't have genetic glitches. Maybe your body doesn't make leptin correctly, or your body has too much cortisol, or you can't get leptin to your brain, or none of your satiety-related hormones work at all. Those are problems no amount of willpower can overcome. Reprogramming your hormonal circuitry is the only solution. You can't beat biology, but you can make it work for you.

One perfect example of hormonal influence comes in the form of the hormone adiponectin, which we talked about in the last chapter. The more adiponectin you have, the lower your weight and body-fat percentages. (And it's directly related to omental fat, your gut fat. If you don't have omental fat, you'll have more adiponectin flying around.) It helps your muscles turn fat into energy and suppresses your appetite. Now get this: When you lose weight, *more* adiponectin is available to your body. **YOU-reka!** It's one of your body's greatest reward mechanisms. The more weight you lose, the better your body is able to deal with the inflammation we talked about in the last few chapters, because of the protective effect of adiponectin. It's one of the reasons why when you gain weight, you start increasing the irritation in your body — you produce less of this natural anti-inflammatory agent.

The Sex Factor

We all know what testosterone and estrogen do for things like body hair, breast size, and the desire to spend Saturday night rampaging between the sheets like a pair of Greco-Roman wrestlers. But your sex hormones can influence more than just the activity that goes on below your waist; they can also influence what happens *to* your waist.

Reproductive-hormone friendly fire: One of the most common causes of obesity in women comes from a condition called polycystic ovary syndrome. In fact, PCOS is responsible for 10 percent to 20 percent of weight problems among younger women and is often diagnosed by irregular periods and by physical appearance: abdominal obesity, acne, thinning hair, and malelike hair growth (for example on the face). In the end, sufferers lose their feminine appearance. What happens is this: Women with PCOS have stingy ovaries — they get an egg all primed and ready to go in its follicle, but they won't hit send and ship the egg out. The follicle, raring to go, keeps sending out its messenger, estrogen. Now, estrogen works great when it gets paired up with, or balanced by, another ovarian messenger called progestin, which gets released from the egg sac (called a corpus luteum) after the follicle ships out its egg. In PCOS, some of that excess estrogen running around gets converted to androgens, or male hormones; these cause that extra hair growth and increased appetite. That's when the pounds add on. To combat this drive for another slice of coconut cream meringue, many women go on the birth control pill, which stops the weight gain by giving finite doses of estrogen and progestin, telling the ovaries to quiet down. The pill alone won't cause you to lose or gain, but having less of a voracious appetite and reversing the hormonal burden of PCOS often will.

Testosterone: It may be what produces chin hair and male egos, but testosterone is also found in women and is another hormone that could play a role in weight gain in both genders. Testosterone levels tend to fall in postmenopausal women and older men; this reduces libido and can lead to weight gain because you have less muscle mass, and more calories get stored as fat. When the cause of weight gain isn't clear from other diagnoses (such as other hormonal deficiencies, including thyroid disease) and the cause of libido loss isn't clear (conflict in relationship, stress, vaginal atrophy), supplementation with testosterone patches or topical testosterone gels or creams could make sense not only to reverse a plummeting libido, but maybe — just maybe — to eliminate a paunch. And some argue that increased sexual satisfaction can help with satiety. Quick note: Testosterone is currently under investigation and not ready for prime-time use. So before you consider treatment, know that testosterone has risk factors and several side effects, including acne, facial hair growth, and rage reactions.

YOU TIPS!

If You Think It's Not You, Find the Cause. For some of you, it doesn't matter whether you eat like a worm or exercise like a thoroughbred; you just can't lose weight. "Hormones" are an appropriate scapegoat for some with knee-tickling guts. If you're convinced that your fat can't be attributed to your lifestyle, it's worth asking your doctor about blood tests that measure hormone and other chemical levels to see what medications may address hormonal issues. These are the levels we'd suggest learning about:

Myth Buster

Test	Desired Level
Thyroid-Stimulating Hormone	Less than 5 mIU/l (milli-international units per liter)
Urinary Cortisol	Less than 100 mg/day
Potassium	More than 3.5 mg
Calcium	Between 8 mg and 10 mg
Luteinizing Hormone/ Follicle-Stimulating Hormone	The individual values aren't as important as the ratio, and you'd like a 3:1 ratio of LH to FSH, no matter what time of the month.
Free Testosterone	More than 200 mg/dl for men; 20–70 mg/dl for women.

Do a Once-over. PCOS can be diagnosed with a blood test that measures total free testosterone. If your ratio of luteinizing hormone to follicle-stimulating hormone is greater than 3:1 (see above), that can also indicate PCOS. Treatment comes in the form of birth-control pills, to regulate the hormonal patterns, and the diabetes drug metformin — Glucophage — to help prevent a cross fire that happens between the ovary and the pancreas, and to calm the inflammatory responses in the liver, so that it helps the body become more sensitive to insulin.

Chapter 7
Make the Move

How You Can Burn Fat Faster

Rectus
Abdomenis
"Six-Pack"

"Lats"

"Glutes"

Diet Myths

- Lifting weights will make you bulky.

- The best exercise for losing fat is cardiovascular training.

- You need weights to build muscle.

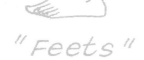

"Feets"

We all know that muscles give us the power to lift boxes and babies. They give us the power to walk around the mall and sprint for the 5:32 train to Schenectady. And depending on your tastes in movie-star muscle, they have the power to make your tongue wag faster than a golden retriever's tail. But you don't have to be an appliance deliveryman, an Olympic shot-putter, or an oiled-up spring breaker to benefit from muscle. When it comes to waist management, the real power of muscles lies in their ability to work like an anatomical pack of wolves. While your hormones are responsible for a large portion of your metabolism, your muscles can expedite the process of burning extra calories.

 YOU-reka! While muscles give us the metabolic ability to burn calories every time we move — during exercise, during gardening, during sex — their true advantage is that they constantly feed on calories, even when you're moving about as fast as a skateboard with a busted wheel. See, every pound of muscle burns between 40 and 120 calories a day just to sustain itself, while every pound of fat feeds on only 1 to 3 calories. Day after day, that's a huge difference in your metabolic rate and your daily calorie burn. When you add a water bottle full of muscle to your body, you're able to burn a refrigerator full of fat.

Myth Buster

When we think about muscles, we tend to think about really big ones (Hulk Hogan's) or really nice ones (Brad Pitt's abs, Hilary Swank's shoulders). Working

FACTOID

Think of exercise as medication. Too much of a stretch? Well, studies show that exercise decreases the risk of depression as well as an antidepressant. Thirty minutes of daily walking has been shown to decrease the risk of breast cancer by 30 percent and increase the rate of survival by 70 percent. Plus, it also improves the survival rates of heart attack victims by 80 percent.

your muscles isn't necessarily about making you big, brawny, and eligible for the NFL draft.

By focusing on the right muscles and following the right plan, you won't add bulk; you'll firm up, and you'll stimulate the amount of growth needed to help burn extra calories. Best of all? You don't need any expensive equipment or a gym membership to see the benefits of adding muscle. You need only one piece of equipment: your own body. Your body is your gym.

Your Muscles:
Strength Builders and Fat Burners

Your skeletal muscles — that is, the muscles attached to your bones by tendons and ligaments, not the involuntary muscles associated with working your organs, like your heart or esophagus — come in pairs. That allows one muscle to move a bone in one direction, while the other moves it in another (when you bend your arm at the elbow, your biceps muscle pulls your upper and lower arm together, while your triceps muscle pushes them away from each other).

Now, we could bore you to a pond's worth of tears by explaining the biology of muscle, so we'll summarize what you need to know: Skeletal muscle is designed to do two kinds of things — to make you fast and strong. It's made up of bundles of fibers, each of which is like a strand of spaghetti.

FACTOID
Starting with the 1960s, the increase in time that the average American spends watching TV perfectly parallels the increase in the average person's waist size. Besides keeping us from running errands outside, TV frees our hands to engage in mindless eating as we plan for the next commercial-break run to the fridge. This is an especially big problem for kids, who on average watch seventeen hours per week.

179

These fibers have filaments that have to slide over each other like an expandable ladder.

When your brain sends the message for your muscles to move — to walk, to lift a couch, to kiss your lover's ear — your muscles contract the way an extendable ladder would contract, by ratcheting the poles up and down. And it uses a catch or hook to stop the muscle and keep it opened or closed (see Figure 7.1). Now, you can build up two parts of that ladder — the actual poles, which give you strength; and the force that it takes to move those poles up and down, which gives you stamina. The force-generating structures act like calorie-guzzling cyclers pedaling furiously to pull together muscle fibers (see Figure 7.1). Elastic recoil generated by the contraction and aided by stretching helps the muscle relax after exercise.

The two main forms of exercise — stamina training and strength training — influence the structure of the ladder differently. Stamina training increases your muscles' capacity to produce and use the energy they need to contract, since you are adding more powerful cyclers, but muscle strength requires strength training that builds up the ladder poles — making for a bigger, stronger, and sturdier muscle fiber structure. How? When you do any kind of resistance training (that is, pulling or pushing some kind of weight) you create tiny tears in your muscle fibers. Your body reacts to those tears by saying, "If you can tear down my ladder, I'm going to build a stronger,

Figure 7.1 **Muscle Makeup** Mitochondria create ATP from energy we consume and feed the muscle fibers. The cells are coupled with tracks and move on one another to shorten (lifting your body) or relax (stretching).

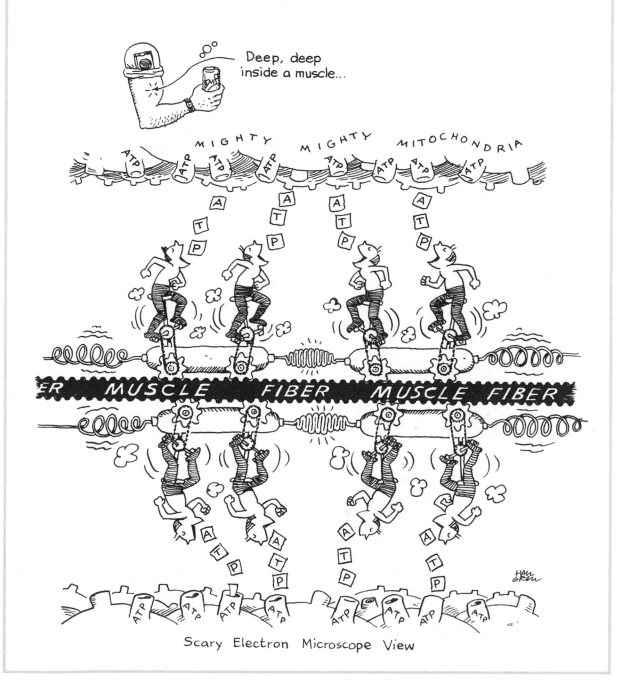

Scary Electron Microscope View

bigger one next time." And your body builds back bigger and stronger ladder poles. (Walking, by the way, increases both your energy capacity and your poles, which is one of the many reasons why it's a central part of this plan.) By regularly doing strength training, you create more muscle mass — muscle mass that you need to help you burn fat. In essence, you make the spaghetti strands a little thicker and stronger rather than making more spaghetti strands.

Muscle serves as a primary energy consumer for your body. Think of it as a raging fire. Toss a log into it, and it'll burn the log up pretty quickly. But your fat is more like one lit match — it would take years for that match to burn the log. In your body, muscle can fry up that cheese dog a lot faster than can fat — thus reducing the amount of fat you store. **YOU-reka!** Add just a little more muscle, and you'll use more energy and store less fat. And that makes it an even more efficient exercise for burning fat than cardiovascular training.

That's pretty crucial when you consider that we lose an average of 5 percent of our muscle mass every ten years after the age of thirty-five — if we don't do anything about it. (Historically, hunters, gatherers, and carriers of children needed their muscular strength until they were about

Myth Buster

FACTOID

Sports drinks may have some of the coolest commercials, but they're necessary only if you exercise for more than sixty minutes. They rehydrate your body faster than water after long periods of exercise because they help you recover muscle power sooner than water does (because they contain minerals in your body called electrolytes that hasten the absorption of water). But if you drink them regularly or after short workouts, you'll end up consuming more calories that won't get burned off.

thirty-five, when kids were able to walk and younger tribesmen could hunt. But after they turned thirty-five, their bodies didn't give two tubers about whether they had any muscle, so their bodies adapted and allowed for that gradual loss.) Today we see drastic effects when we lose muscle — we gain weight. If you don't intentionally rebuild muscle through exercise, every ten years you'll need to eat 120 to 420 fewer calories each day to maintain your current weight.

So if you're at a stable weight at age thirty-five and don't do any kind of resistance training, while still eating the same amount of

FACTOID

Besides the muscles you can voluntarily exercise, there are others in your body that you have no control over — such as the ones around your intestines and esophagus. They're involuntary smooth muscles, and they're the ones that no amount of crunches can ever build up.

How Much Muscle Do You Have?

While some waist-related measurements are easily quantifiable (pounds, waist size, number of pants ripped since 1993), muscle mass is a little trickier to calculate. Sure, you can eyeball yourself in the mirror and see if your abdominals look like an alligator's back. One indirect way to estimate is through knowing your body-fat percentage: The lower your fat percentage, the higher your muscle mass (this percentage can be measured at a gym, or with at-home devices like calipers). The truth is that the amount of muscle mass doesn't matter in terms of health (most of us have between twenty and thirty pounds of muscle) and waist size does. What is important is that you do enough strength-building exercise to maintain your muscle mass, which otherwise decreases as you age.

food, you'll gain weight.

Now, as your muscle ages, you also lose a little bit of the proteins that make up your muscle; they're what give your muscles the ability to have both strength and stamina. Exercise rebuilds and maintains proteins and muscle mass to prevent you from gaining weight. Here's what you need to do:

- thirty minutes of walking *a day* to help rebuild the stamina- and strength-based proteins. That prepares your muscles for . . .
- thirty minutes of strength/resistance training *a week* to rebuild the strength-based proteins. (That's once a week for thirty minutes, or split up into two fifteen-minute sessions or three ten-minute ones.

FACTOID

Doing exercises for a particular body part will not burn fat at that very point. Your body decides where it wants to burn fat, so there's no such thing as spot-reduction through exercise. Otherwise, wouldn't we be seeing people doing double-chin crunches in the gym? Instead, by doing exercises for a specific body part, you're building muscle mass in that area — which, after burning fat, will have the appearance and attributes of lean, strong muscle.

In Chapter 11, we'll outline the specifics of the plan, but we also want to explain that muscle is a heavyweight prizefighter — not just in its ability to clobber fat but also because it's literally heavy. When people start to exercise and eat healthier, their initial reaction is typically frustration, because it seems like their weight doesn't change that much at first. **YOU-reka!** That's because fat floats and muscle sinks; muscle is simply a lot heavier than fat. So as you build a little bit of muscle mass and lose fat, you may not see a dramatic reduction in scale numbers right away, but you will see reductions in waist size and overall shape. After you make it through the initial transition into exercise, chances are that you'll continue to see more dramatic changes in your body composition, your metabolism, your weight, and your waist.

Now, the question is: How do we add more muscle, rather than just maintaining what we've got? And how do we do it without ending up looking like a middle linebacker for the Bears?

The answer, of course, lies in exercise — but perhaps not in the way you might think. Most of us break down exercise into two categories: stamina-based training (*aerobic,* like jogging or swimming) and strength-based training (lifting weights). Any kind of exercise burns calories while you're doing the activity, but the most potent and long-lasting fat burners are created not when you're swimming or running, as you might believe,

FACTOID

Deciding between free weights and weight machines is like trying to decide between salmon and tilapia: They both have their strong points. Free weights (barbells and dumbbells) help you work on balance because your body has to work to balance the weights as well as lift them, while machines can help prevent injuries stemming from poor form because they're built in such a way that they force you to use proper form.

but *after* strength training. That makes muscle one of your body's greatest anatomical allies. Here we're going to show you how to take advantage of your muscles' muscle — the right way, the easy way, the way that will not only get you more stares than a Monet masterpiece but also help you get the waist that you want.

While many diet plans don't discuss the role of exercise, we consider physical activity vital to inflate your health and deflate your waist size. Building muscle is one component, but cardiovascular training and increasing your flexibility are also part of your waist management plan. Together, the three components of exercise will have numerous effects on your body:

- Exercise increases your metabolism so that you burn energy at a higher rate than if you didn't exercise, and it reduces your appetite by turning on your sympathetic nervous system, which activates your fight-or-flight response. Do the experiment yourself. Take a quick walk or jog when you feel the first twinge of hunger. Presto, your hunger is gone when you return.

- Exercise will help you lose the extra weight that's stressing your joints. By dropping weight, you'll feel less pain in your knees, hips, ankles, and back. And that will put you into a positive cycle of behavior, so that you'll have the desire to exercise more.

- Exercise stimulates the release of endorphins, which stimulate the pleasure centers in the brain. When they're stimulated, they give you a sense of control, which is associated with a decreased need to eat out of control.

- Exercise helps decrease depression and increases positive attitude, so you make other positive choices and don't have to use food as your medication. That will also help prevent your couch, chair, and bed from becoming anti–waist management devices.

- Exercise keeps your blood vessels open and clog-free, thus decreasing your risk of obesity-related morbidities like high blood pressure, elevated lousy cholesterol, memory problems, and heart attacks.

We could spend dozens of pages listing all the benefits of physical activity, but we think you get the point. You don't have to be an infomercial beefcake with a shaved chest to make physical activity a priority — and you don't have to spend three hours a day doing it to see the benefits.

In fact, what's so wonderful about exercise is that unlike the things you have to take away from your life (junk foods, excuses), physical activity is something you can *add* (all while watching *Raymond*

FACTOID

Some athletes laud the supplement creatine as a wonderful muscle builder — and the difference between a homer and an out, or the difference between a world record and third place. Some studies show that creatine can increase power and speed as well as cellular energy, but the fact is that most of the gain in muscle size is due to increased water accumulation. Studies show that a simple sugar and some protein can help muscles recover faster after exercise (think apple with a handful of nuts).

Asian Invasion

Wake up any morning in Beijing, China, and you see hundreds of people of all ages greet the sun with awkward movements. They appear to be wrestling demons in the air, but they're practicing tai chi — a form of exercise used to balance, center, and relax the body. You can use tai chi as a meditative form of exercise or as a way to improve your balance.

Have You Gone Too Far?

Exercising is like nuts in at least one way: There is such a thing as too much of a good thing. While exercise has more pluses than a math workbook, you can take it too far. Burning more than 6,500 calories a week through exercise (that's roughly thirteen hours) or doing more than two hours in a row of cardiovascular training not only can stress your joints (depending on the exercise), but it also appears to be the level at which you induce too much oxidative stress in your body, and that decreases your longevity.

reruns). When you get your muscles moving in the right direction, your waist size will follow.

When you first start exercising, your body will respond with very outward signs: You'll sweat, you may feel sore, you may stink like month-old macaroni salad. Your body will also start responding on the inside, with changes in muscle size, blood flow, and blood chem-

FACTOID

As you increase the intensity of your exercise, the typical body utilizes a higher percentage of carbohydrate-fueled energy rather than fat-fueled energy. Some incorrectly interpret this to mean that as you increase exercise intensity, you are no longer burning fat, but burning only carbohydrates. Since the total number of calories burned during higher-intensity exercise is larger than the number of calories burned at lower intensities (even though a slightly higher percentage may come from carbohydrates than fats), you are almost always using (burning) more total fat than if you worked at a lower intensity.

istry. While exercise — even combined with a healthy diet — won't suck fat out of you instantaneously (more on liposuction in the appendix), you will see and feel changes in your body shape even within a week. And with the combined workout and eating YOU Plan, you may see a two-inch reduction in waist size within the first two weeks as your body composition changes. So get up and get moving.

YOU TIPS!

Know Your Fantastic Four. Physical activity and exercise are like vegetables; they come in all shapes, sizes, and tastes, and just about all of them are good for you. Depending on your health level and experience, you need to be thinking about including these components of activity in your life:

■ **Walking:** We do it at the mall, around the house, and back and forth from the fridge to the water bed. And, yes, any walking is healthy (the optimum is to hit at least 10,000 steps a day). But you also need to dedicate a total of thirty minutes a day to walking (broken up into chunks of at least ten continuous minutes if you need to). It's the foundation for all other exercise because it not only increases your stamina but prepares your body for strength training. As a daily routine, walking is the psychological discipline that helps you stick with an activity plan. In fact, it has the highest compliance rate of any exercise. Commit to walking, and you'll start committing to more than just the TV lineup on Thursday nights.

■ **Strength:** Even if the only barbell you've ever seen is the one that's piercing your buddy's tongue, that doesn't mean you should shy away from resistance training. Strength training — whether you use dumbbells, machines, bands, or your own body weight — helps rebuild muscle fibers and increase muscle

Myth Buster

Figure 7.2 **The Tone Zones** Think of yourself as a homunculus with a studly torso, hips, back, and belly — your body's foundation muscles. When it comes to fighting fat, who cares about muscle-bound biceps and calves?

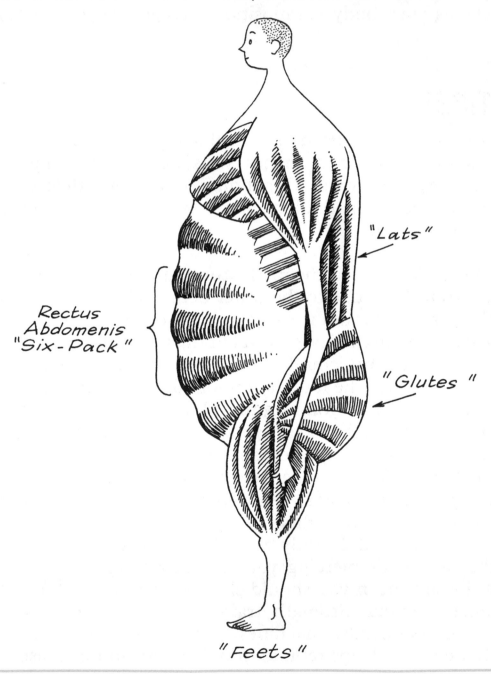

"Lats"

Rectus
Abdomenis
"Six-Pack"

"Glutes"

"Feets"

mass, which will use up all those extra calories that you crave, so you can burn calories more efficiently and help prevent age-related weight gain. Now, here's the key to making it work: Many Americans tend to spend a lot of time working their peripheral muscles (like their biceps or their calves), but efficient strength training comes when you work the big muscles that make up the core axis of your body — your legs, the large muscles of your upper body (like your chest, shoulders, and back), and your abdominals. They're your *foundation muscles.* Best of all, you don't need a single piece of equipment to see the benefits.

One quick note about abdominal exercises: They won't burn fat per se, but they will strengthen your entire core to help flatten and tone your stomach when you do burn fat. And they'll give you a layer of muscular support that will also protect your lower back from injury. The tighter your abs, the less excess strain you'll cause your lower back. You can't build a house from the second floor down, and, in a way, your abdominal muscles and your entire core provide a base foundation that you can build upon.

■ **Cardiovascular Stamina:** By doing cardiovascular exercise — that is, any activity that raises your heart rate for a sustained period of time (sorry, watching George Clooney movies doesn't count) — you'll increase your overall stamina, burn calories, and improve the function and efficiency of your heart, as well as lower your blood pressure. Getting your body to sweat also helps you to release toxins that would otherwise build up in your tissues.

■ **Flexibility:** Being flexible isn't just a good trait for yoga teachers and potential spouses; it's also what you want for your muscles. Good flexibility helps prevent injuries to your joints, because stretching works your muscles through a wide range of motion that you'll go through during exercise and everyday activity. Plus, being flexible just makes you feel better; it keeps your body from feeling stiffer than a week-old roach corpse, helps facilitate meditation, and allows you to center yourself as you focus on your body. Plus, the more pliable and loose you are, the less you're affected when you fall or get into accidents.

The YOU Diet Activity Audit

What You Need to Do	How Much You Need to Do
Walking	Ten thousand steps, total, accumulated throughout the day (with at least thirty minutes of continuous walking)
Muscular strength	Thirty minutes of resistance exercise a week
Cardiovascular stamina	Eighty percent of your maximum heart rate (calculated by 220 minus your age) for twenty minutes, three times a week. For a fifty-year-old, the target would be 0.8 times (220 minus 50), which equals 136 beats per minute. Also, you can measure it through exercise intensity. On a scale of one to ten, rate the intensity of your exercise. You should exercise at about a seven or eight on that scale — 70 percent to 80 percent of your perceived maximum.
Flexibility	Five minutes a day

Excuse-Proof Your Life. When it comes to working out, most of us have two excuse cards we like to play: We have the ace of "no time" and the jack of "it's not convenient." Now, we know you're busy. We know you're juggling more balls than a twelve-armed clown. We know it's easier to sit on the couch than to do a push-up on the floor. But we also know this: Time and convenience aren't excuses. First of all, with this plan, you don't need a whole lot of time (thirty minutes a day to walk and thirty minutes a week to do some resistance training). If you don't have the time to do this, then you have to be willing to admit that the problem is not the fact that you're out of time but the fact that your life is so out of control that you can't budget enough time for your health and well-being.

And second, you don't need a gym or fancy equipment; heck, it takes more time to drive to the gym and change clothes than it does to actually work out. You can do all of this activity at home — with a few modest pieces of equipment or even by making use of items you already have. In fact, in the YOU Workout, you use your body as your weights. It sure beats spending your workout time waiting at the exercise machine for someone to finish her issue of *Quilting Quarterly*. Yes, it's easy to say you're too tired, too stressed, too busy, too this, or too that. We say, too bad. The only way you'll strip away the fat is to start by stripping away the excuses.

You Move, You Lose. One unsung form of exercise: fidgeting. Studies show that fidgety people are simply skinnier people. If you have two people working the same job and eating the same diet, the one who gets up to talk to someone down the hall rather than emailing her will be skinnier. Studies show that it isn't some mysterious food, organ, cell, or gremlin that makes these people burn up fat like an iron skillet, it's these fidgeting movements. Now, that's not to say that if you go on an all-fidgeting, leg-shaking, finger-tapping program (think Robin Williams), you'll be thinner than a Hilton sister. But numerous studies have shown that the more you move — in very subtle ways — the more calories your body will burn throughout the day. Find an excuse to move your muscles wherever you are. Clear the dishes. Stand up and walk in circles while you're on the phone. Walk down the hall to ask a coworker a question, rather then IM-ing her. Tap your toes in a meeting. Take every opportunity to move around, and you'll give your body subtle metabolism boosters that may just have more-than-subtle effects.

YOU Test

How Fit Are You?

There are lots of ways to gauge progress on a weight-loss plan: inches lost, Wendy's coupons tossed. But you can also measure your fitness levels in different areas of activity. Use these tests to see how you stack up. (Before doing each test, make sure to properly warm up by walking or doing light exercise for at least five minutes.)

Cardiovascular: You can measure your heart's efficiency by measuring your heart rate *after* exercise. After exercising for a period of eighteen minutes at 80 percent to 85 percent of your max (that's 220 minus your age), do three minutes at your maximum heart rate, then stop and check your pulse. Your heart rate should decrease sixty-six beats or more after two minutes of stopping. Do not do this without approval of your doctor unless you do it regularly as part of your workout.

Squeeze Yourself. Here's an abdominal exercise you can (and should) do anywhere: Suck your belly button in tight and squeeze your butt in as if you're trying to pull up a pair of too-tight jeans. Pretend the top of your head is being pulled by a string to the ceiling. Now hold that position. Besides putting you into proper posture, it's working your transverse abdominis muscle (your supportive girdle muscles). Do it on the elevator, waiting in line, at work, and anywhere you walk.

Muscular: To gauge upper-body muscular stamina, do the push-up test (men in standard form; women can do it with knees on the floor). A thirty-year-old man should be able to do at least thirty-five (five less every decade after that, until he reaches seventy). A thirty-year-old woman should be able to do forty-five with knees on floor (five less every decade after until she reaches eighty).

Flexibility: Measure lower-back flexibility by sitting on the floor with your legs straight out in front of you and slightly spread apart. With one hand on top of the other and fingertips lined up, lean forward and reach for your feet. Women forty-five and under should be able to reach two to four inches past their feet. Older women should be able to reach to the soles. Men aged forty-five and under should be able to reach to the soles. Older men should be able to come within three to four inches of the soles.

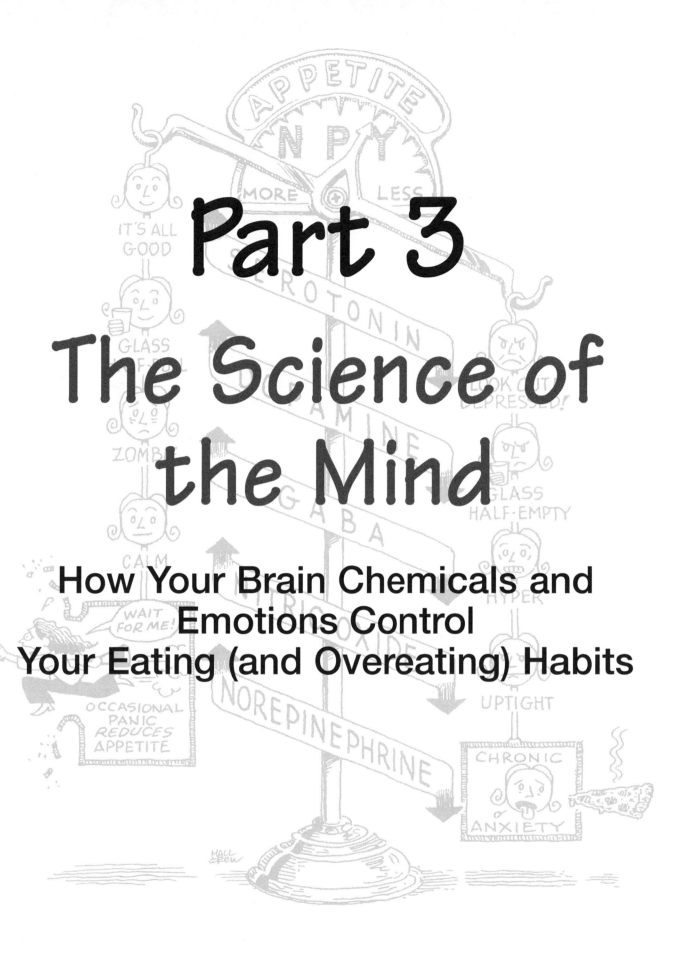

Part 3
The Science of the Mind

How Your Brain Chemicals and Emotions Control Your Eating (and Overeating) Habits

Chapter 8

The Chemistry of Emotions

The Connections between Feelings and Food

Diet Myths

- Hedonistic eating is triggered mainly by extreme hunger.

- Cravings are directed by taste buds.

- The best way to resist temptations is with willpower.

Our ancestors ate to survive; they ate because they were hungry or maybe to celebrate a victory over a warring tribe. Us? We eat because we're angry, bored, stressed, depressed, frustrated, watching a movie, busy, not busy enough, getting together with friends, or PO'd that the Lions lost. What we think of as an emotional reaction — where we substitute chocolate for a conversation, or ice cream for a bath, or chips for a punching bag — isn't always as much about character as it is about chemistry.

Early in the book, you learned about the chemical reactions that take place in your body that stimulate hunger. Leptin and ghrelin are the joysticks that control our eating actions. But oftentimes, the physical action of eating can be triggered by emotions that coax us to wolf down the mustard-smothered dog. In the next two chapters, we'll discuss how the science of your brain and emotions can contribute to what and why you eat. While emotions are the least understood part of the obesity issue, they're also a very real part of overeating for many people. Your hypothalamus (remember, the site of your satiety center) is also the part of your brain where your mind and body literally connect. As the bosom buddy of the hypothalamus, the pituitary gland sends chemicals to talk to the rest of the body. It's really where the whole weight-loss game is won and lost — this connection between physiological and psychological needs for eating.

As you well know, emotional eating isn't about reaching for celery. **Myth Buster** Rather, it's out-of-control, hedonistic eating (that often comes from your food memory), where we eat every cookie in the bag because they look good and taste even better. It's a craving, and usually for something that's starchy, sugary, salty, or loaded with fat. The following five brain chemicals are the ones that primarily influence our emotions, and not only do they provide the foundation for why we eat at certain times, but they're also the key chemicals in many of our current and future weight-loss drugs.

Please know that we're purposely leaving out the intricate web of interactions that take place among these chemicals, and the nonemotional effects. The intricacies of these interactions — fully understood by only a few people in the world — are real but not integral to your understanding of the science of emotions for eating. To deal with some of the emotions and stresses that lead to eating, you have to remember that the brain chemicals that influence our hunger and our moods are our "why" regulators of eating.

Norepinephrine: the caveman fight-or-flight chemical. It's what tells you to tangle with a saber-tooth or hightail it to the safety of your hut.

Serotonin: the James Brown of neurotransmitters. It makes you feel good *(Hyah!)* and is a major target of antidepression drugs.

Dopamine: the brain's fun house. It's a pleasure-and-reward system and is particularly sensitive to addictions. It's also the one that helps you feel no pain.

GABA (gamma-aminobutyric acid): the *English Patient* of amino acids. It makes you feel like a zombie and is one of the

> **FACTOID**
>
> When the level of serotonin in your brain falls, your body senses starvation, and to protect itself, starts craving carbs the way twelve-year-olds crave Hilary Duff sightings. Serotonin levels plummet after you go too long without eating, and that prompts your bodily machine to fill itself with foods. Some have tried to keep their serotonin level up by supplementation with 5-HTP, the breakdown product of tryptophan that converts to and stimulates serotonin. In a six-week study, a group of dieters using 5-HTP lost an average of twelve pounds, while a control group lost an average of four. Although one side effect of the supplement is nausea, about 90 percent of women taking 300 milligrams of 5-HTP reported satiety while on the diet.

Figure 8.1 **A Game of Emotions** Serotonin bounces around your brain, stimulating your pleasure hot spots and hitting your satiety bumpers. But when your emotional and feeding flippers fail to keep the ball in play, your instinctual desire to eat (especially carbohydrates) returns.

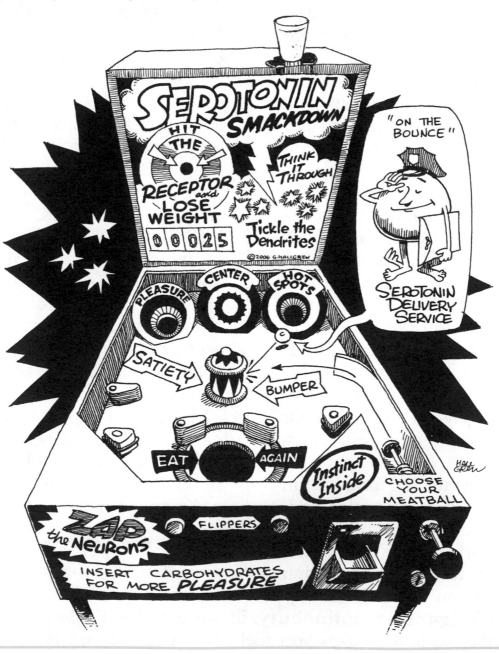

ways that anesthesia may work to reduce your responsiveness to the outside world.

Nitric Oxide: the meditationlike chemical. It helps calm you. This powerful neuropeptide is usually a very short-lived gas that also relaxes the blood vessels of the body.

Mood Foods

Recent research shows what many of us knew all along: Our moods dictate what we eat. Researchers studied the diets of people to show how personality and foods collide — how our moods may steer us to certain foods, on the basis of their physical characteristics. The study theorized that many moods send specific signals; for example, stressed adrenal glands could be sending salt-craving signals. So what does your favorite turn-to food say about you?

If You Reach For . . .	You May Be Feeling . . .
Tough foods, like meat, or hard and crunchy foods	Angry
Sugars	Depressed
Soft and sweet foods, like ice cream	Anxious
Salty foods	Stressed
Bulky, fill-you-up foods, like crackers and pasta	Lonely, sexually frustrated
Anything and everything	Jealous

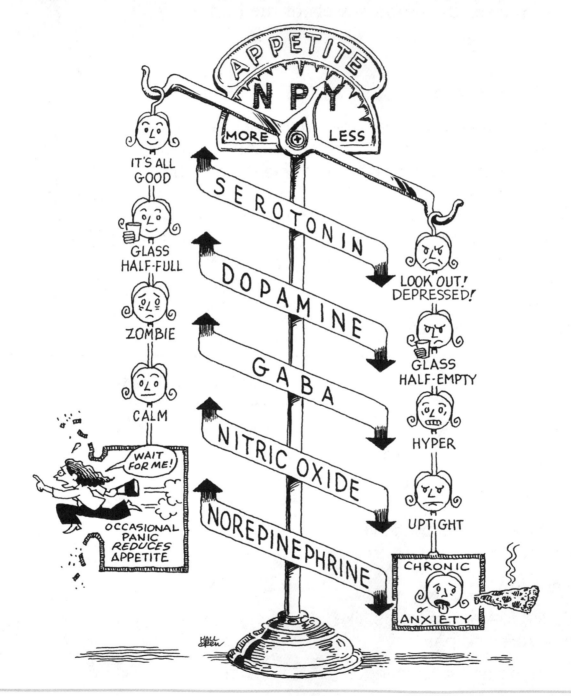

Figure 8.2 **Scale of Injustice** Brain hormones that control emotions also influence appetite. Not having enough of each pulls the scale toward more NPY — and more appetite.

Now, the real question is: What do all these chemicals have to do with whether or not you snack on a Hershey bar or a plum? Probably the best way to think about it is to use serotonin as an example. Picture your brain as a small pinball machine (see Figure 8.1). You have millions of neurotransmitters that are sending messages to and from one another. When your serotonin transmitters fire the signals (from the flippers), they send the message throughout your brain that you feel good; this message is strongest when that feel-good pinball is frenetically bouncing around in your brain, racking up tons of yeah-baby points along the way. But when you lose the ball down the chute (that is, when cells in the brain take the serotonin and break it down), that love-the-world feeling you've just been experiencing is lost. So what does your brain want to do? Put another quarter in the machine and get another ball. For many of us, the next ball comes in the form of foods that naturally (and quickly) make us feel good, to counteract the drop in serotonin that we're feeling.

Unfortunately, the way we typically satisfy our urge to play another ball is to use the foods that provide an immediate rush of serotonin. That rush can come with a jolt of sugar: sugar stimulates the release of serotonin. Insulin facilitates serotonin production in the brain, which in turn boosts our mood, makes us feel better, or masks the stress, pain, boredom, anger, or frustration that we may be feeling. But serotonin is only one ball in play. You have all of these other chemicals fighting to send your appetite and cravings from bumper to bumper.

To see how the total picture works, think of these chemicals as parts of a scale. When the chemicals associated with positive feelings (like serotonin or dopamine) are in the up (or activated) position, you're chemically high. But when they're down, you experience a big chemical downfall (see Figure 8.2). **YOU-reka!** And this puts you in a state of anxiety that sends you searching for the foods, especially those simple carbohydrates, that get you back to the chemical high. That's how illegal drugs work too; users keep seeking the high not always for its own sake but to avoid the lows. You're constantly fighting to get back to that place of neurochemical comfort. When these chemicals are high, your weight gets lower, and when they're lower, you reach for the foods that eventually make your weight higher.

That's the reason why what happens under your skull plays such a vital role in what happens under your belt. Knowing how your emotions can steer your desire to eat will help you to resist your cravings and, ideally, avoid them altogether. Your **Myth Buster** goal: Keep your feel-good hormones level so that you're in a steady state of satisfaction and never experience huge hormonal highs and lows that make you search for good-for-your-brain-but-bad-for-your-waist foods. In the next chapter, we'll explore this further — with the deeper emotions that can contribute to eating, hunger, and weight gain.

YOU TIPS!

Work Foods in Your Favor. Foods all have different effects on your stomach, your blood, and your brain. These are some of the nutrients that may influence your hunger and the brain chemicals that affect it:

- Turkey contains tryptophan, which increases serotonin to improve your mood and combat depression, and help you resist cravings for simple carbs.
- Omega-3 fatty acids, which are found in fish, have long been known as brain boosters and cholesterol clearers, but they've also been shown convincingly to help with depression in pregnant women. Depression, as we'll explain in the next chapter, contributes to he-

donistic and emotional eating. Since many of us have low omega-3 intake, it might explain some other instances of depression as well.

Savor the Flavor. If you're going to eat something that's bad for you, enjoy it, savor it, roll it around your mouth. We suggest taking a piece of dark 70 percent cocoa chocolate and meditating — as a healthy stress reliever and as way to reward yourself with something sweet. We're trying to find small ways to make you feel good and increase serotonin, so you don't plummet and scavenge for anything you can find. It's OK to eat bad foods — every once in a while. It's not the first piece that's going to Shamu you; it's scarfing down the whole bag that will.

Go to Sleep. Getting enough sleep keeps you thin. **YOU-reka!** That's because when your body doesn't get the seven to eight hours of sleep it needs every night to get rejuvenated, it needs to find ways to compensate for neurons not secreting the normal amounts of serotonin or dopamine. The way it typically does that is by craving sugary foods that will give you an immediate release of serotonin and dopamine. The lack of sleep throws off your entire system — even increasing your levels of NPY, which increase your appetite. Lack of sleep can become an even bigger factor as you age. When you get older, the pineal gland in your brain produces less of the sleep hormone melatonin, resulting in a craving for carbohydrates.

Chapter 9
Shame on Who?

The Psychology of the Failed Diet

Diet Myths

- The diet would work if only you had the willpower of a lean person.

- It's better to have dieted and failed than to not have dieted at all.

- You can't make mistakes when you're dieting.

Most diets aren't about action; they're about thoughts. By their very nature, they force us to think, think, think, think. Diets make us think about food more than inmates think about escape. You have to think about calories, or zones, or the hour when you're next allowed to have half a cracker. You think about not having food so much that you develop only two sets of standards when it comes to eating: Either you follow your diet or you don't. It's bean sprouts or it's prime rib. It's carrots or it's cookies. It's cucumbers or it's pepperoni. It's all or nothing.

Myth Buster
In a way, we've all been thinking too much about weight and what to eat, and not enough about how and why we eat. When most of us try to lose weight, we pull out the most powerful weapon we'd like to think we know — our brains — and launch a psychological attack in the form of discipline ("I can resist this food!") and ego ("I'm smart enough to avoid this food!"). But as you'll see in this chapter, the truth is that there are very strong emotional triggers that make us eat — and make most diets fail. In many ways, it's our brains that sabotage our best dieting efforts.

By trying the very thing that's designed to help us lose weight — a diet — we've created a no-win system of failure that spins us into a cycle of blame. And what's not to blame? The experts blame our societal fatness on free restaurant bread and meals with Mount McKinley–size portions. Or we blame our fatness on fast food (for the grease), magazine covers (for the unrealistic body images that taunt us to smear our self-esteem in daily fistfuls of cheesecake), sixty-hour workweeks (for making us sit down all day), cloud-soft recliners and reality TV (for making us sit down all night), sausage *(blech!)*, or an intervention-worthy Velveeta addiction (double *blech!*).

But deep down in your gut (there, over by the sticky buns you ate two weeks ago), there's really only one thing you blame for the size of your gut:

You.

You blame *you.*

You tell yourself it's not the restaurants or food manufacturers or deep-fried cheese-stuffed peppers that are derailing your weight-loss efforts, it's your mind. The entire battle of the broken belt comes down to a flurry of mental "if onlys" — and your perceived inability to control what food you shuttle down your esophagus year after year, day after day, meal after meal, bite after bite. If only you had the willpower to step away from the mayonnaise. If only you could stop after four Pringles. If only you had the power, the strength, the discipline, the chutzpah, the energy, the drive, and the motivation to control your waist, then you'd *finally* have the body you want.

What you're really doing here is laying brain blame. We rely on our minds to resist temptations, to make smart decisions, to eat right, to know better, and to make healthy choices. So we naturally rely on our minds to combat the emotions that we think we should be able to handle — stress, anxiety, depression (studies show that those with higher levels of all these emotions are more likely to be overweight or obese). So when we give up on a diet and balloon to a size that makes doorways cringe, then we automatically think something's wrong with us, that our minds aren't strong enough to win over our waists.

The reason we fail? Researchers theorize that it's your mind that might be crossed up, but not because of anything you're doing. At least scientifically, overeating may work a little bit like drug addiction; in fact, studies show that obese people even have reward centers in the brain similar to those of drug addicts.

So let's say you're stressed. Remember the hypothalamus and the chemicals that change according to your moods. At points of stress, you've activated neurotransmitters from a part of the brain called the locus coeruleus. Your body, in response, tries to calm those neurotransmitters and combat the stress. Some people do it with cigarettes, some do it with food, some do it with sex, some do it with drugs. When you combat the stress with food, you're also activating the reward center of your brain. And then after that initial feel-good system wears off, you'll reach again for the same thing that made you feel good, calm, and relaxed: food. That's why stress and anxiety make it that more difficult, neurochemically, to stick to whatever plan you're trying to follow.

What's especially interesting is that right next to the hypothalamus, where the feeding and satiety chemicals NPY and CART are produced, is a part of the brain called the mammillary body (because it physically looks like a pair of breasts). That's where food memory is stored, so when you get the signal that you're hungry, you're also accessing your memory of and cravings for foods you've eaten in the past — which may have been bad foods. Plus, the parietal region of the brain — the control center of the movement of the tongue, lips, and mouth — acts differently in heavy people than in skinny people. Brain scans show that in heavy people tempted with sugar, this region becomes activated. In skinny people the region stays dormant, showing how sugar can play a role in emotional eating for some people but not others.

If you've struggled with waist issues, you've probably placed all the responsibility for dietary success or failure on your little three-pound brain. You've expected it to go head-to-head with such formidable foes as deep-fried taco shells and Alfredo sauce. But you can't outwit nature. There are simply too many of those hormones and neurotransmitters whose jobs roughly translate to "pass the pound cake." And to expect that your *will* or your *fortitude* can override these chemical messages is the equivalent of trying to stop a train with your pinkie.

Dieting: Avoiding the Issue

For a second, think about one particular kind of person — the extreme example of fat gone wild. These people are often the stereotypical ideal — funny, kind, generous, charming, articulate, creative, and more brilliant than a perfect diamond — except for the fact that they're regularly mistaken for a four-story silo. (We all say it: "He'd be so great, if only he were *thin*.") And that bothers us. It bothers us that we can't figure out the yin and yang of the situation. How can a person smart enough to know the difference between scrapple and

Figure 9.1 **Food for Thoughts** When you eat sugar, you light up the motor cortex of your brain, which controls your lips, tongue, and mouth. The hippocampus, which controls memories of food, lights up when people on rigid diets crave certain foods — overwhelming their willpower and ability to resist.

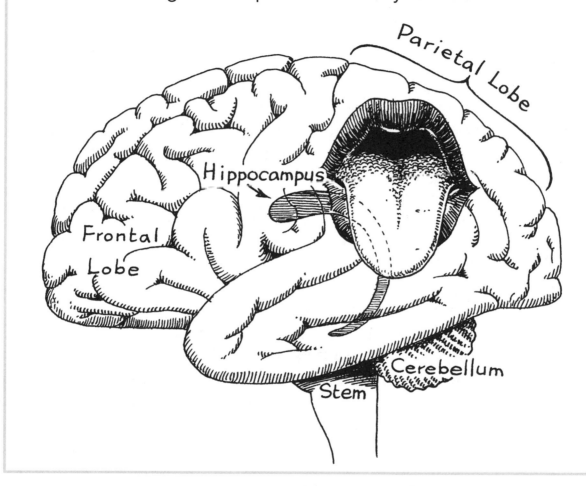

apples or driven enough to have a successful career be the very same person who, night after night, gets clobbered silly by a helpless sleeve of Oreos hiding in the back of the pantry shelf?

Something has to be wrong.

And it is. But it's about as likely to be what you think as you are to find your true love in Las Vegas. The issues aren't at waistband level, they're at brain level. You may know you have health problems and

213

a waist circumference the size of Neptune. And you may even know that you struggle with the emotional issues of confidence and esteem that come as the side orders with the entrée of obesity. **YOU-reka!** But you may not know that you could be what's called an avoider, in that you suffer internally from a tornado of psychological turmoil that comes with the public and private disdain for obesity, and you avoid confronting your situation at all because of the internal fear of not being able to beat it.

Here's how avoiders think (nod if this sounds familiar): Once you deviate — even slightly — from a diet or healthy eating plan, you figure you might as well drop the whole thing. (Nodding?) And this starts a cycle that avoiders can't find a way out of: We're fat, we try to lose weight, we deviate just a little, we fear rejection for the perceived failure, we isolate ourselves from people, we stop talking about it, we stop the diet, we mow through a pound of cheesecake, we get fat. And then we try to lose weight, and the cycle continues.

Avoiders at all levels (from the extreme cases to the milder ones) will see their weight bop up and down like a bull rider. Physiologically, it's a never-ending cycle of weight gain and loss (that's called weight cycling). But the real avoider issues stem from the psychological effects of weight cycling. Instead of avoiding bad foods, avoiders tend to want to avoid other things — like the people who want to help them and the discipline of trying to eat healthfully. Above all, avoiders try to separate themselves from these two strong emotions associated with dieting.

Guilt: "I Hope They Don't Find Out"

No matter what kind of diet you may have tried in the past, you've undoubtedly worked with a list of off-limits foods. High-protein diets might ban potatoes. Low-fat diets might ban cheese. Sugar-busting diets may ban you from ever setting foot in Aunt Thelma's kitchen again. Inevitably, like a child instructed not to touch the champagne flutes, you will want potatoes, you will want cheese, and you will find it incredibly rude to turn down Aunt Thelma's

Figure 9.2 **Swirling World** As we battle with food, the cyclone of guilt and shame touches down on our psychological landscape. The collateral damage: our waistlines.

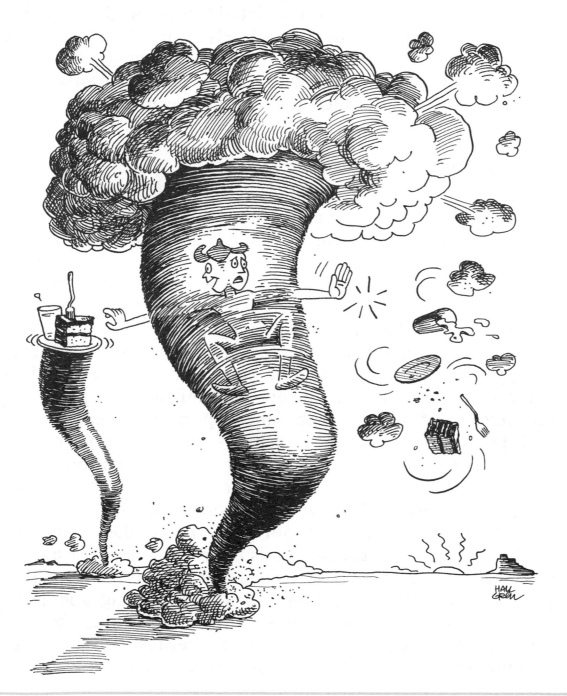

snickerdoodles three times in a row. So you cave. But because you've set yourself up with a list of banned foods, you perceive half a cookie, or a hunk of Gouda, or three measly fries as first-degree diet homicide: The diet's dead. And that's where guilt sets in — from the fact that you know you deviated from a predetermined set of standards. That holds true for all levels of avoiders. We all identify with nutrition-induced guilt, and then we make a subconscious decision that it's easier to deal with the effects of being overweight than it is to feel the boulder-heavy guilt every time we want to smother a carrot in blue cheese.

Shame: "Oh Gosh, They Did Find Out"

For the person who feels he cheated on that diet — whether it was a simple kiss with a Kit Kat or an adulterous romp with a vat of cake batter — there's an even worse feeling than guilt. And that's the shame associated with dietary infidelity. You've cheated, so you now feel you lack the strength to succeed. So what are you going to tell your spouse and all your coworkers who've been watching you feast on iceberg lettuce at lunch for the past eight days? That, yes, you're a failure? You could last on your diet for only a week? You have one little thing you're doing, and by gosh, you can't even keep a stinking croissant out of your mouth? The public humiliation, or just the perceived threat of possible embarrassment, primarily stems from that societal disdain for obesity. This shame — a much more profound emotion than guilt — spins you back into the cycle of avoidance: It's better to not be on a diet and be fat, the avoider calculates, than to be on a diet and eventually prove to the world that you can't succeed.

Research shows it's better for your health not to diet at all than to say you're dieting and steal spoonfuls of crème brûlée during every commercial break. That's because diets typically promote weight cycling and yo-yo dieting (gaining and losing, gaining and losing), which are actually more hazardous to your health than keeping a steady overweight weight. (That's probably because most weight cyclers eventually gain more than they lost and suffer the slings of shame.)

So how does this all work for you, the person who knows she has to lose some weight but isn't necessarily breaking floorboards with every step? Well, if you've spent years struggling with weight, then it's likely you've experienced similar thought patterns of guilt and shame and may even follow the same behavioral patterns: If you can't reach 100 percent compliance on the rules of your chosen diet, then you might as well feast like a piranha in a river full of ankles. Eat as much as you can as fast as you can.

Avoidance is a normal thought process: When you reach an obstacle, you decide that instead of trying to find a way around it, you might as well turn around and go back to the beginning. Four fries lead to a handful. A handful leads to another. And two handfuls lead to, "Britney, sweetie, pass that little ol' bag right over to Mama." Approximately sixteen seconds later, you feel guiltier than an un-neutered dog without a leash. Whether you negated your diet in one bite, one dish, or one meal, your noncompliance ruined everything. One of the strategies for handling emotional eating is to live and eat in the present — not being upset about what you ate in the past and not obsessing about what you'll eat in the future.

Why Our Brains Aren't Equipped for "Dieting"

Unfortunately, the very thing that's designed to help people lose weight is the very thing that promotes this behavioral and psychological pattern: diets that promote the all-or-nothing mentality.

It turns out that much of the diet dogma we've all accepted as fact is more hype than horse sense. Like a tantalizing trailer that creates expectations well beyond what the movie can deliver, the problem with most diets is not with the preview; it's with the plot. The typical diet drama opens to reveal the hero dieter preparing for battle — attacking the enemy head-on. Armed with grit, determination, and little else, the hero prepares for battle against flying chocolate sundaes in a quest for total domination over food. But what our hero doesn't realize is that the secret weapon she was counting on will

Can You Spare Some Change?

We all know that making a change in your life is as mental as it is behavioral. Research shows that this is the best four-step process for making change:

Be Positive. It works for coaches, bosses, and parents, as well as waist managers. If you blame yourself for your weight, if you are depressed about your weight, if your mood is fouler than a subway station in August, then your first job is to refocus. You need to think about what you can do, how you can do it, why it's good for you, and how you'll succeed. In the weight-loss game, poker-faced confidence trumps negativity every time. By stripping yourself of the negative emotions of guilt and shame, you'll make the right rational (and long-term) decisions about your eating obstacles.

Add Some Support. You may not know it, but your world is full of saboteurs — people out to make you fatter than Microsoft's coffers. There's the boss who brings in sweets for every Thursday meeting. The friend who brings you a pie when you're upset. The spouse who suggests pitchers of margaritas and a plate of cheese nachos to celebrate the end of the week. Maybe there's nothing wrong with their intentions, but there is something wrong with the fact that their attempts to appeal to your heart are actually damaging it. What we want you to do — no, *need* you to do — is develop a support system of people who know your goals, know your obstacles, know your weaknesses, and know your strengths. (Don't have anyone? You can hook up on the Internet, including on www.realage.com.) This person will be your sound-

never arrive; the cavalry is nowhere in sight. So the battle becomes grueling, mentally and physically exhausting, and never-ending, and all this hard work tends to create quite an appetite, and the energy halo from yesterday's feast of three stalks of celery and a cherry tomato is quickly fading. Our hero needs a pizza, and fast.

ing board, your comfort system, and your measure of accountability. With public accountability — that is, you reporting in on those daily struggles and successes — you're more likely to make a permanent change.

Make a Gesture. Small gestures (ones not involving individual fingers flung at passing motorists) can be viewed as anything from signs of love to signs of bribery. Token gestures can also help kickstart the psychology of change. Just making a seemingly small change will help determine your long-term success, whether it's buying a pedometer, a health-club membership, or new walking shoes; throwing away the unhealthy foods in your pantry; and even setting up a computer file to record your progress. **YOU-reka!** If you make one small move like this, research shows that you'll be three times more likely to follow through with the specific plan you intend to follow. This small change is your way of putting the key in your waist management ignition (www.mychoicescount.com can help).

Then Do It. Once you start with the small gesture, you're ready. Eat a full day's worth of perfect-for-you food. Walk thirty minutes today, tomorrow, and every day after that. That's right, thirty minutes of walking a day is the minimum commitment. (You can break them up into smaller segments if you can't do it all at once.) Then make a second action commitment: Commit to doubling (or tripling) your daily vegetable intake. With one foot, take one specific first step. The next foot has no choice but to follow.

The camera zooms in tight as our hero quietly prays for the inner strength necessary to fend off yet another attack by the Food Insurgency. But just as she is reaching a state of inner peace, she is jolted back into reality by the unmistakable roar of a rapidly approaching truck. What she had hoped was a Humvee packed with volunteers from the local chapter of foodaholics turns out to be a minivan full of Girl Scouts offering free samples of their new and improved megamint cookies.

Unfortunately, much of the dieting mind-set comes from the initial expectation we set early on. When you're ready to go on a diet, you set the rules, you know the parameters, you know that veggies are nutritional G-men and cookies are nutritional mass murderers. That process and anticipation of going on a diet can work in your favor, as long as you remember that the way your brain works isn't just psychological but chemical as well. The way it works for many of us is that many diets leave you less wiggle room than one of Beyoncé's dresses, so that there are only two options: rewards for compliance and no tolerance for failure.

In just about every other area of our lives, we allow ourselves margins of error. Baseball players who make outs 70 percent of the time are Hall of Famers. Basketball players need to make only half their shots to become all-stars. Lawyers don't win every case. Parents don't **Myth Buster** always make the right decisions. In fact, almost all of us make mistakes in our daily jobs. We learn from them and try to correct them so we don't repeat them again and again, or at least figure how to minimize the damage. But when it comes to diets, we hold ourselves to the precision of a Blue Angels flight team. No errors. No mistakes. Once we've blown it and deviated even an inch from our plan, that's it. We head back into the locker room, take off the uniform, shower, game's over. Diet's dead. Pass the fondue pot.

Through the tips below, you can learn to reprogram your mind to strip away the guilt that comes with eating, the guilt that comes with diets, and the guilt that comes with occasionally enjoying foods that aren't at the platinum level of healthy-eating charts. You also have to realize that it's not the first fry or first slice of cake that will doom your diet. It's the second, the third, and the whole dang shebang that lead to dangerous fat and waist gain.

At the beginning of our plan, you do have to listen to your body and respond intelligently to your cravings and your emotions. But over time, you'll learn how to eat right and manage your cravings. And that's when you'll train your brain to stop obsessing about eating right — and punishing yourself for every obstacle you face. **YOU-reka!** The unrecognized truth is that when you stop overthinking, you'll stop overeating.

The Role of Soul

It's no secret that we use food as a medication for our acute emotional problems. Stress at work directs us to the box of doughnuts. Crazy kids send us to the snack shelf. A downer of a day puts us incisor-deep into a half-pint of Edy's. But to end our discussion of how emotions and obesity collide right there would be like saying that Band-Aids and ice packs can cure all diseases. The reality is that a good number of us with weight problems have emotional issues that run deeper than the middle of the Pacific, and we try to satisfy our need for a higher power by self-medicating with food.

If you're one of those people, you don't much care about leptin, ghrelin, and NP-whatever.

Being overweight is more about self-esteem — about the petrifying fear that you don't *deserve* to be thin. How do we know this? Not through studies or research — but through real-life living, through our patients, through eavesdropping on a cavalcade of doughnut addicts. Here, we have to step out of the safety zone of hard science into an area that's typically not studied by the white-coat-and-goggles set, because the mental, emotional, and deep psychological issues involved with obesity are simply very difficult to "prove" in a Western sense.

So let's start here: Many people — women especially — lack the self-esteem for waist control. (In fact, the most common reason a woman doesn't take care of her own health is because she puts others' needs before her own.) But let's dive deeper: What *is* self-esteem? Let us assume our general sense of self-worth comes from two forces: overcoming obstacles and accomplishing some kind of goal. In the case of waist management, what happens if you don't overcome an obstacle (the box of Ding Dongs) and don't accomplish something (your goal weight by your high school reunion)? Yep, your self-esteem plummets faster than ratings for summer reruns. To resurrect it, you need to find ways to overcome and accomplish — without making the very standards by which you measure your life unrealistic weights, measurements, and stricter-than-boot-camp eating habits.

Now, let's step back to see how the relationship developed between the emotional need for self-esteem and the physical need for baggy clothes. In our youth, many of us long for something in our lives that's deeper and greater than our everyday reality of work, home, sleep, repeat for 29,930 days. Maybe it's religion, or maybe a calling to help others, or maybe a belief that the world revolves around the Cubs. We don't care as much *what* the "It" is as that we *find* the "It" and *explore* the "It."

Now, there are some chemical and biological foundations for that feeling of soul-level satisfaction. Oxytocin, a hormone that is elevated in women after childbirth, also makes you feel a sense of community and pleasure within your family, or during a religious experience, or when you have an epiphany about your existence. When levels of oxytocin increase, you feel calm. Another hypothesis argues that your sense of self-esteem and well-being is influenced by the chemical nitric oxide (not to be confused with the laughing gas nitrous oxide). Traits such as hopefulness and optimism are associated with the release of nitric oxide through the body. In the same way, the release of nitric oxide may serve to help reduce feelings of anxiety and stress. But this chemical effect lasts for only seconds, so you need to continually stimulate your body with the right cerebral karma.

Soul-level satisfaction exists at a biochemical level as well as in your perceptible life. It's your deeper drive — not the drive to fill the needs of your stomach or your muscles or even your mind, but the drive to fill the needs of your soul.

OK, OK, OK, we know what you're saying: What does your soul have to do with the fact that you just mainlined an entire can of whipped cream?

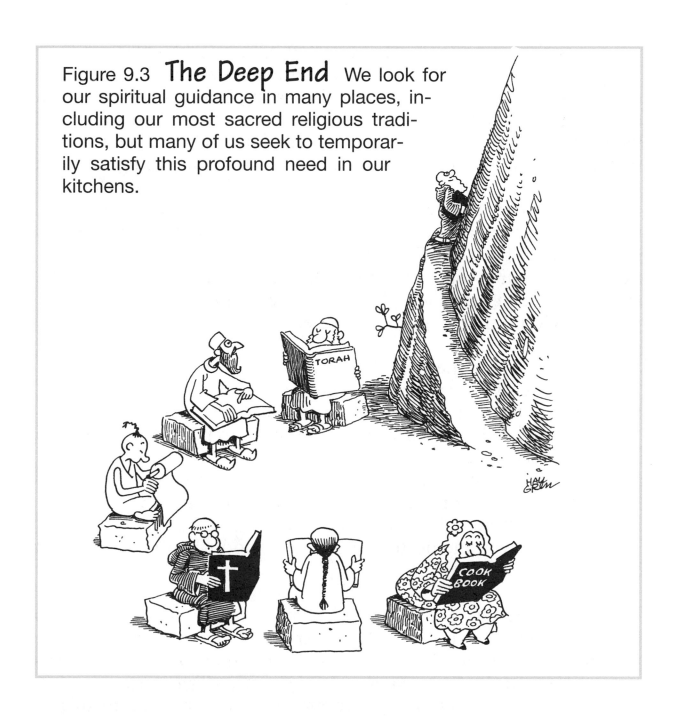

Figure 9.3 **The Deep End** We look for our spiritual guidance in many places, including our most sacred religious traditions, but many of us seek to temporarily satisfy this profound need in our kitchens.

A lot.

For many of you, instead of addressing — or even acknowledging — this deeper longing and the restlessness you feel for never quite fulfilling it, you try to fill the emptiness with food and drink. You use a temporary fix (General Tso's chicken) to satisfy the permanent void caused by not satisfying your spiritual needs (the "It").

Sound familiar? We bet it does. Of all the actions you pursue, one of the few things you totally control is eating. You have the freedom to chow down what you want, where you want, how you want, and whether or not you want to do it with or without clothes on. Because of that freedom, eating makes you feel good. Funny thing, though; food is like the paint you use to cover cracks formed in the foundation of your house. Two coats of robin's-egg blue may hide the flaws temporarily, but they're never going to fix the real root of the problem. **YOU-reka!** If this is you, your cover-up is what starts that tornadolike cycle that keeps you from ever feeling satisfied physically or emotionally. Ask yourself: Could this be part of a cycle?

- You long for something deeper . . .
- And when you can't find it, you eat to feel better . . .
- But you feel lousy because you gain weight . . .
- Then you tell yourself you don't deserve to be thin because you can't keep weight off . . .
- Then your self-esteem drops further because you haven't overcome obstacles or accomplished what you want . . .
- So you self-medicate with food . . .
- And then you medicate yourself with food when you can't find "It" . . .

What's especially interesting is that many people who use food as a cover-up *want* to live life in the tornado. They're terrified by the thought of being thin. Being fat gives them an excuse to fail, an excuse to be depressed, an excuse to tango with a Twix bar.

So what does the theory say about why many people do this to their own bodies? Or *why* you'd do it to your body? You may do it because this thought process is a safe one and because your fat serves as a literal and metaphorical protective layer that keeps you from interacting with reality. You don't have to play the game of life if you're constantly making excuses for living on the bench. If only you could lose weight, if only you could fit into that bikini, if only you could take a hike with the family without breathing heavier than a prison escapee. While some people may say that fat is a failure, the truth is that fat — for many of us — is a way of avoiding failure, because it's an excuse for never competing and engaging in life. (Remember, "if only" are the world's two most dangerous words since "jalapeño popper.")

So where do you go from here, short of self-injecting oxytocin or inhaling high doses of nitric oxide? It's not like you can turn this page and all of your self-esteem issues will vanish faster than Coney Island hot dogs on the Fourth of July. It will take some time, but it also takes some awareness that this tornado may be swirling. We're not asking — or expecting — you to fix it; we're asking you to be aware that this deep, in-your-gut feeling might be the reason why our society's belts are now being used to accurately measure out 5K road races. Simply realizing that you may use food as a psychological painkiller is part of the solution for helping you avoid it. So let's just consider that the warranty on this emotional baggage has run out. Now that you know this baggage doesn't serve you, it's time you dropped it off at a psychological landfill and got rid of it for good.

YOU TIPS!

Make the Split. Clearly, some of us eat for physical reasons (we're just hungry) and some of us gnaw on leftover Halloween candy for emotional reasons (we're steamed at the boss about having to start and finish a new report by 10 a.m., and it's 9:47). But sometimes it's not always easy to figure out the difference. To help, you need to start using the YOU Diet Hunger Test. Throughout the day, record your level of hunger as judged by this scale. Stay tuned to what your stomach is telling you, not what's happening outside with stresses (kids going crazy), emotions (spouse is working late *again*), or habits (Leno equals bowl of Apple Jacks). This process will help you really *feel* your hunger, so that you can let your stomach, not your emotions, dictate your habits.

O Tank = Hungry. It feels as if you haven't eaten since junior year of high school.

1/2 Tank = Edge is off. You're OK, not desperate, like maybe when you're driving home from work.

3/4 Tank = Satisfied and not hungry. You can go much longer without food. You just ate nuts and a drink before dinner.

1 Full Tank = Full and comfortable. It's the way you feel after finishing an average-portion, healthful meal.

Overflow Level S = Stuffed. You could've stopped two scoops of pudding ago.

Overflow Level OS = Overstuffed. Audible groaning detected.

Overflow Level BP = Button Pop/Exploding. It's the typical Thanksgiving gorge. You feel sick, and even take the name of your momma's stuffing in vain.

The way the test works is, every time you find yourself reaching for the cheese sauce or cookie box, rate your hunger. Then think about whether you're reaching for the leftover lasagna because you're truly hungry or for a reason that has absolutely nothing to do with hunger. Ideally, you'll want to stay in the 3/4 to Full Tank range — satisfied at all times. And you'll get there by eating regularly throughout the day. (See Part 4 for details.) After applying these gauges for two weeks, you'll start to instinctively know why you're eating, and, better, you'll train yourself to eat simply to keep your stomach satisfied — and not your emotions.

Pick and Stick. Yeah, sure, variety may be the spice of life, but it also can be the death of dieting. When you have a lot of choices for a meal, it's a lot easier to slip out of good eating habits and into ham-induced bad ones. When you sit down at a diner and are presented with a menu that's the size of a phone book, it's easy to give in. One way to get away from fat bombs is to eliminate choices for at least one meal a day. Pick the one meal you rush through most and automate it. For most people, it's lunch. So find a healthy lunch you like — salad with grilled chicken and olive oil, turkey on whole-grain bread — and have it for lunch every day. Every day. Yes, every day.

YOU-reka! More and more research is showing that putting a cap on the variety of foods and tastes you experience will help you control your weight. (Think of your dog: Penelope stays the same weight when she has her regular food every day. But as soon as she starts gorging on the variety of nightly table scraps, the puny poodle looks more like a massive mastiff.) How does it work? It seems that when you have meals rich in flavor variety, it takes more and more calories to keep you full (think of Thanksgiving, when you eat a lot of different things, stuff yourself, and still have room for pumpkin pie). So when we experience meals with lots of diverse flavors — think Mexican or Indian cuisine — we tend to eat more to satisfy our taste buds. Now, we don't want you to become bored with food, but if you make this a habit for at least one meal a day, it'll decrease your temptations and help you stop thinking about food so often. In fact, we usually prescribe two meals that are the same each day for our patients. It's one of the ways to automate your brain so that your habits follow. Of course, we don't want you to stop enjoying the wonderful diversity of flavors, but it will help control your appetite.

Another trick: Use extra-light virgin olive oil, which has less flavor and may help control taste cravings.

Find a Substitute. For avoiders, we know that eating is about as rational as an inebriated sports fan. If we all had the ability to make rational choices, like zucchini is better for us than fettuccine — then there would be no need for the multibillion-dollar diet industry. Eating is an emotional action, and it's an addictive one. The average person knows doughnuts are hand grenades to health. But we pass by a neighboring cubicle with a dozen cream-filled jobbies, and we've finished three before we've even turned the corner. Add to this the fact that research shows that people under the most work stress gain the most weight, and you've got yourself an obesity double whammy. So the question is really, how you can take irrational, emotional, and addictive actions and turn them into smart, rational, good decisions? For one thing you can develop that list of healthful contingency foods and clear your fridge and pantry of waist-killing foods, which we'll show you how to do in Part 4. For another, you can look for other things to fill the needs that food is currently filling. Traditionally, so much of our self-satisfaction comes from how we see ourselves externally. But that satisfaction is fleeting, and we need to find and focus on the things in life we're truly grateful for — be it our families, our careers, or a hobby that we're passionate about.

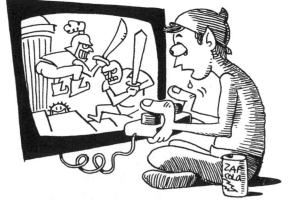

Keep Your Hands Full. You'd think that being plopped in front of a TV playing Xbox would mean that you're destined for a life of fatness. But that's not the case; studies show that playing video games is actually not correlated with obesity. Why? Turns out that when you've got your two hands on the controllers and your fingers moving faster than Liberace's, that means one thing: Your paws won't be knuckle-deep in a bowl of cake batter. (Some games even have foot mats for you to make commands with your feet, too, so you can get a complete workout; ask your kids about the Dance Dance Revolution craze.)

Now, that's not to say that an intimate relationship with Super Mario should be your number-one strategy, but it does prove an underlying point. **YOU-reka!** When you keep your hands and brain occupied — whether it's with video games, gardening, or removing a spleen — it means you're putting your brain in the state you want: not thinking about eating and not automatically reaching for something to put in your mouth.

Walk This Way. The root of the YOU physical activity plan is a minimum of thirty minutes of walking a day (broken up into three segments of ten minutes each if you need to) — and telling somebody about it after you're done (yes, every day, no excuses). You will do it not only for the physical effects, but also (even more so, actually) for the psychological effects. Remember what self-esteem comes from: the ability to overcome obstacles and achieve goals. Walking accomplishes both. **YOU-reka!** Walk for thirty; it's easy, doable, and maintainable — and it's a first step out of the tornado and back into the game of life. A lot of people feel they haven't earned the right to lose weight. Walking every day earns you that right, and telling someone about it helps you feel proud of your accomplishment.

Get Lost in Your Mind. Whenever you feel the urge to eat, just sit and think about your life and what's driving you to pick up a fork or open the fridge. Would you shove that stuff in a friend's or family member's body? It's OK to cry, it's OK to think, it's OK to meditate. In fact, maybe you can learn from your pain — not make it worse by thinking you can pad it with three extra inches of abdominal fat. For some, meditation or prayer enhances their power to satisfy the subconscious drive they have.

Get Touched. Both on a physical level and on a psychological level, seek out positive interactions with other people. (Remember the phone call at the end of your walk.) Evidence shows that increased amounts of oxytocin may be able to decrease blood pressure and lower the

YOU Test

Why Ask Why?

The fact is, you *know*. You know if you need to lose weight. You can tell by the way you look, by the way you feel, and by whether your clothes feel tighter than an unopened pickle jar. But to be able to make changes — sustainable changes — you not only have to know *what* you've done to your figure. You also have to know *why* you're abusing your body, in the form of the emotional and physical triggers that led you to gaining waist. To start, perform a self-administered "why" test — that is, keep asking yourself "why" questions about your weight until you come to the real answer about why you want to lose weight and why you can't. It may go something like this:

Why do you want to lose weight? Because I want to fit into my old pair of jeans.

Why do you want to fit into your old pair of jeans? Because

230

effects of stress. And the way research shows that you increase oxytocin levels is through CCK, which helps control your appetite, and through an increase in social interaction and touch. If nothing else, it's a darn good reason to schedule that weekly massage. And it may help reinforce why things such as meditation and hypnosis — suspected to increase oxytocin — can be helpful with weight loss. Also, while there's as much information on this as on obesity in elite marathoners, the fear of touch and lack of oxytocin release may be one reason why the abused individual often has problems with waist management.

I'd have more confidence.

Why do you want more confidence? Because I'll feel better trying to meet new people.

Why do you want to meet new people? Because I'm recently divorced and hoping to start a new relationship.

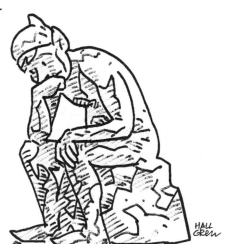

Why do you want to start a new relationship? Because I'm feeling lonely . . .

And that's likely to be where the thread of questions stops — where you can link the first question to the last answer. You want to lose weight because you're lonely, but the likely cause of your weight gain is the very same thing: that you're lonely.

YOU Test

The Personality Test

Yes, you could make the argument that those marshmallow-covered corn dogs at the carnival have a little something to do with your about-to-burst waistband. The more likely saboteur? Your excuses. Here, take this personality test to see what attitudes and behaviors may be preventing you from losing weight and getting healthy (Dr. Robert Kushner's full test is available at www.diet.com). Add up your check marks and see how your attitude toward eating and exercise influences the size of your waist.

Sound Like You?	Then Check Here	Because It Means You're a . . .
EATING PATTERNS		
"Day to day, I change my meal patterns more often than Martha Stewart changes fabric patterns."		**Meal Skipper:** You skip meals and have no pattern or routine to when you eat.
"I eat like a sardine during the day and like a humpback at night."		**Nighttime Nibbler:** You consume 50 percent or more of your calories between dinner and bedtime.

232

Sound Like You?	Then Check Here	Because It Means You're a . . .
EATING PATTERNS		
"The place I'm most likely to eat: one that has a waiter, a drive-through lane, or a delivery dude."		**Convenient Diner:** You're a brand-name eater. All of your meals are packaged, bagged, microwavable, or frozen.
"Fruits and vegetables have the same taste appeal as, oh, sewage."		**Fruitless Feaster:** With few exceptions, you're all about meat and potatoes (or pasta, bread, and desserts).
"I need a dietary restraining order. If there's any food within fifty feet of me, I'll eat it."		**Steady Snacker:** Besides your regular three meals, you snack anytime you come near food.
"My plate's so high, it breaks at least three city codes."		**Hearty Portioner:** You eat a lot, and you eat it quickly, whether it's healthy or not.
"I eat salads when I'm out with friends, then raid the pantry when I'm home."		**Swing Eater:** You eat a strict diet of good foods, but fall off the wagon and then overeat bad foods.

Sound Like You?	Then Check Here	Because It Means You're a...
EXERCISE PATTERNS		
"I enjoy being physically active as much as I do making paper-clip chains."		**Couch Champion:** You don't like to sweat, and you don't really like any physical activity.
"I don't exercise because everyone else at the gym looks like a supermodel or Schwarzenegger compared to me."		**Uneasy Participant:** You hate exercising in public because of your body image.
"I like exercise, but if I have to miss it, I'm like a crashed NASCAR — it's hard for me to get back on track."		**All-or-Nothing Doer:** You work out hard for a few days or weeks, then stop and do nothing for even longer.
"For the past three years, I've been doing the exact same workout without changing it a bit."		**Set-Routine Repeater:** You're on a fixed exercise routine but aren't able to lose weight because your body has adjusted to the routine.

Sound Like You?	Then Check Here	Because It Means You're a . . .
EXERCISE PATTERNS		
"I'm afraid I'll get hurt on the wrong end of the exercise machine, worsen my condition, or have a heart attack if I exercise hard."		**Tender Bender:** You either have an injury that prevents you from exercising or worry that you may suffer one because you're out of shape.
"I'd like to exercise, but I barely have enough time to shave, let alone step on a treadmill for twenty minutes."		**Rain-Check Athlete:** You're so busy and frustrated that you can't make time to exercise.
COPING PATTERNS		
"Ahhh! I find food as comforting as a down pillow."		**Emotional Eater:** You eat when you're stressed, anxious, tired, or depressed.
"As for my clothes, I've got a bigger cover-up plan than a criminal — I'm ashamed of my body and how I look."		**Self-Scrutinizer:** You feel ashamed of your body and have trouble separating body image from self-esteem, and that affects your day-to-day decision making.

Sound Like You?	Then Check Here	Because It Means You're a . . .
COPING PATTERNS		
"I'm the Socrates of diets — I spend more time thinking about what I need to do to lose weight than actually doing it."		**Persistent Procrastinator:** You know the importance of losing weight and say you want to lose, but you never seem to make it happen because something always gets in the way.
"I'm juggling more than a circus performer. Last on my list? Time for myself."		**People Pleaser:** You are a good-natured person with responsibility and commitment to family, friends, and coworkers, but you always put them ahead of you.
"My life is moving fast, my to-do list is the length of a novel, and I can't find the brakes."		**Fast Pacer:** You multitask and don't take the time to think or plan how to improve your lifestyle.
"I've tried everything to lose weight, but nothing ever works. Nothing! Nada! Zippo!"		**Doubtful Dieter:** You say you've tried everything and nothing works, so you develop a self-defeating attitude.

Sound Like You?	Then Check Here	Because It Means You're a . . .
COPING PATTERNS		
"My work? Great. Family life? A blast. I expect the same amazing results from my weight-loss plan — but my progress is never enough."		**Overreaching Achiever:** You're successful at home and work — and expect the same in your weight loss. But you never feel satisfied, and your high expectations make you feel frustrated and discouraged.

Adapted from *Dr. Kushner's Personality Type Diet* (St. Martin's Press) with permission.

Check Yourself: Add up your scores and get a score for food (eating), mood (coping), and movement (exercise). The dimension with the highest score is the category where you need to focus. A score of 4 or more in any one category means you need to focus on that area no matter what. So, if your food score is 6, mood score is 4, and movement score is 2, then you need to focus on food and mood, but don't forget your thirty-minute daily walk — no excuses.

YOU Test

Don't Avoid This Test

It shouldn't come as much of a surprise that avoiders typically have feelings of inadequacy and are hypersensitive to being negatively evaluated. Identifying with four or more of the following statements means you have strong avoidance tendencies.

- I avoid work activities that involve close interpersonal contact — not because of my deodorant level but because I fear criticism or rejection.
- Unless I know I'm going to be liked, I'm hesitant to get involved in relationships.
- When I'm in social situations, I feel more inept than an umpire with a detached retina.
- My shirt's not coming off unless the lights are going off.
- All of my social situations feel like high school; I'm preoccupied with being criticized or rejected.
- I don't engage in risky activities because my biggest fear is the risk of embarrassment.
- In new interpersonal situations, I feel the same way I feel at the beach: shy and inhibited, and I would do anything to be somewhere else.

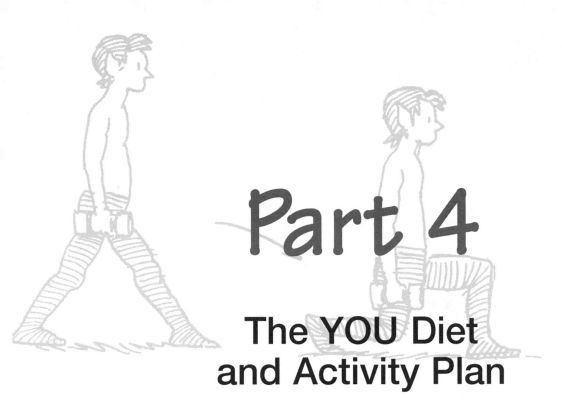

Part 4

The YOU Diet and Activity Plan

The Eating and Activity Plan That Will Become Lifelong and Automatic

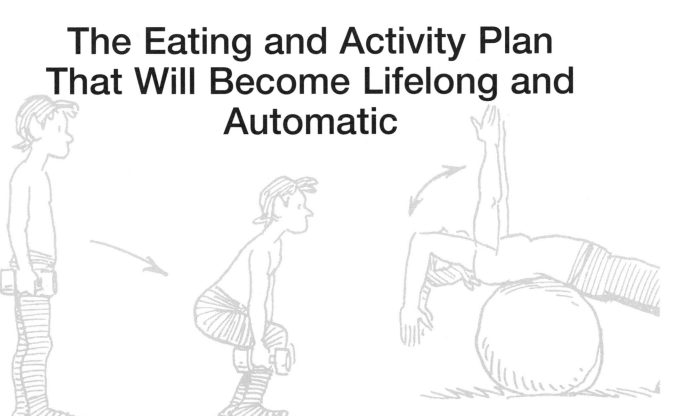

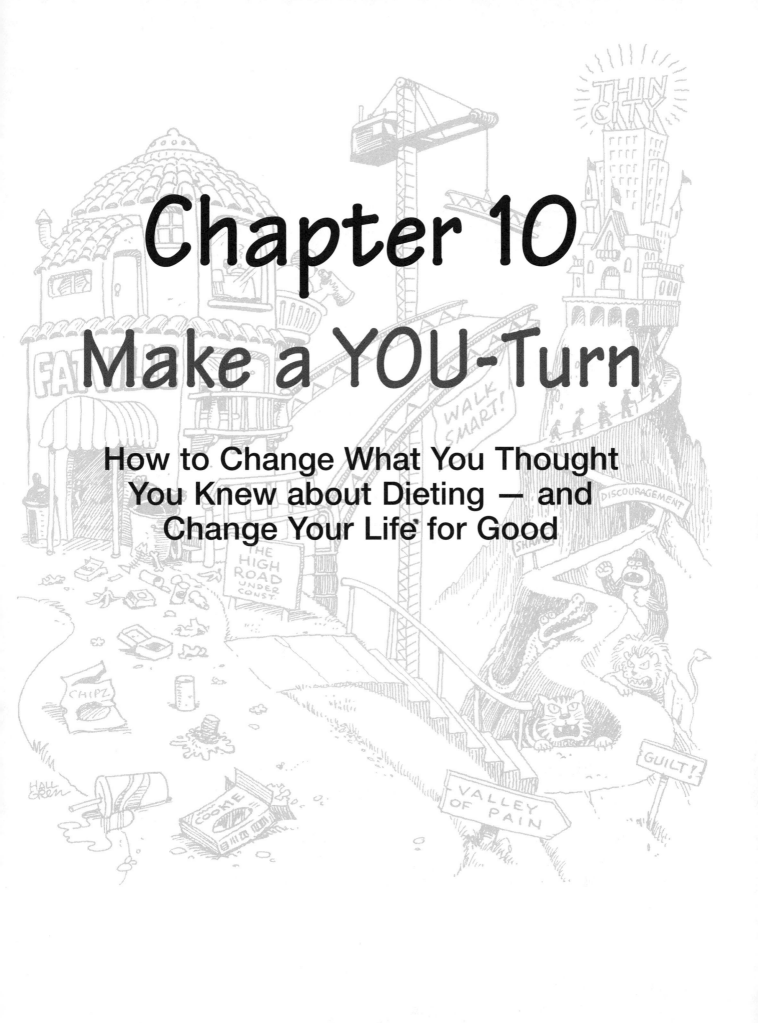

Chapter 10
Make a YOU-Turn

How to Change What You Thought You Knew about Dieting — and Change Your Life for Good

By now, you don't have to be Marie Curie to know the power of chemicals and realize that you're the clear-cut underdog if you try to take them on with brute force. You know that chemical changes in your brain and body play a big role in dictating everything from your actions to your emotions. But you can alter your chemistry in more subtle ways. For instance, take the act of positive thinking and inter-acting in social groups. There's evidence that those kinds of actions change serotonin levels to make you feel better and reduce appetite. That's really how you should be using your mind and all the intangible concepts like willpower, discipline, and motivation — to complement the chemical changes you're making in other, more concrete ways. They're the things that will help you overcome the occasional butter-laced obstacles that you'll face.

To show how you can use emotions to work for you as you're about to embark on the YOU Diet, let's step back into the mind of a typical dieter — let's say a woman. One of the psychological realities of being overweight is that many dieters — that is, people who know they need to lose weight and want to — are somewhat comfortable with their bodies. Yes, that body may be twenty, thirty, forty, or more pounds heavier than it was the day she turned eighteen. But maybe she's used to post-pregnancy weight, she enjoys Friday lunches with her friends, or she can't face a total wardrobe overhaul. **YOU-reka!** It's who she is — and she's more comfortable living her life at that level than going through the struggles and hard work (not to mention the guilt and shame) of trying to shed weight.

So the dieter has two choices: She can remain on top of the hill where she's currently standing and (relatively) comfortable. Or she can try to get to the top of that beautiful mountain in the distance — the ultimate destination for all of her weight-loss goals. There, on the mountain, she'll find smaller sizes, leaf-size bikinis, fewer doctor visits, and probably fewer health risks and an improved quality of life. Maybe that's where she'd *ideally* like to be. But the problem is that there's no easy bridge from the comfort zone of the hill to the peak of the mountain. To get there, she must travel all the way down

Figure 10.1 **The Right Route** Descending into the valley can make the trip up to the promised land daunting. Dieting smartly will build you the bridge you need to transition to your playing weight.

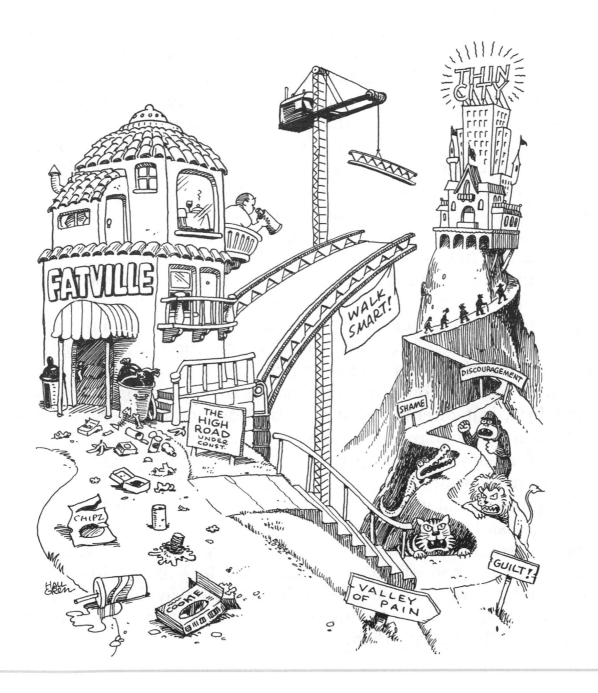

from her current comfort level, hit some rough terrain along the way, and then climb, climb, climb her way up this seemingly insurmountable incline. So she asks: Is it worth it to go through all the hard work to reach the top of the ideal mountain, or am I comfortable enough with where I'm standing right now?

That's how the dieter thinks after trying it once or twice. It's easier to stay at the current comfort level at a less than ideal size than it is go through a short period of somewhat uncomfortable change — doing things like developing a physical activity program, or avoiding drive-throughs, or changing menus, or going through periods of irritability and hunger. For many dieters, that path is hard to navigate, so they return — very quickly — to the original hill, the original place of comfort (often it is an even wider hill, psychologically and waist-size-wise). The fact is, most people aren't willing to face the challenges of finding the mountain peak, even if the peak reveals such vistas as better health and higher self-esteem.

So what we have to do is build that bridge — that bridge of smart food choices, of exercise discipline, or working smart, not hard. And we have to support the bridge with strategies and tactics that allow you to make wrong steps without falling completely into the abyss of chocolate nougat. How do we do it? By getting started. Right now. With small actions that lead to big changes.

Sometimes, we think the motivation to start a program has to come first, but oftentimes, the motivation comes after the action: Make a small change (be it walking thirty minutes a day, or eating nuts before dinner to keep you full), and suddenly you feel motivated to make more changes — and to succeed.

The point is that we want you to make it across the bridge as pain-free as possible, by giving you the tools to avoid the uncomfortable feelings associated with dieting, with hunger, with evil scales. The journey to the top of the mountain may feel like a little bit of a climb, but it shouldn't feel like you're starting way down there at the bottom. We'll build that bridge with these strategies and our YOU Diet and YOU Activity Plan.

YOU TIPS!

Adopt the YOU-Turn Mantra. If you've ever ridden in a car with a GPS satellite navigation system, you know how it works. Plug in your destination, and the system — using satellites to plot your current and final points — tells you exactly what to do when. Turn left after 400 feet. Stay straight. Get in right lane. But let's say you make a mistake and miss a turn or turn onto the wrong street. The GPS doesn't berate you, doesn't scold you, doesn't tell you that you might as well drive off a cliff, since you made a mistake and missed First Avenue. Instead, all it says, very politely, is this: "At the next available moment, make an authorized U-turn." **YOU-reka!** The GPS recognizes the mistake matter-of-factly and simply guides you back onto the right road. The GPS allows for mistakes and tries to help you correct them.

That's the kind of mentality we want you to have. You're going to make wrong turns. You're going to turn left at the hot dogs, make a right at the blueberry pie, and occasionally merge onto the interstate of banana-nut pancakes with a side order of sausage patties. Does that mean you should steer off the dietary cliff and fall into the fatty crevasse of destructive eating? Of course not. What it means is that you need to pay closer attention to the road signs and the instructions about how to make it to your final destination. It also means that you can't beat yourself up with a basket of croissants every time you lick a little whipped cream off your finger. So what you're going to do — right now — is acknowledge that you will face obstacles. And instead of falling into the avoidant and defeatist mentality by drop-kicking healthy eating the moment you make one bad choice,

you will confront it. How? By repeating the YOU Diet Mantra:
"At the next available moment, make an authorized YOU-Turn."
"At the next available moment, make an authorized YOU-Turn."
"At the next available moment, make an authorized YOU-Turn."
Get back on the right road.

What kills any regimen of healthy eating isn't the occasional dessert or slice of pizza; it's the cascade of behavior that happens after the initial indulgence. Use this mantra to steer yourself back — to understand that you can make mistakes but that you can correct and overcome them with some nonjudgmental coaxing. Why does it work?

- It gives you a mental crutch to carry when you're faced with difficult eating situations.
- It reminds you to be confident, to be positive, to know that the harm isn't in the first mistake, it's in not figuring out how to deal with it.
- It reinforces the grand scheme of this whole plan — the reason why you're trying to manage your waist. The long-term benefits to your health far outweigh what you're giving up in your Pyrex dish.

Know Your Fighting Weight. In all likelihood, the most common way you've measured your so-called dietary success or failure is by pounds lost. If you've lost down to your target weight, then you've won. If not, you've lost. But the reality is that over the long term, all of us will intermittently gain and lose small amounts of weight, even when we're trying to lose it. For one, our water weight often fluctuates depending on what we're eating. The reason why so many low-carb dieters lose weight fast is because the lack of carbohydrates causes them to lose glycogen stores from their muscles, and with this loss of glycogen comes a loss of a lot of water; as soon as they reinstate the carbs, the glycogen comes back to the muscles and attracts the water. That adds the pounds right back. So the first five to eleven pounds of weight loss on a low-carb diet is the fake loss due to a temporary loss of water.

Instead of tracking your weight by a single goal weight of, say, 145 pounds, what you're going to do is pick your weight class. You're going to pick a range of weight that's comfortable for you — say, 142 to 148 pounds (or 31 inches to 33 inches of waist size). When you divulge your weight to someone (not that anyone will be asking), it should never be in one number; you need to think of your weight as an ideal range. For one thing, this allows for the natural fluctuations that occur. For another, it also does something even more crucial to your psychological success: It stops you from focusing on some arbitrary number that promotes the idea of all-or-nothing success or failure. And it puts your mind in the right programming mode — to remind yourself that your body is supposed to change.

Stay Accountable. You can use your weight range to tell when you're pushing the upper boundaries of your ideal weight/waist with periodic checks using a measurement too — be it a tape measure around your waist, a scale, or, hey, how about a plastic waistband that you keep around your waist to alert you when you're getting too big, like a large version of one of those Lance bracelets? Whatever your accountability tool, we suggest checking it every Saturday around midday to keep yourself honest with your weight and waist class. Think of your body as a rubber band. Stretch it a little, and it can certainly snap back into shape. But once you stretch it too much, it's going to lose its shape and make it more difficult — if not impossible — to return to the original size.

Plan to Fail — and Develop Contingency Plans for When You Do. We keep tires in our trunks in case one goes flat. We keep candles in our drawers in case the power goes out. We keep backups of files in case our computers crash. (And some of us wish we backed them up more often.) And that's good; contingency plans give you the mental assurance that you'll be able to adapt to unexpected crises. But the one area where we don't make backup plans is in our diets. We eat broccoli, fish, and fruit for three days, then splurge on a double-fat burger with supersize fries on the fourth. For so many of us, that's grounds for euthanizing the diet right away — putting us right back in touch with our three favorite food groups of chocolate, chips, and chocolate chips.

Instead, start carrying a dietary contingency plan — a diet emergency pack for those times when you may experience a crash-causing blowout in one of your meals. Follow this three-step contingency plan to help you cope with occasional mishaps and potential catastrophes. Exercise it the moment you feel you're deviating from your waist management plan:

- **Mental:** Say the YOU-Turn mantra ten times. Let the mantra remind you that it's OK to stray occasionally, that you can take control of the situation and steer yourself back, and that the positive reinforcement and confidence that come with overcoming challenges will give you the mental strength of a tank. Plus, the relaxing aspect of it will help influence your serotonin levels in your favor. And it will help distract you, which is what you need when you're beelining toward the bonbons.

- **Physical:** Do a yoga pose or try the hippie stretch (see the YOU Workout). We suggest the downward dog pose (see below), balancing your weight on your hands and feet with your butt hiked toward the ceiling in an inverted *V.* Not only will it help you refocus, give you a few moments to take deep breaths, and remind you of your goals, but it will also work because it's sort of difficult to eat when you're upside down.

- **Nutritional:** Keep in your fridge a container of baby carrots, celery, or any crisp vegetable of your choice, or a favorite apple type (yes, types matter to our individual taste choices). Carrots and apples are perfect antistress foods because, one, they have just a tinge of sweetness to satisfy that craving, and, two, they give you something to crunch into at times when you really want to sink your teeth into your boss's neck. This will become your turn-to food — that is, the food you turn to when you feel angry, frustrated, mad, sad, or upset — as well as the one that will help you feel better about the nutritional mistakes you may have just made.

Many of us take the mental approach that the only way to "do a diet" is to do it perfectly. But that's a setup for failure and shame, because it never works. Success comes with persistence — persistence to overcome challenges, persistence to see the big picture, persistence to work hard enough in the beginning of the plan so that good habits become automatic.

Make It Automatic. Think of your waist management plan a little like the way you'd drive to work. Maybe the first day on a new job in a new city, you took the highway. But then you found out it was more clogged than Rapunzel's shower drain. So you experimented with a few back roads, shortcuts, and bypasses until you found the very best way to get to work. Now you don't need a map; you do it automatically, and you don't spend a single nanosecond worrying about what turn you take. It's automatic — just the way your approach to eating should be. When you're starting out on this plan, you'll experiment with different routes, get stuck in a few traffic jams, maybe even get a little lost along the way. But if you stick with it and find the right course, you'll automate your habits, regulate your chemicals, and make eating the easiest trip you've ever made.

How do we make it automatic? By using the tools that we've outlined in the book. (For those of you who've skipped ahead, the major ones are listed here.)

The 99-Second Edition

In the dietary gates and can't wait to start the race? Then skim through this cheat sheet of the YOU strategies — big and small — that you'll adopt and automate as your new eating, activity, emotional, and behavioral plan. It's the path to your new life. And your new body.

The Major YOU Principles
YOU Need to . . .

Choose elegance over force.

Dietary battles are won not when you work hard, but when you work smart.

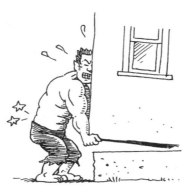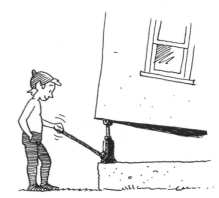

Make your eating plan automatic.

Train yourself over fourteen days to make appropriate choices, and you'll reprogram your body so that you never have to sweat over what you're eating again.

Remember that waist is more important than weight.

Belly fat is one of the strongest predictors of health risks associated with obesity. Ditch the scale in favor of the tape measure.

Know your body.

Understand the beauty of your internal organs to appreciate what you can do to influence them.

Stay satisfied.

To lose weight, you need to eat.

Add support.

Enlist a friend, family member, or new cyber buddy as your partner.

Know that it's OK to make mistakes.

As long as you quickly get back on the right road, you won't travel too far down the wrong one.

Eating Strategies for YOU

- To help make eating automatic, pick at least one meal a day to alter and have the same foods every day for all other meals.
- Eat throughout the day so that you're constantly satisfied. The less you eat, the more likely you are to sink into starvation mode and make your body want to store fat.
- Inspect food labels. Limit saturated fats to less than 4 grams per serving, and avoid all trans fats. Don't buy foods where high-fructose corn syrup (HFCS), or another simple sugar, is more than 4 grams per serving, or one of the first five ingredients. You're avoiding simple sugars in foods not just because of the calories but because they induce highs and lows in blood sugar that put you into a cycle of craving more high-calorie foods.
- Eat foods with fiber, healthy fats (monounsaturated and polyunsaturated), whole-grain carbohydrates, and protein, as well as fruits and vegetables. Eat a little healthy fat before your meal (like one handful of nuts) to allow the satiety signal to go from your brain to your stomach, so you don't overeat during your meal. Eat fiber in the morning to help control afternoon cravings. Eat anti-inflammatory foods to help counteract the effects of obesity. Anti-inflammatory foods include green tea, omega-3 fatty acids (found in fish and walnuts), coffee, vegetables, and fruit.

- Drink a glass or two of water before you eat. Your perception of hunger signals may actually be thirst signals.
- Keep on hand emergency foods and items that can help you kill cravings, like V8, carrot sticks, an apple, or even Listerine breath strips.
- Keep a log of how hungry you are on a scale of one to seven (one being famished, seven being gorged). Try to stay in the three to four range at all times by eating moderate amounts of food throughout the day.
- Two spices have been shown to aid in waist management: red pepper and cinnamon.
- Realize that it's OK to make mistakes. The key is getting back on the right road, not beating yourself up over them. Use YOU-Turns to right yourself as soon as possible.
- Use nine-inch plates for meals. Smaller dinner plates equal smaller portions.

Activity Strategies for YOU

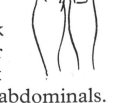

- Walk thirty minutes a day every day. No excuses. Then call your support partner after you do it.
- Start a strength training program focusing on core muscle (legs, abdominals, and upper body) in the form of twenty minutes two or three days a week.
- Stretch every day after physical activity to keep your muscles loose and pliable, to help you prevent injury.
- Do this exercise any time you want: Suck in your belly button and squeeze your butt as if you're pulling up tight jeans. It helps with posture and strengthens your abdominals.

- Get up and go. Anytime you can move at work or at home, do it.

Who Woulda Thunk It Strategies for YOU

- Get seven to eight hours of sleep a night. Lack of sleep promotes hedonistic eating as you search for something to boost chemicals in your brain. Your brain needs sleep to regenerate these chemicals, and sugary foods help release the diminished supply of chemicals you have, to make up for the lack of sleep.
- Play video games. Keeping your hands full keeps them off the coconut muffins.
- Have healthy, safe, monogamous sex. Satisfying one appetite center of your brain can help satisfy another.

Measurement Strategies for YOU

- Measure your waist. Ideal is 32 1/2 inches or less for women, and 35 inches or less for men.
- Ask your family what your parents and grandparents looked like when they were eighteen, to give you a sense of what your ideal body should look like.
- Get tested: blood pressure, cholesterol, blood sugar, and C-reactive protein (a marker of inflammation), and certain hormone levels, depending on your weight situation.

Medicine Cabinet Strategies for YOU

- Take two aspirin (162 milligrams) every day to decrease arterial inflammation and health risks associated with obesity. Consult your doctor first.
- See your doctor about prescription drugs associated with weight loss if you hit a waist plateau on the plan (see appendix).
- The following supplements have been shown to have effectiveness in some aspect of waist management: chromium picoli-

nate, grapefruit oil, Garcinia, Hoodia, 5-HTP, L-carnitine, coenzyme Q10, turmeric, jojoba beans, simmondsin. Consult your doctor about which ones may be appropriate for you.

Chapter 11
The YOU Activity Plan

Physical Strategies for Waist Management

The world has all kinds of gyms: home gyms, hotel gyms, female-friendly gyms, muscle-head gyms, and gyms that look like spas. Though any of them may be perfectly decent places to pump your muscles, work your heart, or admire spandex, there's one gym that gives you absolutely everything you need:

Your own body. Your body can be your best gym.

Really, all you need are two things: your body and the knowledge of how to use it. No barbells, no dumbbells, no balls, no ankle weights, no machines, no infomercial equipment — just your body. By learning and using a plan that requires only your physiological barbells, you have all the tools you need to make exercise easy and automatic. That's because:

- Your body costs nothing to use.
- You eliminate the best excuses for avoiding exercise, like driving hassles or needing to buy equipment.
- Using only your body, you can work all of the muscles necessary for effective waist management — and that's for both beginning and advanced exercisers.

In fact, you can complete an entire workout that hits all three areas of activity — strength, flexibility, and cardiovascular — in one easy twenty-minute workout three times a week (or do it in smaller bits for almost as much benefit). And you can change that workout no matter what your skill level, simply by making small exercise adjustments to perfectly match your abilities.

Before we detail the plan, remember why you're exercising: Adding lean muscle through strength training, working your heart through cardiovascular training, and flexing your body with stretching help burn fat, reduce stress, improve health, and decrease your waist size. All without bulking you up to the size of a Miami condo. The other point of this program: You'll focus on your foundation muscles — the major muscles most responsible for fat burning, waist trimming, and injury prevention. Those key groups: your thighs, chest, back, and abdominals.

Whether you're a newbie to exercise or an old pro, the YOU plan starts with walking for thirty minutes a day — no matter what. Only when you've mastered that, no matter how long it takes, should you begin the rest of this program. Walking thirty minutes a day is as necessary and important as daily sleep, and it benefits you whether your exercise skills are those of a professional athlete or a potato chip. Most of us wouldn't entertain the nightmare of no sleep. From an aging perspective, it's as bad to skip a daily walk as it is to skip a night of sleep. As the nonwalking exercises get easier, and you get stronger and leaner, you'll be able to challenge yourself, too, by adding exercises, or making slight but important variations of the positions.

The YOU Activity Plan

Every Day:

■ **Walk:** Walk thirty minutes. No matter what. No excuses. It doesn't matter if you do this in one whole block or broken up into as many as three shorter sessions.

■ **Stretch:** Once your body is warm (after walking, for instance), stretch for five minutes to help elongate your muscles. You'll find stretches detailed in the You Workout below and the yoga poses we've outlined later.

Three Times a Week:

Do the Twenty-Minute YOU Workout. Do the exercises in this order; in general, you'll strengthen a muscle and then stretch it. If you want to break the workout up into smaller sessions, pick and choose as you like, but always try to match the strength and stretch exercises for a particular body part — that is, work your legs with a strength exercise, then do the stretch exercise immediately after it. Also, on the other four days of the week, you can simply take all the stretches outlined below (denoted by the *S* after the number) and turn them into the three- to five-minute postwalk total-body stretch.

257

Form Fit: How to Exercise the Right Way

1. Look out at eye level or above to spare your neck and keep you from rolling your shoulders forward.
2. Assume the Botox pose: Keep your face relaxed and tension-free.
3. Relax your shoulders and lift up your chest.
4. Pretend the top of your head is being pulled up by a string to elongate your spine and keep you from rolling forward.
5. Count your reps of each exercise out loud; this counting will help you remember to breathe continuously and keep you from holding your breath.
6. Keep your abs tight and pulled in to support your lower back. (Practice sucking in every time you enter a car, bus, train, plane, elevator, escalator — that way it becomes automatic.)
7. Keep your knees slightly bent, so you don't lock them.
8. When doing shoulder exercises, make sure you could always see your hands (if you wanted to).

The Twenty-Minute YOU Workout

Do the following movements in order. Make adjustments to time or repetitions as your ability level dictates. Each strength exercise is followed by a stretch to loosen the same muscle group and keep you limber. On nonworkout days, you can just do the stretches (labeled with an S) after walking for a short flexibility session. See www.realage.com for video of each move.

9. Breathe. Many people hold their breath while doing strength training.

10. Keep moving in between exercises to keep your heart rate fast, or move directly to the next exercise. If you're unable to hold a conversation, you're exercising too hard. If you can keep a conversation going and are able to fill the listener in on all the details, you may not be going hard enough.

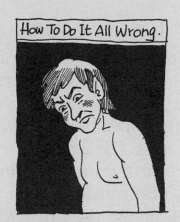

How To Do It All Wrong.

11. As you get stronger, go longer rather than harder with cardio exercises, and stronger with weight exercises. That is, do more repetitions of any non-weight-bearing exercise. That will help prevent injuries from overexertion. If you really feel weak, just hold the exercise position without moving and slowly work up. It's more important to follow perfect form and do fewer repetitions than to do a lot of repetitions with form that's sloppier than spaghetti in a high chair.

1: Roll with It

Allows any kinks in your shoulders to be smoothed out.

Roll your shoulders forward for a count of ten and back for ten. "Swim" shoulders back for ten and forward for ten. Your goal is to get full range of movement with your shoulders. Notice any areas that you don't move fluidly and try to open them up by relaxing as you move your hands in full circles. Between sets, get into the habit of rolling your shoulders five

259

times forward and five times back.

2: The Chest Cross

Strengthens chest and shoulders

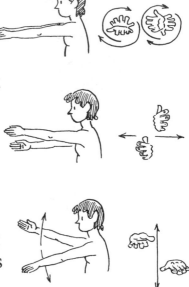

(A) Reach your arms as forward as possible at shoulder height, and twirl your hands back and forth like you have a tennis ball in your hands. (B) Then, cross your straight arms in front of your chest in a series of quick horizontal motions with your palms facing each other (so they provide some wind resistance to your motion). (C) Next move your hands rapidly up and down with your palms facing the floor. Try to do each of these variations twenty-five times.

3 (Stretch): The Clapper

Stretches chest

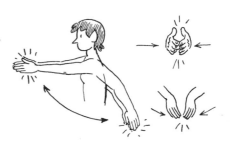

In a standing position and keeping your chest up, clap in front of you; then bring your hands behind your back and clap your hands together. Keep your hands as

FACTOID

You can have 100 percent strength gains within a few months, but it also works in reverse: By not doing strength training every week, you'll start to lose some muscle mass and your strength by up to 50 percent in three months and by up to 80 percent in three years. Look at exercise the way you'd study Spanish — the more consistent you are, the more consistent your results will be. Your muscles forget, just as your mind does.

high as you can in front and back during the movement. Keep your chest lifted when clapping in back. Do ten times.

4 (Stretch): The Hippie

Stretches hips and hamstrings

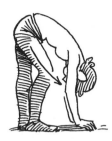
With your feet flat on the ground, bend forward at your waist. Alternate bending one knee and keeping the other leg straight (but still keeping your feet flat), and let your head dangle down, releasing all your tension. Stretch each side for fifteen seconds.

5: Push-up Pride

Strengthens chest

Get in the appropriate "up" push-up position for you by either staying on your toes or keeping your knees on the ground. Lower yourself until your chest nearly touches the ground and push back up. As you straighten your elbows, push your spine toward the ceiling to exercise (to help engage your back muscles as well). Pull your heels away from your shoulders, keeping a long, solid body. Don't let your stomach hang down toward the ground; make your stomach active by pulling it in to support your lower back. This will help release any unnecessary tension on your lower back. Keeping your stomach tight in any exercise strengthens your belly muscles. If your lower back starts to hurt, raise your butt slightly and curl your tailbone by tightening your butt. Keep your chin slightly up and look six inches past your fingertips. This forces you to use your chest and not overextend your neck while doing push-ups. Do as many push-ups as you can (this is called exercising to failure, and it's what helps build strength

Easy

Med.

Hard

Preparation for Perspiration

Before beginning an exercise program, you need more than a Lycra top. Exercise isn't dangerous, but your risk of injury will be less if you live with a few principles to protect your muscles and your entire body.

Warm Up. Before beginning any exercise, warm up your muscles for about five minutes to prevent injury. (The YOU twenty-minute workout includes a warm-up, but if you're doing another activity, follow these guidelines.) Remember, your muscles are like spaghetti strands; they're pliable when they're warm, and more injury-prone if they're not. Jogging, brisk walking, cycling, or doing exercises with light weight or no weight will help prepare your muscles for activity. One good rule: Do the same exercise you will be doing but at a slower pace or with lighter weight. Your goal is to move your joints through the same range of motion as they will do with exercise — to raise your heart rate and to increase the temperature of your muscles, which will make them more viscous and less likely to be injured. Some advocate that at the end of exercise, you should cool down with a light jog, cycle, or walk, but there's no evidence that a cooldown will reduce injury or muscle soreness more than just stretching at the end. But if you are doing intense cardio exercise, you do need to do a cooldown, rather than stopping

proteins in your muscle). If these are too hard, just hold your chest off the ground without moving. Or you can do a pyramid push-up routine: Do five push-ups, then hold in the up position for five seconds. Then do four and hold for four in the up position, all the way down to one.

6 (Stretch): Pecs Flex

Stretches chest and arms

Sit up straight on your heels and interweave your fingers behind

abruptly at the end of the workout. For a cooldown, do the same activity, like running, at a much slower pace than you were maintaining during your workout.

Focus on Your Muscles. Take special notice of where you tense up. You want to release tension in your body, not shift it somewhere else. Most commonly, people shift it to their shoulders and their foreheads. Notice this, breathe, and focus on the muscles you are working.

Listen to Your Body. Throughout stretching, make sure to keep breathing freely and slowly. If you ever feel pain during stretching, stop. (That's different from a little discomfort as you're loosening up; actual pain should be your warning to stop. We *want* burning in the muscles.)

Wear the Right Shoes. You'll need to invest in a good pair of lightweight running shoes for walking (the strength workout you should do barefoot). They're well cushioned and designed to handle the heel-to-toe movements for both walking and running. Best option: Go to a specialty running store, where the often underpaid salespeople are the experts; ask the pro there to analyze your stride and match up the best shoe for your feet.

your butt, while keeping your arms straight. Lift your fingers up, knuckle side facing back, while opening your chest wide. Squeeze your shoulder blades together to open your chest more. Use your breath to your advantage here, by breathing into the muscles being stretched. Another option is to interweave your fingers behind your head and pull your hands away from your head. Face forward for all versions.

Basic Training

Sometimes choosing a trainer can be like buying a car — it sure does look nice, but do you really know how well it runs? While a personal trainer isn't required, many people like working out one-on-one, specifically because of the trainer's knowledge and the accountability of having to regularly report to him or her. To make sure you get one who's qualified, take these steps:

- Make sure trainers are certified by a reputable organization like the American College of Sports Medicine (ACSM), the American Council on Exercise (ACE), the National Strength and Conditioning Association (NSCA), or the National Academy of Sports Medicine (NASM), as well as having Cooper Institute certifications.

- Check to see if they practice full-time, and aren't just doing training between acting jobs.

- Make sure their motivational style (including the voice) matches your workout style; some trainers are more vocal, while others are more soothing. If they're inspiring to *you*, you'll push yourself to get results and to show up, which is nine-tenths of the battle. If cost is a problem, try out our free program with New York City trainer Joel Harper or Tracy Hafen on www.oprah.com or www.realage.com, or create a customized workout with world-class personal trainers delivered to your doorstep monthly by visiting pushtv.com.

7: Steady on the Plank

Strengthens abs and shoulders

Get into a push-up position with your elbows and toes on the floor, while pushing the area between your shoulders toward the ceiling and keeping your stomach pulled in toward your lower back, to support it. Keep your buttocks

264

tight and your eyes looking at the floor (ignore the fact that you suddenly realize you have to vacuum). Hold the position for as long as you can. If you can last more than one minute, make it more difficult by dropping your chin twenty times out in front of interweaved hands, or by trying to balance on one foot.

8: Whose Side Are You On, Anyway?

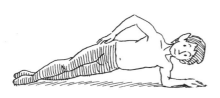

Strengthens obliques (the muscles at the side of your abdominals)

Turn to the side by putting an elbow on the floor and rotating the opposite hip toward the ceiling. Keep your body in a straight line and resist pushing your butt back. Keep your abs tight as you hold the position for as long as you can. Alternate sides. If you can hold for more than one minute, you can increase the difficulty by repeatedly dropping your hip, tapping it on the mat, and bringing it back into the lateral plank.

9 (Stretch): Up, Dog, Up

Stretches abdominals and obliques

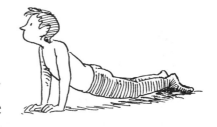

From a down push-up position, with your hands below your shoulders, lift your chest and torso up into the air so that your upper body is nearly perpendicular to the floor as you come onto the tops of your bare feet. Lean backward to stretch your abdominals, but keep your butt relaxed. Hold for ten seconds. Then look over your right shoulder for ten, then your left shoulder for ten, then back to center.

10: The Rickety Table

Strengthens upper back and butt

Put your hands and knees flat on the floor with your fingers spread apart and pointing directly forward. Keep your back flat and parallel to the floor and your supporting elbow slightly bent. Look down six inches above your fingertips. Reach your right hand forward and your left foot back and stretch them as far away from each other as possible, keeping your right hand higher than your head. The higher your arm goes up, the more work your back has to do, and the more effective the exercise. Now bring your right elbow to your left knee. Do twenty on this side, then alter- 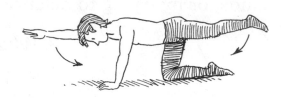 nate and do it with the other leg and arm. For more advanced exercises you can move your arm and leg out at a right angle from your body, keeping them above your spine, and hold them there for twenty seconds. Your stomach should be pulled in the entire time, supporting your lower back.

11: Superman

Strengthens lower back

Lie flat on your stomach, reaching your arms out in front of you with the palms down. Spread your extremities straight out in all four directions and lift your arms and legs simultaneously for enough rep- 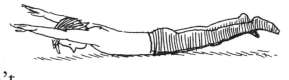 etitions to cause some mild fa- tigue. Continue to look down dur- ing the movement, and don't overextend your neck up. This exercise is about how long you can make your body stretch — not how high you can get it. Focus on squeezing your butt as you lift. Try to make it to one minute.

12 (Stretch): The Seated Pretzel

Stretches lower-middle upper back and hip

Sit down with your legs stretched in front of you. Bring your right foot up and set it down on the outside of your left knee. For back support,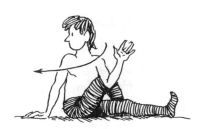

FACTOID

It shouldn't be a surprise that the exercise and movements that require the most intensity are the ones that burn the most calories. Some samples of exercise and activities and how much energy they burn per minute for typical people (with a weight of 200 pounds for men and 150 pounds for women):

Exercise	Calories Burned per Minute (Male)	Calories Burned per Minute (Female)
Running, 9 min/mile	22	17
Swimming, moderate	16	12
Stationary cycling, moderate	16	11
Weight lifting, vigorous	12	9
Walking 4 mph	10	8
Activity		
Chopping wood	12	9
Shoveling snow	12	9
Gardening	9	6
Playing with kids	8	6
Watering plants	5	4
Job		
Firefighting	24	18
Construction	12	9
Masseur/Masseuse	8	6
Nursing	6	5
Computer work	3	2

Top of the Morning

Coffee, roosters, and shock jocks aren't the only things people wake up with. Many people enjoy starting their day with yoga's sun salutation: a series of movements that strengthen, stretch, and energize your body. Consider it your caffeine-free way to start the day. Do the sequence twice, switching legs on the second repetition.

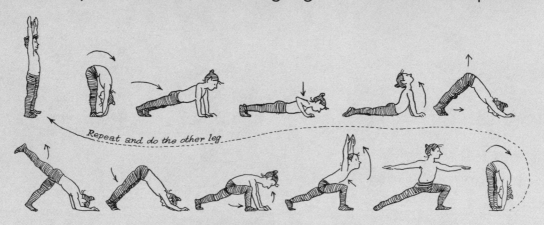

Repeat and do the other leg

Sun Salutation

1. Stand with feet touching. Bring your hands together, palm to palm, fingertips pointing upward. Make sure your weight is evenly distributed. Exhale. Raise your arms upward. Slowly bend backward, pulling your abs in and up, stretching arms above the head. Relax your neck. Inhale.

2. Exhale while you slowly bend forward until your hands are in line with your feet, touching your head to your knees if possible. Press your hands down, fingertips in line with toes (bend your knees if you have to), and touch the floor. Maintain a slight bend in the knees to take pressure off your back through your hamstrings, and extend and elongate your back, rather than arching it, to avoid lower-back issues. Relax your neck and shoulders; let them dangle down toward the ground. Use their weight to stretch your spine.

3. Move into an up push-up position with your hands and toes

on the floor and your back straight.

4. Lower your body to a down push-up position with your elbows bent and your body remaining in a straight position from your legs to your head.

5. As you inhale, raise your head and bend backward as far as possible, while straightening your arms. To go deeper as you lift, arch backward and pull the top of your head up and out and come onto the top of your feet as you lift your pelvis off the ground. The four points would be your two palms and two tops of your feet.

6. Keeping your arms straight, raise your hips into down dog, pressing your armpits toward your knees, and align your head with your arms. Exhale throughout movement.

7. Keeping your leg straight, raise your right leg so it stays in line with your spine. Raise the left leg your second time through the sequence.

8. Return transiently to down dog position. Lunge your right leg forward.

9. As you inhale, keep your hands and feet on the ground, with your right foot between your hands. Reverse legs the second time through.

10. Raise your head and lift your hands straight up to the sky while maintaining the lunge position.

11. Open your hips by turning to the left and outstretching your arms right side forward and left side back so that they're parallel to the floor.

12. Bring feet together and stand up straight. Keeping your legs straight, bend at the waist and lower your upper body. Touch your head to your knees if possible. Exhale.

13. Return to position 1 by slowly rising, straightening your back into a standing pose. Stretch your arms above your head as you inhale. Exhale and then repeat the sequence so you can work the opposite muscles.

put your right hand behind your right butt cheek. Bring your left toe straight up. Reach your left hand up as if indicating "stop" and drop your chin. Then twist to the right and bring your left triceps to the outside of the right thigh. To go deeper, twist more to apply pressure against your right thigh. Act like a string is pulling the top of your head up to elongate the spine. Breathe by expanding your rib cage like you are blowing up a balloon. Really concentrate on taking deep breaths every time.

Note for exercises 13 and 14: For all reclining abdominal exercises, keep your lower back flat on the ground. Pretend a quarter is trapped between the floor and your lower back, and keep your belly taut to train your stomach to be flat. As soon as you feel your lower back tenting up, stop and pull it back down as flat as possible before continuing. If this gets too hard, stop and hold it down as flat as possible for thirty seconds. Pretend there is a dumbbell tied to a string attached to your belly button, and it is pulling your stomach down toward the quarter.

13: Leg Drop

Strengthens entire abdominal area

Lie on your back with your hands on your chest and put your knees at a 45-degree angle and your feet in the air. Drop your heels down, tap the mat, and bring back up to 45 degrees. Do as many as you can (to failure). As soon as your lower back starts to arch up, return back to 45 degrees; keep pushing yourself a little bit further each time with your back glued to the quarter. Beginners, do one leg at a time. Advanced: Do it with straight legs.

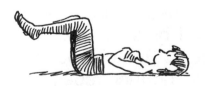 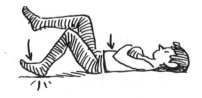

14: X Crunch

Strengthens upper abdominals

Lie on your back with your feet on the ground and your knees at a 45-degree angle. Cross your arms behind your head, putting your opposite hand to the opposite shoulder to form an X behind your head. Rest your head in this X and keep your neck loose (in the beginning, you can put a tennis ball under your chin as a reminder). Using your abdominal muscles, crunch up about 30 degrees from the floor. Without holding your breath, you need to suck in your belly button to the floor to tighten the natural girdle you have (it's a muscle called the transverse abdominis) to keep the entire six-pack tight. Also pull up your pelvic muscles (like when you are holding in your pee) to strengthen the bottom of the natural girdle. Do as many as you can, looking up toward the ceiling the entire time. Then repeat Up, Dog, Up (exercise 9) to stretch your abdominals.

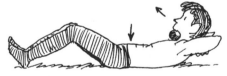

> ## FACTOID
>
> In any ab exercise, pull your stomach muscles in. If you push your stomach out, then that is how your muscles will form. Relax your face and don't furrow your brow. This can also help avoid a future plastic surgery consultation.

15: Seated Drop Kick

Strengthens quadriceps

Sit with your legs straight out in front of you. Bend your right leg up with the knee pointing toward the ceiling. To keep your back straight, interweave your hands around this knee. Act like there is a string pulling from the top of your head, elongating your spine (and don't bob your head). Lift your straight left leg six inches off the ground, keeping your left toe pointed toward the ceiling. Lift twenty-five

Exercise Anywhere, Anytime!

Practice perfect posture — while sitting, standing, or walking — by tightening your abdominals (suck your belly button to your spine). Visualize a straight line from the top of your head down to your hamstring muscles in the back of your legs, making sure to keep your neck and shoulders back and relaxed down away from your ears. Visualize a string pulling you up from the top of your head, elongating your spine. Engaging in good posture not only will strengthen your core but will also add a small extra-calorie burn because you're working slightly harder to maintain the position. If you find your shoulders rolling forward, practice interweaving your hands behind your butt as you talk to people.

times, then switch legs. Do each leg twice. The only body part that moves is the leg; for variation, lift leg and move side to side.

16: Invisible Chair

Strengthens entire leg

Sit in a chair position (with no chair!) with your back against a wall, and with your palms resting on your knees. Ideally, have a stool below you, so you can grab it or sit on it when you're done. Keep your heels directly below your knees and at a 90-degree angle; your relaxed shoulders should be rolled back and the back of your head should be against the wall. Hold for as long as you can, and try to work up to two minutes. Keep your face relaxed and breathe.

17 (Stretch): Nice Thighs

Stretches quadriceps

While standing on one leg, bend the knee of the opposite leg and grab the foot behind your back with interweaved fingers (or use one

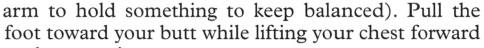

arm to hold something to keep balanced). Pull the foot toward your butt while lifting your chest forward and squeezing your shoulder blades together. Keep your knees together. Switch legs. Keep your abs pulled in the entire time, to support your lower back. Hold each for twenty seconds.

FACTOID

You can add a balancing element to almost any exercise by tweaking it slightly. Try doing two-legged exercises on one leg, or do an exercise lying on a stability ball instead of a bench.

273

Figure 11.1 **Picture this** To remove every possible excuse from your repertoire, the YOU Workout is summarized in three pages that you can post wherever you need to facilitate exercise. Remember, your body is your gym.

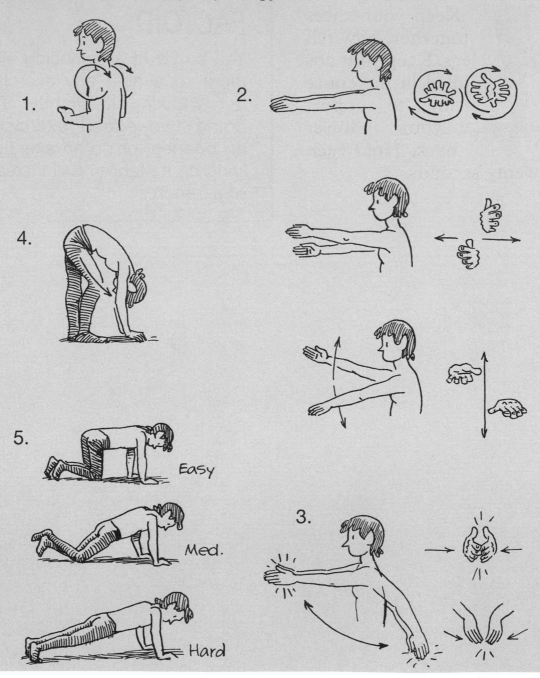

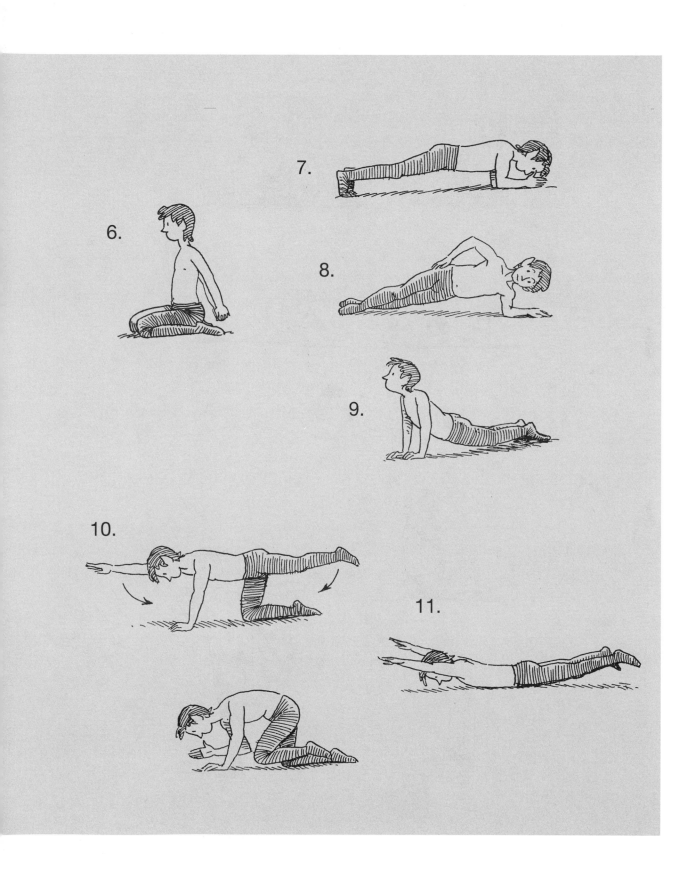

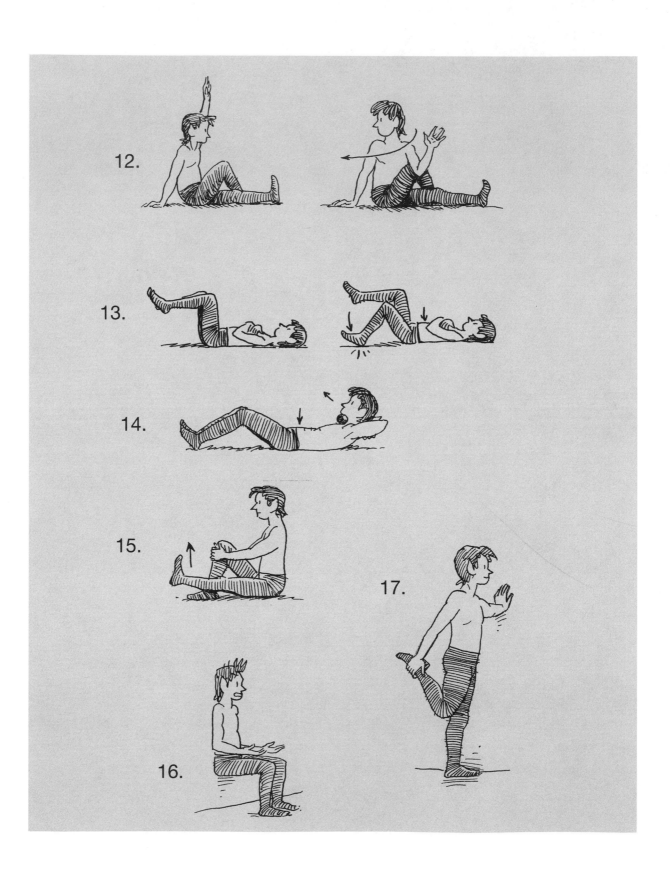

Are You Well Equipped?

Hooked on sweat? Then consider these add-ons to your physiological gym.

As You Get Stronger: Weights

Though you can use household objects for resistance exercises, it can be worth investing in a pair or two of dumbbells to use for lunges, squats, and other exercises as you get stronger. Weights usually cost about fifty cents per pound.

Great Addition to a Home Gym: Exercise Ball

Once you establish a fitness foundation, these large, inflatable balls are wonderful to use for crunches and any other exercise in which you sit on the bench or floor. They help you develop balance and work your stabilizing muscles in your abdominal section. They are also great stretching devices. See www.realage.com for examples.

For the Traveler: Bands

Resistance bands allow you to increase resistance as you get stronger, and they're also small, so you can take them as you travel.

For Balance and Agility: Jump Rope

They're cheap, and easy to use. While raising your heart rate, they'll also test and improve your agility.

For At-Home Cardio: Rebounder	Versatile Bonus: Weighted Vest
Once you progress to doing cardio exercise, you can jog, swim, row, cycle, or do whatever you like to get your heart pumping. If you're one of our highly coordinated readers, one of the easiest ways to work your heart is with either a jump rope or a minitrampoline called a rebounder. You know about the jump rope, but for a rebounder, you can store it under your bed, pull it out, and do mini joint-safe cardio sessions by hopping and jumping on it for the allotted time. (Take a quick lesson before using it, so you can learn the safety rules.)	This vest carries extra weight to give you resistance (many are adjustable so you can change the weights in one-pound increments), and you can use it for all of the central exercises, like lunges, squats, crunches, and push-ups.

Cardiovascular Workout

In a week, you need sixty minutes of an activity that raises your heart rate to 80 percent of maximum (220 minus your calendar age). You can choose from such activities as running, cycling, swimming, rowing, or using an elliptical trainer. (Vigorous sex also counts, but here it has to be continuous minutes, bucko, so it's unlikely this'll be a good alternative.) For the last one to four minutes, raise the intensity to the highest level you can for the maximum benefits. Then cool down for five to ten minutes on low intensity of the same exercise. If you do the YOU Workout above at a level that raises your heart rate, these twenty minutes of sweating can count toward your weekly cardiovascular exercise total of sixty minutes a week.

Note: When doing exercises with your own body weight feels too easy, you can add resistance by holding dumbbells or milk jugs filled with pebbles, sand, or water, or using other household products, like soup cans.

Amp It Up: Bonus Moves!

While the body-weight-only YOU Workout is a total-strength and total-stretch workout, we also believe that some of you may be looking for — or ready for — extra-credit moves. The following moves are ones you can do in addition to the basic twenty-minute workout, and are broken into the foundation areas of legs, chest, back, and abdominals. You can swap them in for similar exercises in the twenty-minute workout or add them in as extras. For you gym goers or home-gym owners, use dumbbells or other equipment. Aim for ten to twelve repetitions unless otherwise noted.

Legs Options

Lunges

Stand with your feet shoulder width apart, with your hands on your hips or holding weights. Take a long step forward with your left foot, like you're stepping over a puddle or stream. Now, for the best muscle burn, bend your left knee so that your thigh is parallel to the floor. (Make sure your knee doesn't extend past your toes.) Pause, then step back into the original standing position. Repeat, by stepping forward with your right foot. This move will also build strength needed for better balance. If you have trouble balancing, turn the toes on your forward foot

279

slightly inward, so you're not on such a tightrope. While doing lunges, pretend you have a broomstick attached to your spine so that you stay straight to the ground throughout the entire movement. You can also do these without alternating legs — do a certain number on one leg, then switch legs. That makes it a little easier on the knees.

Squats

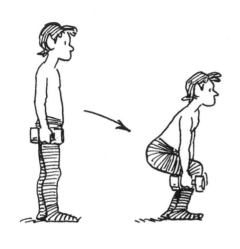

Stand with your feet a little wider than shoulder width apart and with your hands holding weights or in *I Dream of Jeannie* style (elbows in line with shoulders, and hands crossed to opposite upper arm). Throughout, keep your elbows in line with your shoulders. Without curling your back, squat down to the point where your thighs are approximately parallel to the floor (or before that if you have knee or lower-back pain). It should feel like you're about to sit on the toilet seat, but just before your buns touch down. Pause, then rise up to the original starting position. Look forward throughout the movement. Keep your shoulders back and in line with your hips. Breathe in on the way down; breathe out on the way up. You can add resistance by holding dumbbells or other objects. You can do squats over a chair or sofa for safety in case you fall back. For variety, hold the lowermost position and pulse for a count of thirty and then continue your reps.

Step Taps

Stand in front of a set of stairs. Place one foot two steps up; leave it there as you raise the

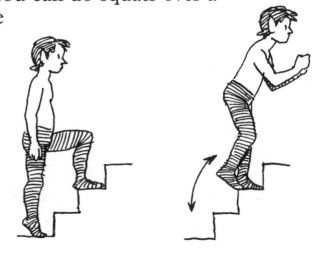

280

other foot, tapping that step twenty consecutive times and then switching legs. Use your arms to propel you up, as a sprinter would do. You barely want to hear your foot tap back down and back up. The softer it hits, the more burn you get, and the less impact on your knees.

Chest Options

Push-up Variations

As you get stronger, you can try these add-ons:

- Get in down-dog position: hands and toes on the floor and butt high in the air, like an inverted *V.* Look two inches above your shoulder-width hands and bend your elbows only, dropping your forehead to where your eyes are looking. Then straighten your arms. Keep your body in down dog the entire time.
- Wear a weighted vest (available at most sports-equipment stores, or try something like the ones at www.thexvest.com), which will increase the amount of resistance during the movement.

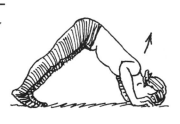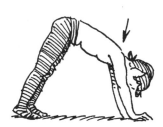

- Alternate lifting each foot a few inches off the floor and bending your knee on each repetition to incorporate balance into the exercise.
- One-arm push-ups. *Hooyah!* (If you can do this, uh, what are you doing reading this chapter, Rocky?)

Back Option

Bent-over Back Rows

Stand behind and to one side of a chair, bend over, and place one hand on the seat, and put a dumbbell (or water bottle) in your free hand. Keeping your back flat, pull the weighted hand up toward the 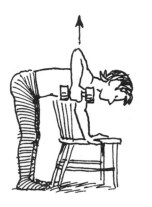 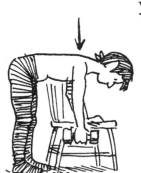 outside of your chest, reaching your elbow toward the ceiling. Then lower your weighted hand as far as you can, keeping it extended to elongate the muscle, and repeat. As you're pulling up, keep your back parallel to the ground and your feet flat, not rocking, with your knees slightly bent. To get your heart rate up and an amazing burn, do 100 with a lighter weight. If it gets too hard, lower the weight and keep going. But you have to maintain good form throughout. Better to use proper form than to do a lot of reps.

Abdominals Options

Crunch Variations

■ At the same time you crunch your body up, curl your legs off the ground toward your head and squeeze your belly button to the floor. (Works the entire six-pack in three sets of two-packs: the upper, lower, and middle, respectively.)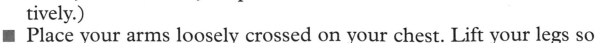

■ Place your arms loosely crossed on your chest. Lift your legs so that the soles of your feet are facing the ceiling. Keeping your legs straight, lift your tailbone one inch off the ground and then slowly lower it. (Works lower region of your abdominals.)

Exercise Ball Moves

■ Lie back on an exercise ball. Reach your arms straight up toward the ceiling with your palms together. Keeping your arms straight, bring your biceps down to the sides or your ears praying hands way above head and back up. The only thing that is moving is your arms.

■ Do a plank (face-down) with your elbows on an exercise ball and keeping your navel in the same spot. Alternate swiveling each hip down two inches toward the ground and then back to plank.

Bicycle

Lie on the floor with your hands resting lightly behind your head. Raise your feet off the ground and bend your right knee and pull it toward your chest. Simultaneously twist your opposite shoulder toward this knee, keeping your elbows out of your line of vision. Switch sides back and forth. Keep your lower foot suspended in the air as you switch sides. Then hold to one side, reaching your shoulder toward the opposite knee for thirty seconds. Switch and then hold to the opposite side for thirty more. The more you pull your stomach in, the more you can lift yourself up. For a harder version, stay in this last position, take the straight leg, and raise and lower it one inch for thirty times.

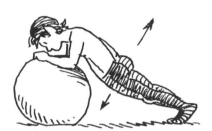

Remember, don't fall into the trap of thinking, misguidedly, that strength exercises are for *increasing* your size. You can do resistance exercises without making your muscles bulge more than a pug's eyes. The true payoff for strengthening your muscles is that you'll build a little more lean muscle mass, which will help you burn more calories throughout the day and speed your metabolism. The trick is to reduce your excuses (which we've done by eliminating equipment in the YOU Workout) so that you devote those sixty minutes a week to building, maintaining, and maximizing your body's natural fat burners.

Chapter 12
The YOU Diet

The Waist-Management Eating Plan

BABY LEAF

Baby GREENS

VEGGIE SPRING

with BROCCOLI · PEA PODS · ALGAE

CARROT

2 oz

IT'S CURLY LETTUCE!

Whether or not you're the kind of person who skips the plot to get to the ending, you've arrived. Welcome to the YOU Diet — our re-programming plan provides you with the tools to make smart choices and with the strategies that allow you to make YOU-Turns after you've made bad choices. The specific program starts on page 294, but first, let's go over a few of our principles.

Whether it's at work, in school, or with sports, we praise the hard workers. If you bust your tail with hustle and sweat, then we'll want you to proceed immediately to the pedestal. You may not always score the promotion, the dean's list, or the championship, but, as a society, we place more value on effort than just about anything else (except maybe a 7 a.m. cup of Starbucks coffee). It's too bad that's the very reason why our societal waistband has exploded to the size of Saturn's rings. We expect that a little of X (hard work) and a lot of Y (suffering) should automatically lead to the promised land of Z (skinny waist). But our bodies don't work that way. In fact, you can't win the battle over waist size with do-or-diet effort: The harder you try to diet (with deprivation, with willpower, with the sheer stubbornness to avoid pork rinds), the more likely it is that you'll drown in an industrial-size jar of Marshmallow Fluff.

There are many solid, smart diet plans available to you. *YOU: On a Diet* is meant not to compete with these worthy programs but rather to give you the tools to succeed no matter what you try. That's because the raw data from current research offer insights into the biology of your body that should enhance your decisions about food and exercise. Let the science-based explanations we offer serve as your operating system to which future diet and activity plans can be added like software programs. After reading *YOU: On a Diet,* you'll know enough to evaluate them all, and you shouldn't have to worry about yo-yo dieting ever again. No matter what your plan, you should know by now that waist management isn't about hustle. It's about the following two things:

Automation. The first thing you need to do is stop trying — and start living. Normally. Automatically. Intelligently. You can do that

A Portion of the Plan

Many experts will tell you that the key to successful dieting comes from two words: *portion control.* That makes sense, but not in the way you might think. We emphasize that you eat healthy portions of food (about a fistful per serving) and use nine-inch plates not to restrict your calories per se but to slow you down. If you can slow your calorie intake, you'll give your brain a chance to keep up — and activate the right amounts of leptin and ghrelin to keep you satisfied. So, start with the right servings of food, take your time eating them, then gauge your levels of satiety (using our fullness gauge on page 226). If you're still hungry, then have another serving (the size of a fist, not the size of a head) of a good-for-you food.

by reprogramming your body with the tools we provide you throughout this book (and the fourteen-day program that follows) so that your decisions, food choices, and lifestyle become an enjoyable, invigorating, energizing routine, not a burden.

Adjustment. To make the transition from a thick waist to a thin one, you also have to acknowledge that waist management isn't a success-or-failure proposition. It's a journey with some side streets, some dead ends, and a few metaphorical and literal forks in the road. That's why you must practice the psychological and behavioral actions that will help you develop routines to help you go from side-

Fill 'Er Up

About twenty minutes before dinner, eat 1/2 ounce of walnuts with 1 cup of your favorite YOU Soup. Or drink at least 8 ounces of water with 1 tablespoon of psyllium. Either will help fill you up so you won't want or need to eat as much to feel satisfied.

287

The YOU Diet Crib Sheet

Meal Strategy	Three main meals plus snacks, so you're never hungry. No eating within three hours of bedtime. Consider dessert an every-other-day treat.
Waist Foods (Eat 'em)	Whole-grain carbohydrates; fiber; nuts, which include healthy monounsaturated and polyunsaturated fats; protein such as lean meats (two-legged preferred) and fish.
Waste Foods (Trash 'em)	Added sugars, simple carbohydrates, fructose as in high-fructose corn syrup, trans fat, saturated fat, non-whole-grain flour, and enriched and/or bleached flour.
In a Hunger Emergency	Apples, almonds, walnuts, edamame (soybeans), sugarless gum, water, cut-up veggies, low-fat yogurt and cottage cheese, or premade YOU soup.
Substitution Foods	In any recipe or meal plan, you can replace any fruit or vegetable with another to make recipes to your taste.
Meal Journal	You can keep track of what you eat at www.mychoicescount.com.

tracked to on track. That's our YOU-Turn — knowing that it's OK to face obstacles, and it's OK that sometimes they'll pound you square in the mouth. As long as you know the way back to the right road and can make YOU-Turns faster than a mouse darts from a cat,

Supplements	Once a day, take a multivitamin as an insurance policy against less-than-perfect food choices. (It's even better if you split the pill and take half twice a day.) Through food and the multivitamin, you need to get a total of 1,200 milligrams of calcium, 600 IU of vitamin D, 400 milligrams of magnesium, and 300 milligrams of pantothenic acid (vitamin B5). Also, take 2 grams of distilled fish oil for omega-3 fatty acids and 1/2 teaspoon of cinnamon daily. And make sure you get 10 tablespoons of cooked tomato sauce weekly.
The Team	Don't be afraid to enlist advice from qualified nutritionists and trainers. But one of your most important team members will be your support partner — someone who can encourage you and be a deterrent to failure, too (you won't want to report to that person a four-doughnut binge).
The YOU-Turn	It's OK to make mistakes. The important thing is to catch them, recognize them, control them, and allow yourself the opportunity to get back on the right (waist management) road

then you can plan for a lifetime of successful waist management.

To go along with that foundation of a dietary operating system, we also want to offer you one "software" option — the YOU Diet, the food plan that can help reboot your body so that you learn to eat smart, not hard. With this plan, you can expect to lose up to two inches of your waist size within two weeks.

As you launch into this fourteen-day rebooting program (it's actually so easy that it's one seven-day plan done twice, so you can do it perfectly and learn to do it automatically), remember this: Your body is made up of hundreds of beautiful biochemical instruments, and they all play different notes, melodies, harmonies, and chords within your anatomical orchestra. As the conductor, you direct how those notes are played and what kind of sound they'll make. Like any new piece of music, the YOU Diet will take a week or two for you to learn it, for you to feel it, for YOU to become ingrained. But once all this happens, your orchestra will play like never before.

The YOU Diet: Before YOU Start

Before you start anything — whether it's a new job, or a 5K race, or putting together your daughter's 547-piece Barbie house — it always pays to prepare. You read the short form of the employee manual, you study the course route, you lay out the plastic pieces all over the floor while silently cursing the world's toy manufacturers. And before you start the YOU Diet, the same applies (minus the cursing). If you've skipped the intro, then we'll do a quick review here of the pieces you'll need to know before you begin. (If you've read the book, then this is just a quick refresher course.)

YOU Change the Inside to Change the Outside: This diet is about understanding and automating your biology to reboot your body back to its original factory settings that make you lean and healthy, not the settings that have caused an alarming increase in yearly Santa applications. This diet is about eating the foods that help all of your organs and systems function the way that they should. By focusing on the recommended ingredients and nutrients, you'll be helping your body's chemicals and hormones do what they want to do: get you to your ideal size. They're the ones that will make

Best Blade Plans

When following any eating plan, what you do and don't do with your fork and spoon are your most crucial actions. But don't underestimate the power of a great knife — to make what you do in the kitchen as enjoyable as what you do at the table. Overpay to buy the best eight-inch chef's knife (without serrations) you can afford. And follow these rules, to avoid leaving a finger in the guacamole: Always keep the pointed edge on the cutting board; just lever from the point and cut sliding away from you under the back end.

Always cut away from yourself.

As you're lining up foods with your noncutting hand, tuck the tops of your fingers under the bottoms, so you let your knuckles, not your whole fingers, be the guide.

See www.realage.com for more cutting instructions.

your body want to burn fat, not store it. And they're the ones that will make your body feel satisfied, not hungry. We call these YOU-th-FULL foods, because they keep you satiated and less likely to gorge on bad-for-you foods. Put together, that's the real recipe for a lean waist and a healthy body.

YOU Better Identify the Problem So You Can Better Solve It: We've tended to treat weight loss as more art than science: more trial and error than predictable cause and effect. Through recent advances in molecular genetics, neurology, and biochemistry, we're finally able to learn what really causes us to gain weight and lose it, and what causes us to stay full and become hungry. Because of that, weight loss is revealing itself as a complex yet predictable and controllable process. Simply put, working smart means clearly defining the problem — that is, by understanding how your body works — before you set about solving it. A problem well defined is half-solved.

YOU Automate the Process: One of the reasons why we're a society of shot-putters instead of a society of milers is that we have millions of choices about what to eat. And while that variety is a win for the food industry, it is a miserable defeat for our waists. One of the ways that you'll be able to reboot your body is by stripping away the thinking and debating about eating. For a few meals a day, you'll take away the millions of choices to automate your actions. You'll eat essentially the same meals for breakfast, lunch, and snacks, and change up options for dinner. By decreasing the variety of foods eaten throughout the day, you'll decrease the chance for the hedonistic rampages that can be so dangerous.

YOU Stop Beating Yourself Up for Every Mistake: Somewhere and sometime, you've been led to believe that the only way you can lose weight is to eat perfectly all the time. That's not realistic. That's not fair. And that's why almost all diets fail. Perfection is impossible. One of the ways you can avoid the all-out Alfredo-fest is to activate your contingency plans: ready-made meals and snacks that you can turn to when you're stressed, tired, or bored. These foods will help you through cravings, they'll help you make YOU-Turns, and they'll help you make good decisions to avoid bad foods.

YOU Make It Easy on Yourself: We all know that the only way you'll be able to automate eating is if it's easy and fast. Almost all breakfast, lunch, and snack recipes take less than ten minutes to make, and no dinner takes more than thirty minutes of prep time.

YOU Eat to Stay Full — Not to Hit a Specific Calorie Count. Before we outline the meals, recipes, and strategies for succeeding on the YOU Diet, we want you to remember this one principle of eating: Eating isn't all about calories, it's about staying satisfied. The key to this program is eating nutritionally rich foods, avoiding the toxic ones, and using your body's clues about satiety to help you stop eating when you should.

It's about eating the foods that will help keep you full — and what "feels right," so that you can achieve and maintain your ideal playing weight. That said, we know some of you are members of the math/stat/calorie squad, so we'll indulge your number-loving selves for a moment.

We've designed this diet and its serving sizes based on a person with a metabolic rate of 1,700 calories. That is, the person who burns 1,700 calories a day through normal processes and activities can eat this to maintain his or her weight. To lose weight, this person would have to have a slightly smaller portion for dinner, for instance. If you burn 2,000 calories a day, you'll lose weight using these portion sizes, but if you burn only 1,400 calories a day, you'll consume more calories than you burn. To find your approximate no-waist-loss point, find your resting metabolic rate and add your physical activities.

- An easy way to estimate your resting metabolic rate is to multiply your desired weight in pounds by 8 and add 200, but this is very variable, so if anyone ever offers to measure your real metabolic rate, accept the offer.
- To find the calories you burn from physical activity, multiply the number of minutes you walk by 4, and your cardiovascular and strength minutes (not the time watching others) by 8. So that's about 300 calories for 30 minutes of walking and 25 minutes of strength or cardiovascular exercise. You can also use the readouts from cardiovascular machines you use if the machines have them.

So let's see how it works.

Say you want to weigh 150 pounds and do an average of 300 physical activity calories per day — about what you do on our plan (more on some days and fewer on others). That means:

Your basic calories used are 8 x 150 = 1,200
+ 200 = 1,400
+ 300 in activity = 1,700

So to maintain your desired weight, you'd need about 1,700 calories a day. To lose a pound a week, you'd need to decrease that by

Be Prepared

Here's a waist management fact: Bad foods aren't bad just because of the ingredients they contain but also because many of them are fast and easy, which are the exact traits that can get you into a whole lot of trouble. The key to successful dietary contingency plans is to have premade foods ready for those times when you've been conditioned to reach for bags of sugar-containing waist killers. Instead, choose your favorites of these options to make once a week so you'll have something to grab when you need it.

Cut-up Vegetables: Your choice. Cut them, bag them, eat them. Nothing wrong with baby carrots, grape tomatoes, and broccoli florets, but if you prefer jicama, sugar snaps, and orange pepper strips, go for it.

Sautéed Vegetables: Your choice. Sauté them in olive oil with chopped garlic, red pepper flakes, or a good dash of tumeric. Refrigerate and use for side dishes or hot (microwaved) snacks.

about 500 calories a day, or increase your physical activity by 500 calories a day, or a combination of the two. But tracking calories is a lot of work if you do not automate your eating. (There are also programs for handheld devices that can do it for you, such as at www.mychoicescount.com.) The point, though, isn't to track calories; it's to let your body, your stomach, and your brain give you the signals to stop when you're satisfied, and not stuffed.

The YOU Diet Meals: YOUR Choices

Think of this rebooting program as the training wheels in waist management. It will help you find your eating balance. The plan is all about using body chemistry, not willpower, to succeed. For exam-

Soups: Make one or more of our filling YOU Soups (see recipes) once a week and store them in serving-size cups in the refrigerator. Eat 1 cup as a predinner appetizer, to take the edge off, or have a cup of soup as a snack.

Steel-cut Oats: If you're worried about time, cook up one week's worth of oats per directions and store in the refrigerator for up to a week. For some people, that may seem as appetizing as a slice of baked wrapping paper, but reheated oats actually taste great.

Emergency Foods: Every house needs fire-extinguisher foods — good-for-you foods that will put out three-alarm starvation fires. Our list of foods that you can reach for when you're hungry include any of the above foods as well as a handful of almonds, peanuts, or walnuts; bags of store-bought, prechopped fruits and veggies; dried fruit (apricots, cranberries); and edamame (soybeans — look for microwave bags in the frozen food section). In a real pinch? Pop one of those mint breath strips — they can help turn off appetite by making food less appetizing.

ple, lots of fiber and lots of protein are included in the morning. (In case you skipped from the first chapter to this one, fiber in the morning helps control afternoon cravings. Extra protein decreases appetite.) More body-chem help comes from all the good fats — nuts, olives, olive oil, omega 3-rich fish oils — which help keep your sense of fullness and healthy HDL cholesterol up and your lousy LDL cholesterol down. We've limited simple sugars because they set off sharp swings in blood sugar levels that put you into a cycle of craving high-calorie foods. Plus all of these food-moves fight the destructive inflamma-

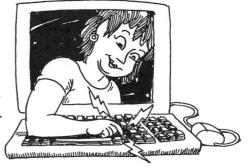

tory effects that make you hungry, your arteries unhealthy, and your waist larger, not smaller.

At a glance, you'll see lots of raw veggies and whole wheat toast. In fact, the same-old-same-old routine actually is the point. Studies show that people who eat the same meal for at least one meal a day lose more weight than those who have more variety. And if you're like our patients, you won't be hungry on this plan. Having a lot of food choices is what makes us live life like we're in a never-ending speed-eating contest. But decrease your food choices, and you'll automatically decrease your appetite and waist size. Pick the one meal you rush through most and automate it. For most people, it's lunch. So find a healthy lunch you like — salad with grilled chicken and olive oil, turkey on whole-grain bread — and have it for lunch every day. Every day. Yes, every day.

Below, we've listed your options for every food moment of the day (except dinner, which you'll find outlined specifically in the daily schedule). You can choose any of the options listed, but ideally choose just one or two to eat on most days. We've found that the most successful people are those who pick just one — and stick with it.

YOUR Breakfast Choices

For Cereal Lovers	For Egg Lovers	For Bread Lovers	For Breakfast Haters
Cooked oat cereal with 4 ounces of skim milk, or soy milk fortified with vitamin D and calcium, and 1 fistful of your favorite fruit OR 1 cup Kashi high-fiber or cold-oat cereal (like Cheerios) with 1 fistful of your favorite fruit, with 4 ounces of skim milk, or soy milk fortified with vitamin D and calcium	Egg-white omelet (3 egg whites and 1 whole egg), plus cut-up mixed veggies OR 2 scrambled, poached, or hard-boiled eggs with 2 pieces of lean turkey sausage or tofu sausage	1 slice toasted whole wheat bread with 1 teaspoon peanut butter, or 1 teaspoon apple or walnut butter or avocado spread	Magical Breakfast Blaster (see recipe, page 330) OR Pineapple-Banana Protein Blaster (see recipe, page 329)

YOUR Lunch Choices

Meal-Size Salad	Soup and Salad	Healthy Burger	Fast Food
Chopped salad: 6 chopped walnuts, chopped veggies (your choice), and chopped mixed greens tossed with 4 ounces of salmon, turkey, or chicken breast; with balsamic vinegar (2 parts) and olive oil (1 part) dressing OR One of the YOU Salads (recipes follow)	1 cup of one of the many hearty YOU Soups plus any of the YOU Salads (recipes for both follow) or a non-Caesar salad using olive or canola oil, or balsamic vinegar and olive oil dressing	Veggie burger or Boca Spicy Chik'n Patty on a toasted whole wheat English muffin with 1 tablespoon of fructose-free olive oil–based marinara sauce, sliced tomato, romaine lettuce or spinach leaves, plus slices of red onion	See best options for fast-food meals on page 322.

YOUR Morning and Afternoon Snack Choices

Fruit and Nuts	Grains and Berries	Revved-up Veggies	Fruit and Yogurt
1/2 ounce raw nuts with an apple, banana, plum, pear, orange, wedge of melon, cup of berries, 2 kiwis, 1/2 grapefruit, or any other fruit	1/2 cup whole-grain cereal mixed with 1/4 cup almonds and 1/4 cup dried berries, apricots, or raisins	1 cup of cut-up sautéed veggies, warmed in microwave and stuffed into small whole wheat pita OR Cut-up veggies dipped into 4 ounces plain yogurt or low-fat cottage cheese mixed with lots of dill, chives, ginger, red pepper flakes, or other spices (your choice) OR Just plain cut-up veggies	Low-fat probiotic (live culture) yogurt covered with 1/2 cup of canned, unsweetened peaches or mandarin oranges and some raisins

YOUR Dessert Choices

Eat Every Other Day

Cinnamon Baked Apples with Tangerine and Cranberries (see recipe)

OR

Cinnamon Apple Sauté à la Mode (see recipe)

OR

Roasted Pear with Raspberry Coulis, Chocolate, and Pistachios (see recipe)

OR

Sliced Peaches with Raspberries, Blueberries, and Chocolate Chips (see recipe)

OR

1 ounce of dark chocolate (made with real cocoa), approximately three or four bites

YOUR Evening Snack Choices

(But Don't Eat after 8:30 p.m.)

Simon's Popcorn (see recipe)

OR

Any snack option

OR

Whole wheat pita toasts and Tomato-Avocado Salsamole (see recipe)

YOUR Drink Choices

Plain or sparkling water (with fruit slice if desired), skim milk, coffee, hot or iced tea (decaffeinated is best if you have problems sleeping), diet soda (but only 1 to 2 a day)

For breakfast, you may include an 8-ounce glass of fruit or vegetable juice, such as tomato juice or 100 percent grapefruit juice or orange juice with pulp, fortified with calcium and vitamin D

For dinner, you can include one glass of alcohol, which we prefer you to drink toward the end of the meal so it does not hinder your satiety center's ability to slow your voracious appetite. If you're a nondrinker, it's OK to swap for a teetotaler's cocktail made with low-sugar grape juice, sparkling water, and lime

Dish List

Nowadays, foods have more labels than a clothes rack, ingredient names look like the names of Greek goddesses, and cunning marketing lingo makes sugar-drenched cereal appear as if it's healthier than a bundle of prunes. And that's just not the case. Prince Nutrition sounds great until you read the label and find no nutrient other than sugar and saturated fat neatly disguised. The trick to navigating through store aisles is not only to shop for value and whisk the kids past the Admiral Nutrition candy bars and potato chips but also to shop for content — for the ingredients and nutrients that allow you to eat smart, not diet hard. Here is our guide for ingredient inspection:

Look for less. Generally, fewer labels and ingredients equal better foods. Natural foods that come directly from the ground generally don't require labels. (Ever seen a marshmallow bush?) That's why any produce is generally OK for you. (One caveat: Make sure it has a great feel, a healthy smell, and has not been waxed; waxed versions are like a Barbie doll — look great, but not much substance. These versions often have less taste and less nutrition.)

Turn the package. Ignore what's on the front of the package and go directly to the food label and ingredient list. "Fat-free!" or "zero trans fats" may sound like a dieter's dream, but fat-free foods (especially salad dressing) can be loaded with more sugar than a baker's bowl. Another caution: Just because something "contains whole grains" doesn't mean it's made entirely or even mostly with whole grains (more on deciphering "whole grains" on page 319). Bottom line: The front of the package isn't even as revealing as the outside of a new car. It might look seductive, but you really have to check what's under the hood to see what it's all about. The ingredient list is where all the answers are.

Beware of the imposters. Many foods contain cheat words in their ingredient list — the words don't clearly scream "imminent heart attack!" as some other words may, but they indicate danger all the same. Some notable clues to watch for:

For sugar: Dextrose, sucrose, or anything with "ose." And mannitol, or anything with "ol." Those are alcohols that are quickly converted to sugar. Stay away from foods that have more than 4 grams of sugar in them. Even natural sugars such as maple syrup and molasses are sugar, so you should also keep them to fewer than 4 grams per serving, unless it's pure fruit (we make that exception because fruit has so many nutrients).

For fats: Besides saturated fats (fewer than 4 grams per serving) and trans fats (avoid them all), you should avoid foods with other fat code words, like partially hydrogenated, palm, and coconut oil.

Relax. We don't want you to spend more time in the store than you did in freshman economics class. If you haven't inspected labels before, it'll just take some time before you know exactly how to ID the nutritional heroes and the imposters. We also don't want you to be paranoid shopper or paranoid about eating — some dangerous-sounding foods such as walnuts or real peanut butter or even honey (fewer than 4 grams per serving here) are OK in moderation.

The Fourteen-Day YOU Diet

During these two weeks, we'll give you the meal guidelines, the tools, the strategies, the tricks, the plan, and the help you need to change your diet into a live-it. By the end of the fourteen days, you'll have developed eating patterns and behavioral habits that will help get you on your way to changing your body from the inside out. Here we outline the seven-day plan and strategies for making smart decisions about food and eating. In week two, you'll repeat the first week, making appropriate food substitutions where you wish.

Day One: Saturday

1. **Walk:** Thirty minutes. Walking — whether you do it by yourself, with a friend, with your dog (only actual walking time

counts, not time spent waiting for the dog to sniff), or around the dining room table — gives you your first dose of physical success. Walk every day for 30 minutes, and you'll establish the behavioral and motivational foundation for the YOU Diet.

2. **Stretch:** Do three to five minutes of stretching after your walk. See Chapter 11. While stretching keeps your muscles limber and flexible to help prevent injury, it also has a meditative element to it, helping you refocus and cope with cravings, as we explain on page 249. "No pain, no gain" does not apply here.

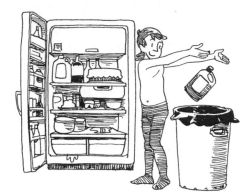

3. **Dump Your Fridge:** To make room for all the new, good food you're about to buy, it's time to rid your kitchen of the nutritional felons. The appeals are up; it's execution time. Read the label of everything in your kitchen cupboards, your refrigerator, your secret boxes, and everywhere else you stash food. If something has any of the following in one of the first five ingredients, throw it out:

- Simple sugar. This includes brown sugar, dextrose, corn sweetener, fructose (as in high-fructose corn syrup), glucose, corn syrup, honey, invert sugar, maltose, lactose, malt syrup, molasses, raw sugar, and sucrose. Keep a little table sugar handy, and honey, and maple sugar, because you'll use some for recipes. (See our box on other sweeteners on pages 131–132.)

- Saturated fat. This includes most four-legged animal fat, milk fat, butter or lard, and tropical oils, such as palm and coconut.

- Trans fat. This includes partially hydrogenated fats, vegetable oil blends that are hydrogenated, and many margarines and cooking blends. (If you must, use cholesterol-fighting sterol spreads such as Promise and Benecol.)

■ Enriched flours and all flours other than 100 percent whole grain or 100 percent whole wheat. This includes enriched white flour, semolina, durum wheat, and any of the acronyms for flour that is not whole wheat — they should not be in your kitchen.

4. **Go Food Shopping:** Your current kitchen is most likely like a prison — it's filled with a lot of bad dudes. We want to turn your kitchen into a nutritional honor society, so that it's filled with good-for-your-waist foods that make it easy (and automatic!) to eat right. The first week, you'll have a larger-than-normal shopping list because you'll stock up on essentials as well as ingredients you'll need for this week's recipes. For a specific shopping list that works with our suggested seven-day schedule, see page 314.

5. **Make Your Weekly Staples:** Your choice of vegetables or soup. See above.

Eat!

Follow guidelines for breakfast, lunch, and snacks. For dinner, have . . .

Asian Salmon with Brown Rice Pilaf

Day Two: Sunday

1. **Walk:** Thirty minutes.
2. **Stretch:** Do five minutes of stretching.
3. **Partner Up:** If you try to undertake this alone, there's a much higher risk that you'll end up lips-first in a bowl of creamed corn. Find your YOU partner — be it a spouse, a friend, a coworker — someone you can talk to about your goals, your meals, your new plan. Make a plan to talk (or email) five minutes every day — to tell him or her that you walked that day and to tell about your day's meals. If you prefer a cyber friend, log on to www.realage.com and match up with a partner there.

   Better yet, try to find a partner or partners who are in this *with* you. Share this book; share the knowledge you've learned; embark on a "work smart, not hard" journey together. It's one thing to lose three, four, or five inches yourself, but quite another when you can help contribute to America's collective loss in waistband size. After all, what's better than experiencing the satisfaction of helping yourself achieve your goal? Helping others do the same.

Eat!

Follow guidelines for breakfast, lunch, and snacks. For dinner, have . . .

Spicy Chili or Stuffed Whole Wheat Pizza

Day Three: Monday

1. **Walk:** Thirty minutes.
2. **Do the YOU Workout:** Follow the twenty-minute no-weights YOU Workout, which includes both strength and stretching exercises, on page 258. Strength training helps you add muscle, which will help speed your metabolism and burn fat. Also start tightening your abs when you walk, which will help improve your posture and make your clothes fit better. Walk at a pace that raises your heart rate, or include twenty minutes of another cardiovascular exercise.
3. **Write It Down (or Type It In):** Generally, we're into guilt trips as much as we're into bourbon as a topical anesthetic, but we also think there's a fine line between guilt and motivation. One of the ways you can help reprogram yourself is by writing down (or recording, for you technophiles) everything that you eat. In a way, it holds you accountable; you won't want to eat bad foods, because you won't want the visual reminder that you ate them. For these two weeks only — just to establish your new routine — write down everything you eat. Yep, even the three M&M's you just swiped. (For the technically savvy, some handheld devices have programs that allow you to scan the bar codes of the foods you eat. You enter the quantity you eat, and the program will keep track of your calories — see www.realage.com or www.mychoicescount.com.)

4. **Go Shopping:** With three days of walking under your soon-to-be-loose belt, it's time you made another trip to the store. This time, make it the sports store — for a good pair of running shoes. Use them for walking only. Running shoes are light-weight, and they provide lots of heel cushioning (because they're made for people who pound the ground with more force). Your best bet: Go to a running specialty store, where the staff can not only measure your feet but analyze your stride and determine what kind of walker you are. (Note: Go shopping in the late afternoon when your feet are more likely to be swollen, to ensure the best fit.) If you like, you can also add these to your list:

- Socks with extra padding on the bottom. (Avoid cotton; you need socks that wick moisture away from your feet.)
- A yoga mat, so you don't slip and slide while enjoying the deep poses (and dumbbells or resistance bands if you're already advanced enough to use those; see page 277).

Eat!

Follow guidelines for breakfast, lunch, and snacks. For dinner, have . . .

Mediterranean Chicken with Tomato, Olives, and Herbed White Beans

Day Four: Tuesday

1. **Walk:** Thirty minutes.
2. **Stretch:** Do five minutes of stretching.
3. **Make Any Needed YOU-Turn:** It's not uncommon at this point for you to have already dabbled in the neighbor's cake, picked at the kids' chips, or snuck a few bites of a butter-covered pretzel from the mall. And that's OK. Just get yourself back together.

   At the next available moment, make an authorized YOU-Turn.

   The next time you find yourself dancing with the Devil Dog,

try these coping strategies:

- ***The Lip Lick.*** Breathe in, lick your lips, swallow, and breathe out slowly, saying "ohm." Let the cool air flow across your lips. The soothing move — which takes all of about three seconds — helps you to reset, calm down, and refocus.

- ***The Waist Hang.*** Stand up straight, bend over at your waist, and let your lower back relax. Reach for the floor, grab your elbows, or hold the back of your knees. The important thing is to let all of the tension you have stored in your back and hips unwind. Relax your neck completely. If you feel tight, don't straighten your knees.

Eat!

Follow guidelines for breakfast, lunch, and snacks. For dinner, have . . .

Royal Pasta Primavera Provençale

Day Five: Wednesday

1. **Walk:** Thirty minutes.
2. **Do the YOU Workout:** Follow the twenty-minute no-weights YOU Workout, which includes both strength and stretching exercises, on page 258.
3. **Call Your Doctor:** Remember, waist management is a team game, and your doctor is one of your MVPs. So schedule an appointment for 30 days from now (or sooner if you have a great relationship). You can use him or her to help you in many different ways:

   - Update your vitals such as blood pressure, waist size, and heart rate. If you need a baseline for such numbers as HDL and LDL cholesterol (HDL is more important for women), now's a good time to schedule a physical, get a few blood tests, and talk to your doctor about your new plan.
   - Having a physical will also prove helpful when you reach a

plateau — when your waist and weight loss will seem to have stalled. (Your doctor may then be able to prescribe medication that can help you get over a hump; see appendix A.)

Eat!

Follow guidelines for breakfast, lunch, and snacks. For dinner, have . . .

Apricot Chicken and Green Beans with Almond Slivers

Day Six: Thursday

1. **Walk:** Thirty minutes.
2. **Stretch:** Do five minutes of stretching.
3. **Do a Little Bragging:** If you go public with your success, it makes turning back more difficult. Tell a friend or a coworker about the progress you've made and the changes you've noticed.

Eat!

Follow guidelines for breakfast, lunch, and snacks. For dinner, have . . .

Turkey Tortilla Wraps with Red Baked Potato

Day Seven: Friday

1. **Walk:** Thirty minutes.
2. **Do the YOU Workout:** Follow the twenty-minute no-weights YOU Workout, which includes both strength and stretching exercises, on page 258.
3. **Restock Your Kitchen:** Check your pantry for ingredients you've run out of and make a shopping list for next week's recipes.
4. **Grade Yourself:** Whether it's with work or a first date, it's always nice to have some way to know how you're progressing. Now is the time to take your waist measurement and weigh yourself, just to see what changes you've made. In your first week, you may see up to a one-inch waist reduction and a two-

to four-pound weight reduction. You might even be able to drop one clothing size.

Eat!

Follow guidelines for breakfast, lunch, and snacks. For dinner, have . . .

Broiled Trout, Orata, or Branzini with Rosemary and Lemon

Day Eight to Forever: Your Reprogrammed Body

There you have it. We've given you all the tools, actions, and adjustments you need to take your body back to its factory settings, with a healthy waist and a healthy weight. Now just repeat the steps for the second week, making meal substitutions as you like (see additional recipes starting on page 329). Work smart, not hard. Week one puts you in motion and allows your body to adjust. Week two gives you seven days to practice the plan, feel what it's like to eat well, and figure out what to do if you don't. Research shows that it takes two weeks of repetitive action to make the action become automated, so now you can take the plan and tweak it. Or repeat it. Or try new dinner recipes that you can find on our website, www.realage.com. Make adjustments based on our nutritional guidelines as well as your tastes. This isn't the end of your waist-management plan; it's just the beginning.

Somewhere between the second and third week of the program, data shows that the behavior changes that are crucial for sustained waist loss will start to become ingrained in you. About the same time, your newly detoxified body will become more sensitive to poor-quality foods. Instead, as you adopt the *YOU: On a Diet* habits, you will crave the foods similar to the ones we list. Your liver will enjoy not having to manage toxic elements and will pass along the love to the rest of the body by reducing inflammation. All the data we have on folks who have lost a lot of weight and kept it off points to using a steady, resilient program. You can make mistakes but still bounce back if you keep moving and keep making calm YOU-Turns without a lot of emotional baggage. The types of foods we advocate will always come to your rescue even if you make a few wrong turns, anyway.

When you reach a plateau — which you will — you will have three choices: drop another few calories from your daily intake, increase your physical activity, or see a physician about extra help if appropriate. But remember that the purpose of losing weight is to gain health, so when you reach your playing weight and your body is loving the feeling, just stay the course.

Sample Eating Schedule

Above, we've given you all the tools you need to reprogram your kitchen, your body, and the biochemicals that will keep you from going hungry and that will keep you from storing fat. Below, we put it all into action by giving you a sample week showing how the YOU Diet works. Want a plan that requires absolutely no thought at all? Then follow this schedule and the shopping list on page 314.

Note: Because we all have higher or lower caloric needs (depending on genes, metabolic rates, activity levels, and other factors), we do not dictate serving sizes here. Your goal is to eat the amount that makes you satisfied — that's a level three or four on our satiety scale (see page 226), not feeling more bloated than a puffer fish. For some people, portions may be a little more than a traditional serving size. For others, they may be a little less.

Sunday

Breakfast: Egg-white omelet; juice and coffee or tea
Morning Snack: Revved-up Veggies with dip
Lunch: Healthy Burger with the works
Afternoon Snack: Yogurt with fruit
Dinner: Asian Salmon with Brown Rice Pilaf
Dessert: 1 ounce dark chocolate with orange slices
Drinks: Water, coffee, tea, etc., as you wish (see proposed broader list)

Monday

Breakfast: Magical Breakfast Blaster

Morning Snack: 1/2 ounce raw nuts

Lunch: Chopped salad of walnuts, veggies, greens, and salmon/turkey/chicken

Afternoon Snack: Yogurt with fruit

Dinner: Stuffed Whole Wheat Pizza

Evening Snack: Simon's Popcorn

Drinks: Water, coffee, tea, etc., as you wish

Tuesday

Breakfast: Cheerios with skim milk; juice and coffee or tea

Morning Snack: Apple

Lunch: Cup of Garden Harvest Soup; Cranberries, Walnuts, and Crumbled Cheese over Greens

Afternoon Snack: Yogurt with fruit

Dinner: Mediterranean Chicken with Tomato, Olives, and Herbed White Beans

Dessert: Cinnamon Apple Sauté à la Mode

Drinks: Water, coffee, tea, etc., as you wish

Wednesday

Breakfast: Magical Breakfast Blaster

Morning Snack: 1 ounce raw nuts

Lunch: Chopped salad of walnuts, veggies, greens, and salmon/turkey/chicken

Afternoon Snack: Yogurt and fruit

Dinner: Royal Pasta Primavera Provençale

Evening Snack: Tomato-Avocado Salsamole and pita toasts

Drinks: Water, coffee, tea, etc., as you wish

Thursday

Breakfast: Cheerios with skim milk; juice and coffee or tea
Morning Snack: Plum
Lunch: Cup of Garden Harvest Soup: Cranberries, Walnuts, and Crumbled Cheese over Greens
Afternoon Snack: Revved-up Veggies in 1/2 whole wheat pita
Dinner: Apricot Chicken and Green Beans with Almond Slivers
Dessert: 1 ounce dark chocolate with a sliced orange
Drinks: Water, coffee, tea, etc., as you wish

Friday

Breakfast: Magical Breakfast Blaster
Morning Snack: 1 ounce raw nuts
Lunch: Chopped salad of walnuts, veggies, greens, and salmon/turkey/chicken
Afternoon Snack: Yogurt with fruit
Dinner: Turkey Tortilla Wraps with Red Baked Potato
Evening Snack: Simon's Popcorn
Drinks: Water, coffee, tea, etc., as you wish

Saturday

Breakfast: Cheerios with skim milk; juice and coffee or tea
Morning Snack: Yogurt with fruit
Lunch: Cup of Garden Harvest Soup; Cranberries, Walnuts, and Crumbled Cheese over Greens
Afternoon Snack: Revved-up Veggies with dip
Dinner: Broiled Trout, Orata, or Branzini with Rosemary and Lemon; Rock Asparagus
Dessert: Cinnamon Apple Sauté à la Mode
Drinks: Water, coffee, tea, etc., as you wish

Your Shopping List

The first week, you'll be buying more stuff than all other weeks, as you're gathering the building blocks for your new fridge and pantry (including spices, oils, and other long-term ingredients). We believe in working from the inside of the store out so that heat and bacteria have less time to grow on your produce before you get it home. This list includes both your staples and your ingredients for the recipes on our seven-day sample schedule (see page 311 for two people). You can make weekly or biweekly shopping lists for any of the recipes and snack choices and for any number of people (one to twenty-four) at www.realage.com.

Shopping List Basics

Serves two for one week:

- The shopping list has been subdivided into categories to make shopping easier (grains, refrigerated items, protein, dried fruits and nuts, fresh veggies, and so forth).
- A general condiment list has been included below for seasonings, spices, oils, and so on, needed to complete the recipes. You may already have many of these items in your pantry.
- Tomato or cranberry juice can be substituted for any or all of the orange juice.

Inside Aisles: Grains

1 box cold oat cereal (Cheerios)

1 package 100 percent whole wheat or 100 percent whole-grain English muffins (try to find without sugar, honey, or high-fructose corn syrup added)

One 12-inch or 10-ounce prepared thin 100 percent whole-grain pizza crust

1 box short-grain brown rice

1 box 100 percent whole wheat rigatoni or linguine pasta

1 box steel-cut oatmeal

1 bag small 100 percent whole wheat pitas

1 bag 100 percent whole wheat tortillas

Inside Aisles: Canned/Jarred Items

2 quarts (8 cups) low-salt vegetable or chicken stock or broth
1 can (15 or 16 ounces) white beans
2 cans (14 1/2 ounces each) stewed tomatoes
1 can whole, crushed, or diced tomatoes
16 ounces tomato sauce (with olive or canola oil and less than 4 grams of sugar per 1/2 cup)
1 jar kalamata olives, halved
1 jar olive relish or tapenade
1 can sun-dried tomato bits or finely chopped sun-dried tomatoes (not in oil)
2 cans unsweetened peaches or tangerines
1 small can jalapeño peppers
1 jar popping corn (enough to make 8 cups)
1 jar unsweetened apple juice or cider (preferably organic)
1 jar apple butter (keep in fridge)
1 jar all-natural peanut butter (no trans fat, no added sugar or fructose)

Inside Aisles: Dried Fruits and Nuts

1 bag raw walnuts (at least 8 ounces)
1 bag raw hazelnuts (at least 4 ounces)
1 bag raw almonds (at least 4 ounces)
1 bag slivered almonds (at least 1/4 cup)
1 bag dried cranberries (at least 3/4 cup)
1 bag dried apricots
1 package chopped pistachios (enough for 1 1/2 tablespoons)

Staple Condiments/Spices: Buy these or make sure you have them in your pantry. Refill as needed.

Olive oil
Canola oil
Salt

Pepper

Fresh garlic

Low-sodium soy sauce

Balsamic vinegar

Wine vinegar

Maple syrup (look for a brand that doesn't have high-fructose corn syrup listed in the first four ingredients)

Marinara sauce or other red tomato sauce

Dijon mustard

Hot red pepper sauce

Pam spray-on canola oil

Nutmeg

Cinnamon

Your favorite coffee or tea

Dark chocolate bar with at least 70 percent cocoa, or 1 small bag mini semisweet all-cocoa chocolate chips (not milk chocolate and without milk fat)

Refrigerated Items

1 half gallon skim milk or low-fat soy milk fortified with calcium and vitamin D

1 quart 100 percent orange or grapefruit juice with pulp, fortified with calcium, magnesium, and vitamin D

1 1/2 cups (6 ounces) crumbled farmer cheese

6 eggs

1 bag finely shredded part-skim mozzarella cheese (enough for 2 ounces)

eight 4-ounce containers of probiotic low-fat yogurt

Chicken/Turkey/Fish

2 bone-in chicken thighs without skin

2 skinless, boneless chicken breast halves (about 4 ounces each)

12 ounces sliced cooked salmon (or white turkey or chicken from deli)

8 ounces skinless salmon fillets (or skinless chicken or turkey breasts)

1 whole fish (trout, orata, or branzini, about 4 ounces per serving)

Frozen Food

1 box Boca Spicy Chik'n Patties
1 bag frozen unsweetened blueberries
1 bag frozen unsweetened raspberries
1 small container nonfat or low-fat vanilla frozen yogurt

Health Food Aisle or Health Food Store

Soy protein (like Nature's Plus Spiru-Tein)
Psyllium
Flaxseed

Other

1 bottle white wine

Produce Area (shop last)

Wild Card: If you especially like particular fruits or vegetables, buy them in whatever quantities you want and eat them as substitutions or additions to your recipes (especially in season).
three 10-ounce bags of salad mix (classic romaine or other mixed-green salad)
10 cups mixed mesclun or spring greens
1 pound cut-up stir-fry veggies (asparagus, broccoli, cauliflower, mushrooms, multicolored bell peppers, red and white onions, zucchini)
Sliced carrots, apples, broccoli and/or celery in a package
2 pounds other veggies (your choice) to sauté, dip, mix into omelets, chop into salads
5 small apples (Jonagold or Ambrosia)
2 small plums
3 tomatoes
1 bunch of carrots
1 bunch bananas
2 red bell peppers

1 yellow or orange bell pepper
1 small head cabbage
1 cup thin green beans
1 pound asparagus spears
1 small eggplant
3 shallots
2 large cloves garlic
3 medium yellow onions
1 red onion
1 small bunch green onions
1 small dried ancho or pasilla chili pepper
1 large russet baking potato
1 bunch each fresh parsley, basil, rosemary, thyme (or lemon thyme), chives, oregano, and chervil
1 piece gingerroot
1 lime
1 avocado
1 small basket fresh raspberries (if available; if not, substitute frozen)
1 small basket fresh blueberries (if available; if not, substitute frozen)

The Whole Truth

It used to be that the only thing with a hole in it was a doughnut. Now, it seems, everything is touted as "whole" this or that. Whole grains, whole wheat, a whole lot of health: It's the latest in food marketing. Why? Because food manufacturers know that whole grains are, in fact, one of the healthiest ingredients you can eat. Surely, more and more foods are made with them, but that doesn't mean all are created equal. Why? Because those marketing words don't always present an accurate picture of what's inside the food.

To decipher the whole mess, you first need to understand what exactly whole grains are and how they work. "Whole grain" means the grain still has all three of its original elements: the outer shell or bran, which contains fiber and B vitamins; the germ, which contains

318

phytochemicals and B vitamins; and the endosperm (what a name), which contains carbohydrates and protein. The key is that they're "whole" and not "refined," by stripping away the bran and germ, which leaves you eating only the aptly named endosperm. Instead, the whole grain should be left intact — meaning you get more fiber and more micronutrients that help protect against disease. These whole grains are also healthy for you because

> To make sure you receive the health and dietary benefits of whole grains and wheat, the labels should read "100 percent whole grain" or "100 percent whole wheat." Anything else means that the food is also made with the less-beneficial enriched or refined flour. Remember to avoid those with added sugars like high-fructose corn syrup or honey.

they're absorbed more slowly than enriched or bleached flour and thus raise glucose and insulin levels less — keeping you fuller longer and slowing your digestion. But not all foods that tout whole grains or whole wheat are the healthiest form. Some fake-out words you should watch out for:

Made with: It may have a drop of whole grains, but unless it's made entirely with them, you won't reap all the potential benefits.

100 Percent Wheat: This means it could have some or a lot or no "whole" wheat.

Multigrain: This tells you nothing about whether the grains are whole or refined. Even if you're getting 38 grains, that isn't much good if they are all refined.

Whole Grain: If the label doesn't say "100 percent whole grain," it may have many blends. Bad words to see: *enriched, bleached, unbleached, semolina, durum,* and *rice flour.*

Blends: "Whole grain blend" means it usually doesn't have much whole grain at all.

Good Source: This means it has 8 grams of whole grains per serv-

ing or as little as 13.5 percent. Don't confuse whole
grain with fiber; 8 grams of
whole grain may have less
than 1 gram of fiber.

Excellent Source: This means
it has 16 grams per serving
or as little as 27 percent.

Supports Heart Health: Any
food can say that it "supports" an organ. What you
want to see on the label:
"May reduce the risk of . . ."
This means that the food
has ingredients clinically
shown to be effective in reducing the risk of, say, heart
disease or high cholesterol,
depending on the
food.

FACTOID

To ensure that a whole grain
food has a slower absorption
in your digestive system and
thus lowers your sugar and insulin levels, eat a little fat with
it — in the form of 1/2 tablespoon of olive oil with your
bread. Alternatively, eat six
walnuts, twelve almonds, or
twenty peanuts about twenty
minutes before you eat the
whole grain.

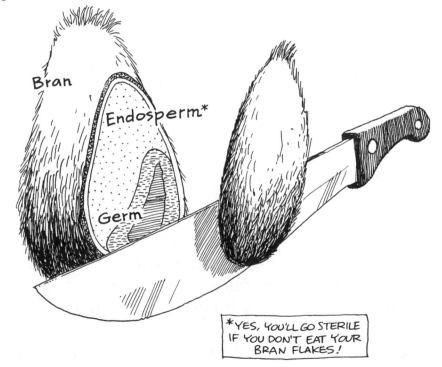

Bran

Endosperm*

Germ

*YES, YOU'LL GO STERILE
IF YOU DON'T EAT YOUR
BRAN FLAKES!

The Perfect Eating Environment

Research shows that your surroundings may play a role in determining how much you eat. Specifically, the more comfortable and relaxed you are, the more you lower your inhibitions. If you want to create the mood to keep you the fullest, make this your dining-room feng shui:

- Choose bright lights over soft lights.
- Choose a warm room temperature over cold.
- Choose conversation over music or TV, which can distract you into eating more.

When You Need the Fast-Food Fix

We understand how it is. Sometimes you need the absolute quickest path from food to belly. While most fast-food options are more destructive than a 4 a.m. vandal, you can still make smart choices in the drive-through lane. Some things to remember:

- There are some main dishes that can be good for you, but you have to be careful. Some slight name variations can make the difference between causing your fat and keeping you flat.
- Avoid side dishes and desserts unless indicated below. They're all loaded with bad fats and simple sugars, and they often have more calories than the main dishes.
- Choose low-calorie dressing, not low-fat. Low-fat dressings are steeped in HFCS, which has plenty of calories, and the fructose

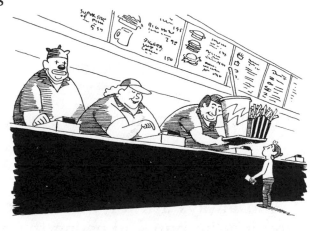

tricks your body into staying hungry.

■ Don't eat breakfast at fast-food places. There are virtually no healthy options on any breakfast menu we could find.

When life steers you out of the kitchen, these are your best bets at these places, which offer some decent alternatives.

	Main Dishes*	Best Salad Dressing	Best Sides
Wendy's	Mandarin Chicken Salad with roasted almonds (but without the crispy noodles)	Reduced-fat creamy ranch	Plain baked potato (ask for marinara sauce to top it), mandarin orange cup, Caesar side salad without croutons, chili
McDonald's	Fruit and walnut salad Caesar salad with grilled chicken	Newman's Own Cobb dressing	Fruit and yogurt parfait
Burger King	BK Veggie Burger (without cheese) Tendergrill Chicken Sandwich (without sauce)	Ken's light Italian dressing	Side garden salad
Taco Bell	Spicy Chicken Soft Taco	Bring your own	None at this time
Arby's	Arby's Chicken Breast Fillet	Raspberry vinaigrette	None at this time
Domino's Pizza	Pizza with green pepper, onions, mushrooms with crunchy thin crust	Use your own	None at this time

* And always ask for whole wheat buns. If not available, consider ditching the bun and eating the meat with a knife and fork.

Restaurant Tricks

Eating out can be a great experience — for everyone except your gut. With Rushmore-sized portions and dietary disasters in every plate, basket, and spoonful, restaurants are dangerous places. While you should always follow our guidelines for good foods (the waist foods, not the waste foods, in our crib sheet), you should also know that most dietary mistakes are made within the first and last ten minutes of any restaurant experience. Some tips for bookending your meal the right way:

- Return the free bread and ask if you can have cut-up raw vegetables instead. (Do this four times in a three-week period, and we've found that most good restaurants remember the trick and automatically make that change every time they see you — if they see you at least once a week.)
- Order oil and vinegar in separate containers and on the side for salad dressing, and put a little on. (You have to do this; relying on the waitstaff or chef to do so gets you about 400 extra calories per side salad.)
- Ask to replace the potato or rice with sauteed vegetables.
- If you're going to have dessert, order one for the table and have just a few bites.
- For a quick guide, use this chart to make smart eating-out choices:

Menu	Order It	Avoid It
American	Salad with oil and vinegar; veggie burger; grilled chicken; any vegetables, boiled and seasoned or sautéed with onions and garlic; baked potato with marinara sauce	Hamburger, grilled cheese, fries, anything that has *fried* in the name
Italian	Sautéed vegetables, salad, seafood salad, fish with olive oil, whole wheat pasta in small amounts with marinara sauce	Fried calamari and zucchini, stuffed mushrooms, baked ziti, fettuccine Alfredo, anything with bread crumbs, pizza with meat toppings and lots of cheese
Eastern Mediterranean	Hummus (chickpeas), tahini (sesame paste), tabbouleh (parsley salad), bean soup, lentils	Phyllo dough, meatballs, fried and breaded meals
Asian	Seaweed salad; sea vegetables; miso soup; edamame; sashimi; any vegetables that are not fried, such as bok choy, bamboo	Tempura; noodles (most are drenched in saturated fat); white rice; smoked foods; anything described as "fried" or "crispy," including fried rice, General Tso's chicken, fried

Menu	Order It	Avoid It
Asian (cont.)	shoots, sautéed green beans; green beans with snow peas and water chestnuts made without lard; broiled chicken; fresh spring rolls; moo shu chicken or vegetables; spicy eggplant; tofu (not fried); whole steamed fish; chicken soup; drunken chicken	noodles, and fried egg rolls; pickled food; food with too much soy sauce; egg dishes, such as egg foo yong, salty soups and monosodium glutamate on dishes for anyone younger than fourteen or any pregnant woman
Mexican	Fajitas, black beans, refried beans cooked without lard, guacamole as a condiment, brown rice, jicama, grilled chicken or fish, ceviche, avocados, chicken enchiladas without cheese, arroz con pollo (request brown rice), camarones	Fried flour or corn items such as tortillas, taco shells, sour cream, cheese, quesadillas, chalupas, nachos, ground beef or pork

Ready-made Meals

Sometimes it's easier to reach into the freezer than it is to pull out the pots, even when you do have drag-race-worthy recipes. That's OK. Plenty of ready-made choices are available for you to sub for one of your lunches or dinners, if that's easiest for you. You should still follow guidelines we've outlined (look at labels to avoid high levels of waist-busting ingredients, like more than 4 grams per serving of sugar or saturated fat and any trans fat). These are some of the ones we favor.

Soups:

Check sodium to make sure it's less than 400 milligrams per serving, and avoid soups with noodles, since they may be cooked in saturated or trans fats.

Dried: Health Valley and Fantastic Always Natural

Canned: Eden Organic, Health Valley, Amy's Organic Soups, Muir Glen Organic, Wolfgang Puck

Snacks:

Low-calorie cheese: Horizon Organic part-skim mozzarella sticks and veggie singles

Meals:

Check to make sure a meal is low in trans and saturated fats.

Lean Cuisine, Healthy Choice, Amy's Kitchen

The YOU Diet Troubleshooting Guide

If YOU...	Then YOU...
Eat something you shouldn't	Don't worry, but don't keep eating. Use one of our YOU-Turn techniques (a stretch, a meditation technique, or the lip lick) to refocus so you don't turn one mistake into a buffet-clearing gorge.
Stall with weight/waist loss	Talk to your doctor about using medication to help you get past the plateau to lead to further weight/waist loss (see page 377, appendix A).
Can't find a support partner	If you can't blackmail a partner with all the benefits she'll also receive (she too will learn about elegant solutions she can apply to her own life), then match yourself with one at www.realage.com.
Have a family that decides to go to the buffet tonight	Before you go, have a cup of soup, a handful of nuts, and one glass of water. That will fill you up before you eat, so you eat sensibly and automatically. And limit yourself to one trip with a seven- or nine-inch plate, and keep it to single-story servings.
Feel foot pain and find it hard to walk	Stop walking and find an alternative activity such as biking or swimming. See a podiatrist to diagnose your ailment.

The YOU Diet Troubleshooting Guide

If YOU . . .	Then YOU . . .
Travel all the time and have to eat on the road a lot	Rely on more snacks rather than gorging on big meals. Travel with easy-to-carry (in plastic baggies) snacks such as nuts and cut-up apples and carrots to take the edge off your hunger.
Are diagnosed with a serious illness	It's not always the time to lose weight when you're sick, but it is the ideal time to get food on your side. But if you're prescribed a drug that may slow weight loss (like a beta-blocker), talk to your doctor about a more aggressive weight-loss approach that's ailment-appropriate, since subsequent weight loss is more difficult.
Might have a food allergy (for example, irritable bowel syndrome or unexplained lethargy)	Do the elimination diet found on page 129.

The YOU Diet Recipes

YOU Drinks

Pineapple-Banana Protein Blaster
2 servings ■ 207 calories per serving

1 large ripe banana
1/2 cup low-fat (1 percent) soy milk
1 can (4 ounces) crushed pineapple in juice, undrained
1/2 cup "pineapple-passion" sorbet, such as Select brand
  (a Safeway brand)
1 tablespoon soy protein powder (8 grams protein)

Peel banana; break into chunks. Combine all ingredients in blender. Cover; blend until fairly smooth.

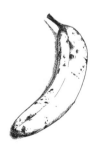

What's in it for you?	
Total fat	2 g
Saturated fat	0.8 g
Healthy fats	1.1 g
Fiber	2.1 g
Carbohydrates	38 g
Sugar	17 g
Protein	11 g
Sodium	31 mg
Calcium	39 mg
Magnesium	40 mg
Selenium	1 mcg
Potassium	428 mg

Magical Breakfast Blaster

2 servings ■ 136 calories per serving

1/2 large ripe banana (or other fruit of your choice)
1 scoop (1/3 cup) Soy Protein (like Nature's Plus Spiru-Tein: natures
   plus.com)
1/2 tablespoon flaxseed oil
1/4 cup frozen blueberries
1/2 tablespoon apple juice concentrate or honey
1 teaspoon psyllium seed husks
8 ounces water

Peel banana; break into chunks. Combine all ingredients in a blender. Optional: Add a few cubes of ice, as well as powdered vitamins. Cover; blend until fairly smooth.

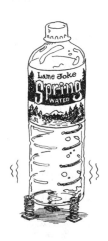

What's in it for you?	
Total fat	2.6 g
Saturated fat	0.3 g
Healthy fats	2.4 g
Fiber	6.3 g
Carbohydrates	16.8 g
Sugar	11.1 g
Protein	29 g
Sodium	380 mg
Calcium	93.5 mg
Magnesium	33.1 mg
Selenium	1.8 mcg
Potassium	195 mg

Garden Harvest Soup

10 servings (about 1 cup each) ■ 176 calories per serving

1 tablespoon olive oil
1 medium onion, chopped
1 carrot, chopped
4 garlic cloves, thinly sliced
1 red bell pepper, chopped
2 quarts (8 cups) low-salt vegetable or chicken stock or broth
1 can (28 ounces) whole, crushed, or diced tomatoes, undrained
2 cups water
1 small head cabbage, thinly sliced
1/2 teaspoon hot red pepper sauce (optional)
Salt and freshly ground black pepper (optional)
Optional garnishes: chopped fresh parsley, chopped fresh cilantro

Heat a large saucepan over medium-high heat. Add oil, then onion; cook 5 minutes, stirring occasionally. Stir in carrot, garlic, and bell pepper; cook until tender. Add stock, tomatoes, water, and cabbage; simmer uncovered 20 minutes. Season to taste with hot sauce and salt and pepper if desired. Garnish with parsley or cilantro if desired.

What's in it for you?	
Total fat	4 g
Saturated fat	0.8 g
Healthy fats	2.85 g
Fiber	3.6 g
Carbohydrates	15.9 g
Sugar	4.6 g
Protein	7.1 g
Sodium	374 mg
Calcium	73 mg
Magnesium	35 mg
Selenium	5.6 mcg
Potassium	631 mg

Lisa's Great Gazpacho

4 servings (about 1 cup each) ■ 120 calories per serving

1 can (28 ounces) crushed or diced tomatoes, undrained
1 cup tomato juice
1 cup *each:* diced (1/4 inch) red or orange bell pepper, unpeeled cucumber
1/4 cup finely chopped red onion
2 green onions, finely chopped
1 bunch cilantro leaves, chopped
3 tablespoons red wine vinegar or apple cider vinegar
3 tablespoons extra-virgin olive oil
2 dashes (or to taste) hot red pepper sauce
2 garlic cloves, minced
Salt and freshly ground black pepper (optional)
Optional garnishes: chopped fresh parsley, diced avocado

Place all ingredients except salt, pepper, and garnishes in large bowl and combine. Coarsely puree about half the mixture in a blender or food processor and return it to the bowl; stir well. Season to taste with salt and pepper if desired. Refrigerate for at least 2 hours and up to 8 hours before serving. Garnish as desired.

What's in it for you?	
Total fat	12.1 g
Saturated fat	1.8 g
Healthy fats	10.2 g
Fiber	4.6 g
Carbohydrates	19.2 g
Sugar	5.2 g
Protein	4.4 g
Sodium	207 mg
Calcium	74 mg
Magnesium	53 mg
Selenium	0.9 mcg
Potassium	780 mg

Spicy Vegetable Lentil Soup

10 servings (about 1 cup each) ■ 94 calories per serving

1 tablespoon olive oil
1 medium onion, chopped
1 carrot, chopped
1 red bell pepper, chopped
5 garlic cloves, sliced
2 quarts (8 cups) water
1 cup dried lentils
1 can (28 ounces) crushed tomatoes, undrained
2 bay leaves
2 tablespoons balsamic vinegar
Salt and freshly ground black pepper (optional)

Heat oil in a large saucepan over medium-high heat. Add onion; cook 5 minutes, stirring occasionally. Stir in carrot, bell pepper, and garlic; cook 3 minutes. Stir in remaining ingredients except salt and pepper; bring to a boil over high heat. Reduce heat; simmer uncovered 18 to 20 minutes, or until lentils and vegetables are tender. Season to taste with salt and pepper if desired. Remove bay leaves before serving.

What's in it for you?	
Total fat	1.6 g
Saturated fat	0.2 g
Healthy fats	1.4 g
Fiber	2.8 g
Carbohydrates	8 g
Sugar	1.6 g
Protein	1.9 g
Sodium	82 mg
Calcium	26 mg
Magnesium	16 mg
Selenium	0.6 mcg
Potassium	228 mg

Two-Onion Delight

8 servings (about 1 cup each) ■ 129 calories per serving

1 tablespoon olive oil
2 onions, sliced
2 shallots, sliced
1 leek (white and light-green part only), sliced
2 quarts (8 cups) low-salt chicken stock or broth
Salt and freshly ground black pepper (optional)
1/2 cup (4 ounces) grated low-fat Swiss cheese
1 bunch chives, finely chopped

Heat oil in a large saucepan over medium-high heat. Add onions; cook 5 minutes, stirring occasionally. Stir in shallots and leek; continue cooking until golden brown, about 5 minutes. Add stock; simmer uncovered 15 minutes. Season to taste with salt and pepper if desired. Ladle into shallow bowls; garnish with cheese and chives.

What's in it for you?	
Total fat	5 g
Saturated fat	1.2 g
Healthy fats	3.4 g
Fiber	0.3 g
Carbohydrates	12.3 g
Sugar	5.7 g
Protein	8.5 g
Sodium	385 mg
Calcium	84 mg
Magnesium	16 mg
Selenium	6.4 mcg
Potassium	321 mg

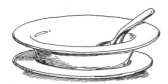

Curried Split Pea Soup

8 servings (about 1 cup each) ■ 155 calories per serving

1 tablespoon olive oil
1 onion, chopped
1 carrot, chopped
4 garlic cloves, sliced
1 quart (4 cups) low-salt vegetable stock or broth
1 quart (4 cups) water
1 cup dried yellow split peas
1 teaspoon curry powder
1 teaspoon ground cumin
1/2 bunch parsley, chopped

Heat oil in a large saucepan over medium-high heat. Add onion; cook 5 minutes, stirring occasionally. Add carrot and garlic; cook until softened, about 5 minutes. Add remaining ingredients except parsley; bring to a boil. Reduce heat; simmer uncovered 30 minutes, or until peas are tender. Ladle into shallow bowls; garnish with parsley.

What's in it for you?	
Total fat	3.6 g
Saturated fat	0.7 g
Healthy fats	2.7 g
Fiber	6.8 g
Carbohydrates	22 g
Sugar	5.1 g
Protein	9.5 g
Sodium	183 mg
Calcium	30.8 mg
Magnesium	38 mg
Selenium	3.4 mcg
Potassium	432 mg

Quick Black Bean Soup

8 servings (about 1 1/4 cups each) ■ 445 calories per serving

1 tablespoon olive oil
1 onion, chopped
3 garlic cloves, sliced
1 carrot, chopped
2 stalks celery, chopped
2 quarts (8 cups) low-salt vegetable stock or broth
2 cans (15 or 16 ounces each) black beans, rinsed and drained
1 teaspoon ground coriander
1/4 teaspoon cayenne pepper
1 tablespoon balsamic vinegar
1 bunch cilantro leaves, chopped

Heat oil in a large saucepan over medium-high heat. Add onion; cook 5 minutes, stirring occasionally. Add garlic, carrot, and celery; cook until soft, about 5 minutes. Add stock, beans, coriander, and cayenne pepper; simmer uncovered 10 minutes. Stir in vinegar. Transfer to blender or food processor; process to desired consistency. Reheat if necessary. Ladle into shallow bowls; garnish with cilantro.

What's in it for you?	
Total fat	6 g
Saturated fat	1.4 g
Healthy fats	2.8 g
Fiber	15.3 g
Carbohydrates	71.8 g
Sugar	7.4 g
Protein	27.4 g
Sodium	360 mg
Calcium	139 mg
Magnesium	180 mg
Selenium	1 mcg
Potassium	1,771 mg

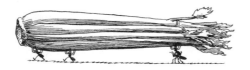

Minted Fresh Pea Soup

8 servings (about 1 cup each) ∎ 157 calories per serving

1 tablespoon olive oil
1 onion, chopped
1 carrot, chopped
2 garlic cloves, minced
2 cups frozen or fresh peas
2 quarts (8 cups) low-salt vegetable stock or broth
1 cup low-fat plain yogurt
Salt and freshly ground black pepper (optional)
1 small bunch mint leaves, chopped

Heat oil in a large saucepan over medium-high heat. Add onion; cook 5 minutes, stirring occasionally. Add carrot and garlic; cook until soft, about 5 minutes. Add peas and stock; simmer uncovered 20 minutes. Transfer in batches to blender or food processor and add yogurt; puree until smooth. Season to taste with salt and pepper if desired. Reheat if needed; ladle into shallow bowls; garnish with mint.

What's in it for you?	
Total fat	4.8 g
Saturated fat	1.1 g
Healthy fats	3.5 g
Fiber	2.3 g
Carbohydrates	18.2 g
Sugar	9.5 g
Protein	10 g
Sodium	376 mg
Calcium	84 mg
Magnesium	30.3 mg
Selenium	7.3 mcg
Potassium	466 mg

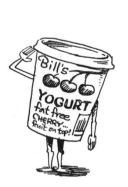

Japanese Ginger Salad with Pumpkin Seeds and Sprouts
8 servings ■ 230 calories per serving

Dressing Ingredients
1/2 cup olive oil
1/2 cup rice vinegar
1 small sweet onion, quartered
1 large carrot, chopped
1 tablespoon orange juice
1 tablespoon grated fresh ginger
1/4 teaspoon soy sauce
Salt and freshly ground black pepper (optional)

Salad Ingredients
2 large heads romaine lettuce, torn
1/2 cup fresh bean sprouts
1/4 cup pumpkin seeds

Combine all dressing ingredients except salt and pepper in blender or food processor; puree until smooth. Season to taste with salt and pepper if desired. Toss lettuce with dressing; top with sprouts and seeds.

What's in it for you?	
Total fat	22 g
Healthy fats	12.1 g
Fiber	6 g
Carbohydrates	16.8 g
Sugar	4 g
Protein	6.4 g
Sodium	53 mg
Calcium	79 mg
Magnesium	74 mg
Selenium	2 mcg
Potassium	499 mg

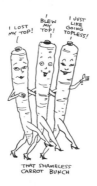

I LOST MY TOP! BLEW MY TOP! I JUST LIKE GOING TOPLESS!

THAT SHAMELESS CARROT BUNCH

338

Spinach-Walnut-Citrus Salad

2 servings ■ 246 calories per serving

Dressing Ingredients

1 tablespoon olive oil
1 tablespoon white wine vinegar
1 teaspoon honey
Dash of cayenne pepper
Salt and freshly ground black pepper (optional)

Salad Ingredients

1 large bunch spinach, washed and trimmed
1/4 cup walnut halves, raw or pan-roasted (beware of smoke-detector sounds if you do this like Dr. Mike and answer the phone when it rings only to forget what is in pan roasting)
1/2 orange, cut into segments
1/2 grapefruit, cut into segments
2 green onions, chopped

Combine oil, vinegar, honey, and cayenne pepper; mix well. Season to taste with salt and pepper if desired. Toss spinach with dressing and walnuts. Arrange orange and grapefruit sections on top and garnish with green onions.

What's in it for you?	
Total fat	17 g
Saturated fat	1.9 g
Healthy fats	14.4 g
Fiber	6.8 g
Carbohydrates	21 g
Sugar	7.6 g
Protein	8 g
Sodium	138 mg
Calcium	218 mg
Magnesium	169 mg
Selenium	3.6 mcg
Potassium	1,203 mg

Cranberries, Walnuts, and Crumbled Cheese Over Greens
2 servings ■ 304 calories per serving

Dressing Ingredients
1 tablespoon olive oil
1 tablespoon balsamic vinegar
1/2 teaspoon Dijon mustard
1 garlic clove, minced
1/4 teaspoon soy sauce
Salt and freshly ground black pepper (optional)

Salad Ingredients
3 cups packed mixed mesclun or spring greens
1/4 cup dried cranberries
1/4 cup walnut halves, raw or pan-roasted
1/2 cup (2 ounces) crumbled farmer cheese

Combine oil, vinegar, mustard, garlic, and soy sauce; mix well. Season to taste with salt and pepper if desired. Toss greens with dressing, cranberries, and walnuts. Arrange on serving plates; top with cheese.

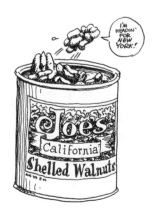

What's in it for you?	
Total fat	22.7 g
Saturated fat	6 g
Healthy fats	15.6 g
Fiber	4.7 g
Carbohydrates	19.6 g
Sugar	11.9 g
Protein	10 g
Sodium	183 mg
Calcium	146 mg
Magnesium	57 mg
Selenium	3 mcg
Potassium	391 mg

Arugula, Watermelon, and Feta Salad

2 servings ■ 190 calories per serving

Dressing Ingredients

1 tablespoon olive oil
1 tablespoon balsamic vinegar
1 small shallot, minced
Salt and freshly ground black pepper (optional)

Salad Ingredients

1 large bunch of arugula (3 cups packed), washed and dried
1 cup cubed seedless watermelon
1/2 cup (2 ounces) crumbled low-fat feta cheese

Combine oil, vinegar, and shallot; mix well. Season to taste with salt and pepper if desired; let stand 5 minutes. Arrange arugula on two serving plates. Arrange watermelon and cheese on top of arugula; drizzle with dressing.

What's in it for you?	
Total fat	13.3 g
Saturated fat	5.3 g
Healthy fats	7.3 g
Fiber	1.1 g
Carbohydrates	13 g
Sugar	6.9 g
Protein	6.4 g
Sodium	334 mg
Calcium	235 mg
Magnesium	41.8 mg
Selenium	5 mcg
Potassium	377 mg

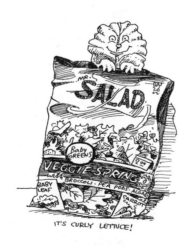

IT'S CURLY LETTUCE!

Greek Feta Salad with Peppers and Olives

2 servings ■ 305 calories per serving

Dressing Ingredients

1 tablespoon olive oil
1 tablespoon red wine vinegar
1 tablespoon lemon juice
1/2 teaspoon dried oregano
1 garlic clove, minced
1/2 teaspoon honey
Salt and freshly ground black pepper (optional)

Salad Ingredients

1 head romaine lettuce, torn
1 tomato, quartered
4 pepperoncini peppers
1 small cucumber, sliced
1/2 cup (2 ounces) crumbled low-fat feta cheese
Several sprigs fresh dill, chopped
1/2 green bell pepper, sliced into rings
8 calamata olives

Combine all dressing ingredients except salt and pepper; mix well. Season to taste with salt and pepper if desired; let stand 5 minutes. Combine all salad ingredients in large bowl; toss with dressing.

What's in it for you?	
Total fat	16 g
Saturated fat	5.7 g
Healthy fats	9.6 g
Fiber	10.9 g
Carbohydrates	35.8 g
Sugar	17.9 g
Protein	12 g
Sodium	510 mg
Calcium	324 mg
Magnesium	108 mg
Selenium	619 mcg
Potassium	1,593 mg

Turkish Shepherd Salad

2 servings ■ 153 calories per serving

1 small cucumber
1 tomato
1 small sweet onion
1 teaspoon olive oil
1 tablespoon red wine vinegar
Salt and freshly ground black pepper (optional)
1/2 cup (2 ounces) crumbled low-fat feta cheese

Coarsely chop cucumber, tomato, and onion; transfer to a bowl. Add oil and vinegar; toss well. Season to taste with salt and pepper if desired. Transfer to serving plates; top with cheese.

What's in it for you?	
Total fat	8.6 g
Saturated fat	4.6 g
Healthy fats	3.6 g
Fiber	2.2 g
Carbohydrates	14.7 g
Sugar	9 g
Protein	6.1 g
Sodium	329 mg
Calcium	186 mg
Magnesium	39 mg
Selenium	5.1 mcg
Potassium	479 mg

Orient Express Salad with Chopped Peanuts
2 servings ■ 200 calories per serving

Dressing Ingredients
1 tablespoon olive oil
2 tablespoons orange juice
1 tablespoon rice wine vinegar
1 teaspoon grated fresh gingerroot
1 teaspoon soy sauce
1/2 teaspoon toasted sesame oil
Salt and freshly ground black pepper (optional)

Salad Ingredients
2 small heads Boston lettuce, torn
1 small cucumber, sliced
1 small bunch cilantro, coarsely chopped
1 carrot, shredded
2 tablespoons chopped peanuts
2 green onions, chopped

Combine all dressing ingredients except salt and pepper; mix well. Season to taste with salt and pepper if desired. Toss lettuce, cucumber, cilantro, and carrot with the dressing. Transfer to serving plates; top with peanuts and green onions.

What's in it for you?	
Total fat	13.1 g
Saturated fat	1.8 g
Healthy fats	10.6 g
Fiber	5.1 g
Carbohydrates	17.7 g
Sugar	7.9 g
Protein	7.1 g
Sodium	458 mg
Calcium	121 mg
Magnesium	72 mg
Selenium	2.3 mcg
Potassium	936 mg

Mediterranean Cauliflower Salad

4 servings ■ 94 calories per serving

1 head cauliflower, blanched for 5 minutes
1 small can anchovies, drained, chopped (optional)
1 tablespoon drained capers
2 tablespoons fresh lemon juice
1 tablespoon olive oil
1 garlic clove, pressed or minced
1 tablespoon chopped fresh oregano or 1 teaspoon dried

Drain cauliflower and break into small pieces. Combine cauliflower, anchovies if desired, and capers in a medium bowl. Combine remaining ingredients; toss with cauliflower mixture.

What's in it for you?	
Total fat	4.6 g
Saturated fat	0.7 g
Healthy fats	3.7 g
Fiber	3.8 g
Carbohydrates	8.8 g
Sugar	3.7 g
Protein	6.2 g
Sodium	519 mg
Calcium	63 mg
Magnesium	31 mg
Selenium	8.7 mcg
Potassium	514 mg

Sweet Beet and Gorgonzola Salad
4 servings ■ 106 calories per serving

6 medium beets, trimmed
1 tablespoon olive oil
1 tablespoon balsamic vinegar
1 teaspoon honey
1 garlic clove, pressed or minced
1/2 teaspoon soy sauce
1/2 bunch of chives, finely chopped
2 tablespoons crumbled gorgonzola cheese

In large saucepan, simmer beets in water to cover until tender but still firm, about 30 minutes. Drain, cool, and remove skin. Meanwhile, combine oil, vinegar, honey, garlic, and soy sauce in a medium bowl. Cut beets into 1-inch cubes; add to bowl. Toss with dressing and chives. Transfer to serving plates; top with cheese.

What's in it for you?	
Total fat	4.8 g
Saturated fat	1.3 g
Healthy fats	3.3 g
Fiber	3.5 g
Carbohydrates	13.7 g
Sugar	9.8 g
Protein	3.1 g
Sodium	239 mg
Calcium	45 mg
Magnesium	31 mg
Selenium	1.6 mcg
Potassium	424 mg

Hearts of Palm Salad with Tomato and Mushrooms

2 servings ■ 132 calories per serving

1 can (16 ounces) hearts of palm, drained
1 tomato, chopped
1 shallot, chopped
6 button mushrooms, sliced
1 small bunch parsley, chopped
2 tablespoons red wine vinegar
1 tablespoon olive oil
Salt and freshly ground black pepper (optional)

Slice hearts of palm in half lengthwise; arrange on a serving platter. Combine remaining ingredients except salt and pepper; mix well. Season to taste with salt and pepper if desired. Spoon mixture over hearts of palm.

What's in it for you?	
Total fat	8 g
Saturated fat	1.2 g
Healthy fats	6.2 g
Fiber	5 g
Carbohydrates	12.2 g
Sugar	2.6 g
Protein	6.2 g
Sodium	632 mg
Calcium	102 mg
Magnesium	72 mg
Selenium	6 mcg
Potassium	632 mg

Carrot, Raisin, and Yogurt Slaw

2 servings ■ 193 calories per serving

4 carrots, shredded
1 small bunch cilantro, chopped
1 cup low-fat Greek-style yogurt
1/4 cup golden raisins
1 garlic clove, minced
1 teaspoon lemon juice
Dash of Worcestershire sauce
Salt and freshly ground black pepper (optional)

Combine all ingredients except salt and pepper in a bowl; mix well. Season to taste with salt and pepper if desired.

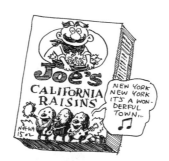

What's in it for you?	
Total fat	4.5 g
Saturated fat	2.7 g
Healthy fats	1.4 g
Fiber	5.1 g
Carbohydrates	35 g
Sugar	23 g
Protein	6.5 g
Sodium	166 mg
Calcium	2.5 mg
Magnesium	41 mg
Selenium	3.3 mcg
Potassium	850 mg

Sesame Cucumber Salad

2 servings ■ 187 calories per serving

1 tablespoon rice wine vinegar
1 teaspoon olive oil
1/2 teaspoon toasted sesame oil
1/2 teaspoon soy sauce
Dash cayenne pepper
2 cucumbers, cut into 1/4-inch-thick slices
1/2 bunch chives, minced
1 teaspoon sesame seeds

Combine vinegar, olive oil, sesame oil, soy sauce, and cayenne pepper in a medium bowl; mix well. Add cucumbers, chives, and sesame seeds; mix well.

What's in it for you?	
Total fat	6.8 g
Saturated fat	1 g
Healthy fats	5.3 g
Fiber	3.2 g
Carbohydrates	29 g
Sugar	8.2 g
Protein	6.2 g
Sodium	180 mg
Calcium	90 mg
Magnesium	85 mg
Selenium	18.1 mcg
Potassium	750 mg

YOU Dinners

Asian Salmon with Brown Rice Pilaf
4 servings ■ 674 calories per serving

Brown Rice
1 tablespoon olive oil
1/2 onion, chopped
1/2 red bell pepper, chopped
2 cups water
1 cup uncooked short-grain brown rice
1/4 cup finely chopped parsley
Salt and freshly ground black pepper
  (optional)

Salmon Ingredients
4 skinless salmon fillets (about 4
  ounces each)
1 tablespoon olive oil
1 garlic clove, pressed or minced
1 tablespoon grated fresh gingerroot
1 teaspoon soy sauce
1 teaspoon maple syrup
2 green onions, chopped

What's in it for you?	
Total fat	20.5 g
Saturated fat	3.4 g
Healthy fats	15 g
Fiber	2.6 g
Carbohydrates	45.9 g
Sugar	4.9 g
Protein	71 g
Sodium	411 mg
Calcium	81 mg
Magnesium	165 mg
Selenium	145 mcg
Potassium	1,421 mg

To make the rice, heat oil in a medium saucepan. Add onion and bell pepper; cook 3 minutes. Add water and rice; bring to a boil. Reduce heat; cover and simmer 50 minutes, or until rice is tender and liquid is absorbed. Fluff with a fork; stir in parsley. Season with salt and pepper if desired. Meanwhile, place salmon in a pie plate or shallow dish. Combine remaining salmon ingredients; mix well. Pour marinade over salmon; let stand 15 to 20 minutes. Heat a ridged grill pan over medium heat until hot. Add salmon, discarding marinade; cook 3 to 4 minutes per side, or until salmon is opaque and firm to the touch. Serve with brown rice.

Spicy Chili

4 servings ■ 390 calories per serving

1 tablespoon olive oil
1/2 pound ground turkey or ground meat substitute
   (such as Boca Crumbles)
1/2 onion, chopped
2 garlic cloves, minced
1 can (28 ounces) crushed tomatoes, undrained
1 can (16 ounces) kidney beans, drained
1/2 teaspoon chili powder
Pinch of cayenne pepper
1 teaspoon maple syrup
1 teaspoon wine vinegar
1/2 teaspoon ground coriander
1/2 teaspoon turmeric
Brown Rice Pilaf (recipe on page 350)

Heat oil in a large saucepan. Add turkey, onion, and garlic; cook 5 minutes, stirring frequently. Add remaining ingredients; simmer uncovered 25 minutes. Serve over Brown Rice Pilaf.

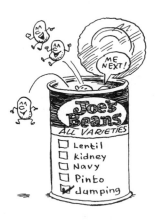

What's in it for you?	
Total fat	8.9 g
Saturated fat	1.9 g
Healthy fats	6.2 g
Fiber	10.7 g
Carbohydrates	31.5 g
Sugar	2.2 g
Protein	18.8 g
Sodium	646 mg
Calcium	86 mg
Magnesium	73 mg
Selenium	13.3 mcg
Potassium	838 mg

Trust Crust

To bake your own whole wheat pizza crust, the recipe will require 25 to 70 extra minutes from start to finish, including time for yeast to do its thing. In a small bowl, combine about 1 tablespoon of dry yeast and 1/8 teaspoon of sugar with 1 1/2 cups of warm water. Let that sit for 10 minutes. In a separate large bowl, combine 1 1/2 cups whole wheat flour and 1 1/2 cups all-purpose (enriched) flour. (After you've tried this on your family several times, you can gradually increase in 1/2-cup lots the ratio of whole wheat to all-purpose flour to 2 1/2 cups whole wheat to 1/2 cup all-purpose.) Add 1 teaspoon ground kosher salt to this. Mix well. Then add the yeast mixture and mix by hand thoroughly. Add 1 tablespoon olive oil. Knead for about 2 minutes until dough is smooth. Cover bowl and let rise in warm area until dough has doubled in size (20 to 60 minutes). Punch down dough with your fist and knead for 1 to 2 minutes. Divide into 4 equal portions (extra portions can be stored in your refrigerator). Roll into balls and preheat oven to 450°F. Lightly coat a baking sheet with olive oil. With a rolling pin, roll one of dough balls on rolling board or on baking sheet (add flour if dough sticks to pin too much) and flatten into 10- to 12-inch pizza crust circle. Poke with a fork 4 to 6 times. Bake for 5 minutes. Remove from oven, then add ingredients.

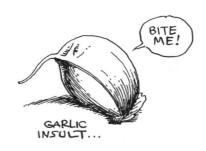

GARLIC
INSULT...

BITE
ME!

Stuffed Whole Wheat Pizza

4 servings (2 slices per serving); for the first two weeks, you can have up to half of the pizza, but most will not need that much to be filled ■ 322 calories per serving

Cooking oil spray
1 pound fresh stir-fry vegetables such as asparagus, broccoli, cauliflower, mushrooms, multicolored bell peppers, red and white onions, and zucchini, cut up
2 garlic cloves, minced
Salt and freshly ground black pepper (optional)
1 cup pizza sauce or tomato sauce
2 tablespoons olive relish or tapenade
2 tablespoons sun-dried-tomato bits
One 12-inch or 10-ounce prepared thin whole wheat pizza crust
1/2 cup (2 ounces) finely shredded part-skim mozzarella cheese

Heat oven to 425°F. Heat a large non-stick skillet over medium-high heat until hot; coat with cooking spray. Add vegetables and garlic; stir-fry (really sauté) 2 to 5 minutes, or until vegetables are crisp-tender. Season to taste with salt and pepper if desired. Combine pizza sauce, olive relish, and sun-dried-tomato bits. Spread over pizza crust; top with cooked vegetables and cheese. Bake pizza directly on oven rack 10 to 15 minutes, or until crust is golden brown and cheese is melted. Cut pizza into 8 wedges.

What's in it for you?	
Total fat	11.5 g
Saturated fat	3.5 g
Healthy fats	7.9 g
Fiber	5.7 g
Carbohydrates	44.2 g
Sugar	3.5 g
Protein	12.2 g
Sodium	682 mg
Calcium	151 mg
Magnesium	44 mg
Selenium	2.9 mcg
Potassium	481 mg

Mediterranean Chicken with Tomatoes, Olives, and Herbed White Beans
2 servings ■ 567 calories per serving

Chicken Ingredients

2 bone-in chicken thighs without skin

1 tomato, chopped

1/2 onion, chopped

8 pitted kalamata olives, halved

1 tablespoon olive oil

1 teaspoon wine vinegar or balsamic vinegar

1 small bunch fresh basil, chopped

Bean Ingredients

1 tablespoon olive oil

2 garlic cloves, minced

1 can (15 or 16 ounces) white beans, rinsed and drained

1 tomato, chopped

1/4 cup chopped fresh mixed herbs

1 teaspoon red wine vinegar or balsamic vinegar

Salt and freshly ground black pepper (optional)

What's in it for you?	
Total fat	19.2 g
Saturated fat	3.1 g
Healthy fats	15 g
Fiber	15.2 g
Carbohydrates	67.4 g
Sugar	5.1 g
Protein	34.4 g
Sodium	313 mg
Calcium	243 mg
Magnesium	171 mg
Selenium	14.3 mcg
Potassium	1,715 mg

To make the chicken, heat oven to 375°F. Place each chicken thigh on a large square of aluminum foil. Combine remaining chicken ingredients; spoon over chicken. Fold foil up and over chicken, sealing edges and forming a packet. Bake 25 minutes, or until chicken is cooked through. Meanwhile, to prepare the beans, heat oil in a medium saucepan over medium heat. Add garlic; cook 2 minutes. Add remaining bean ingredients; cook 5 minutes, or until heated through. Carefully open chicken packets and transfer mixture to two serving plates; serve beans alongside chicken.

Royal Pasta Primavera Provençale

2 servings ■ 451 calories per serving

6 ounces whole wheat rigatoni or linguine pasta
1 small dried ancho or pasilla chili pepper
1 cup (4 ounces) diced (1/2-inch cubes) unpeeled eggplant
1 teaspoon olive oil
1 small yellow onion, coarsely chopped
1 yellow or orange bell pepper, coarsely chopped
3 garlic cloves, sliced
2 cans (14 1/2 ounces each) stewed tomatoes, undrained, coarsely chopped
1 cup packed mesclun or mixed spring salad greens
1 teaspoon chopped fresh thyme or lemon thyme
Salt and freshly ground black pepper (optional)

What's in it for you?	
Total fat	4.3 g
Saturated fat	0.6 g
Healthy fats	2.9 g
Fiber	6.3 g
Carbohydrates	95.2 g
Sugar	15.4 g
Protein	17.6 g
Sodium	533 mg
Calcium	179 mg
Magnesium	183 mg
Selenium	65.5 mcg
Potassium	1,163 mg

Cook pasta according to package directions, omitting salt and fat. Meanwhile, heat a large, deep skillet over medium heat until hot. Add the chili pepper; cook, turning occasionally until fragrant and toasted, about 2 minutes. When the chili pepper is cool enough to handle, discard its stem and set the seeds aside for a garnish. Chop the chili pepper. Add eggplant to hot skillet; cook until browned, about 4 minutes, stirring frequently. Add oil, then chopped onion, bell pepper, and garlic; cook 3 minutes, stirring occasionally. Add tomatoes and chopped chili pepper. Reduce heat; simmer uncovered 10 minutes, or until vegetables are tender and sauce thickens. Remove from heat; stir in salad greens and thyme. Season to taste with salt and pepper if desired. Drain pasta; transfer to two serving plates and top with sauce.

Apricot Chicken and Green Beans with Almond Slivers

2 servings ■ 430 calories per serving

Chicken Ingredients

2 skinless, boneless chicken breast halves (about 4 ounces each)
(or substitute pork)
4 dried apricots, chopped
2 tablespoons white wine
2 shallots, chopped
1 tablespoon olive oil
1/8 teaspoon ground cinnamon

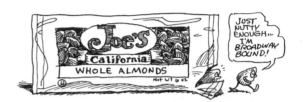

Green Bean Ingredients

1 cup thin green beans
3 shallots, thinly sliced
1 tablespoon olive oil
1 teaspoon wine vinegar
1 teaspoon maple syrup
1/4 cup slivered almonds
Salt and freshly ground black pepper
(optional)

What's in it for you?	
Total fat	22 g
Saturated fat	2.8 g
Healthy fats	18.1 g
Fiber	4.6 g
Carbohydrates	25 g
Sugar	3.5 g
Protein	32.7 g
Sodium	89 mg
Calcium	95 mg
Magnesium	100 mg
Selenium	22.4 mcg
Potassium	813 mg

To make the chicken, heat oven to 375°F. Place chicken in a glass baking dish. Sauté remaining chicken ingredients together until tender; transfer to blender or food processor and puree. Spoon over chicken and bake until chicken is cooked through, 15 to 20 minutes. Meanwhile, to prepare the beans, steam or blanch beans until tender but still firm and bright green. Sauté shallots in olive oil, vinegar, and maple syrup until translucent. Add almonds and brown slightly; toss with beans. Season to taste with salt and pepper if desired. Serve alongside chicken.

Turkey Tortilla Wraps with Red Baked Potato
2 servings ■ 497 calories per serving

Red Potato Ingredients
1 large russet baking potato, washed, pierced with tip of knife
2 tablespoons marinara sauce or other red tomato sauce

Turkey Wrap Ingredients
Two 6-inch whole wheat flour tortillas
4 slices deli roast turkey breast
4 romaine lettuce leaves
4 slices tomato
2 thin slices red or yellow onion
Mustard or hot peppers (optional)

To make the red potato, cook in microwave on high power 8 to 9 minutes or until fork-tender. Slice lengthwise in half; spoon 1 tablespoon sauce over each half. Meanwhile, to prepare the turkey wraps, layer all turkey wrap ingredients on tortillas; roll up.

What's in it for you?	
Total fat	14.5 g
Saturated fat	4.5 g
Healthy fats	10 g
Fiber	7 g
Carbohydrates	64 g
Sugar	6.5 g
Protein	28.5 g
Sodium	1,654 mg
Calcium	180 mg
Magnesium	71 mg
Selenium	11.3 mcg
Potassium	1,596 mg

Broiled Trout, Orata, or Branzini with Rosemary and Lemon
2 servings ■ 182 calories per serving

8 ounces whole fish (trout, orata, or branzini)
Salt and freshly ground black pepper (optional)
2 garlic cloves, sliced
4 sprigs of fresh rosemary
1 lemon, sliced

Preheat broiler. Open fish like a book; season to taste with salt and pepper if desired. Arrange garlic, rosemary, and lemon slices on one side of each fish; close other side and transfer fish to greased rack of broiler pan. Broil 5 to 6 inches from heat source 5 minutes. Turn fish over; continue to broil 4 to 5 minutes, or until fish is opaque throughout.

What's in it for you?	
Total fat	7.3 g
Saturated fat	1 g
Healthy fat	4.9 g
Fiber	2.7 g
Carbohydrates	10.3 g
Sugar	4.9 g
Protein	15.8 g
Sodium	126 mg
Calcium	76 mg
Magnesium	43 mg
Selenium	10.7 mcg
Potassium	688 mg

Lemon Caper Chicken with Sweet Potato Puree

2 servings ■ 273 calories per serving

Chicken Ingredients

2 skinless, boneless chicken thighs (about 4 ounces each)
Juice of 1 lemon
1 tablespoon olive oil
2 shallots, minced
1 tablespoon capers, drained
1 teaspoon Dijon mustard

Sweet Potato Ingredients

2 sweet potatoes, microwaved or baked
2 tablespoons orange juice
1/4 cup golden raisins
1/2 teaspoon ground cinnamon
Salt and freshly ground black pepper (optional)

To make the chicken, preheat broiler. Place chicken in a shallow roasting pan. Combine remaining chicken ingredients and pour over chicken. Broil 6 inches from heat source 12 to 15 minutes, or until chicken is cooked through. To prepare the potatoes, scoop hot sweet potato pulp into bowl. Add remaining sweet potato ingredients except salt and pepper; mix well. Season to taste with salt and pepper if desired. Serve with chicken.

What's in it for you?	
Total fat	10.9 g
Saturated fat	2 g
Healthy fats	7.9 g
Fiber	1.4 g
Carbohydrates	20.6 g
Sugar	12.7 g
Protein	24.7 g
Sodium	336 mg
Calcium	39.5 mg
Magnesium	41 mg
Selenium	16.5 mcg
Potassium	494 mg

Chicken Kabobs with Tabbouleh

2 servings ■ 397 calories per serving

Chicken Ingredients

2 skinless, boneless chicken breast halves (about 4 ounces each),
   cut into 1-inch cubes
1 teaspoon dried oregano
1/2 teaspoon dried sage
1 red chili pepper, crushed (optional)
1 onion, quartered
1 tomato, quartered
1 bell pepper, seeded, stemmed, quartered
4 button mushrooms

Tabbouleh Ingredients

3/4 cup bulgur wheat
1 1/2 cups boiling water
1 tomato, chopped
1 bunch green onions, chopped
1 large bunch parsley, finely chopped
1 small bunch fresh mint leaves, finely chopped
2 tablespoons lemon juice
1 tablespoon olive oil
Salt and freshly ground black pepper (optional)

To make the chicken, prepare grill. Toss chicken with oregano, sage, and, if desired, chili pepper. Alternately thread chicken, onion, tomato, bell pepper, and mushrooms onto metal skewers. Cook on covered grill 3 to 4 minutes per side, or until chicken is cooked through and vegetables are tender. Meanwhile, to prepare the tabbouleh, place bulgur wheat in medium bowl; add boiling water and mix well. Let stand until all water is absorbed, about 30 minutes. (Pour off any excess water.) Add remaining ingredients except salt and pepper; mix well. Season with salt and pepper if desired. Serve tabbouleh with grilled chicken and vegetables.

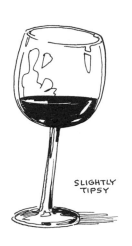

SLIGHTLY
TIPSY

What's in it for you?	
Total fat	9.4 g
Saturated fat	1.5 g
Healthy fats	7.1 g
Fiber	5.6 g
Carbohydrates	72.1 g
Sugar	12.1 g
Protein	14.2 g
Sodium	22.4 mg
Calcium	93 mg
Magnesium	148 mg
Selenium	68 mcg
Potassium	1,121 mg

Hot Wild Salmon

2 servings ■ 384 calories per serving

2 wild salmon fillets with skin (about 4 ounces each) or salmon steaks
 (preferably line-caught)
2 tablespoons finely chopped fresh ginger
1 tablespoon wasabi paste
1/4 teaspoon turmeric
Rock Asparagus (recipe on page 301)

Prepare grill or preheat broiler. Brush skinless side of salmon with combined ginger, wasabi paste, and turmeric. Grill or broil 4 to 6 inches from heat source 10 to 12 minutes without turning, or until salmon is opaque in center. Serve with Rock Asparagus.

What's in it for you?	
Total fat	14.5 g
Saturated fat	2.3 g
Healthy fats	10.6 g
Fiber	0.4 g
Carbohydrates	2.7 g
Sugar	0.2 g
Protein	45.2 g
Sodium	11 mg
Calcium	31 mg
Magnesium	73 mg
Selenium	82.5 mcg
Potassium	1,176 mcg

Grilled Peanut Shrimp with Sesame Snow Peas

2 servings ■ 163 calories per serving

Peanut Sauce Ingredients
1 tablespoon natural peanut butter
1 tablespoon canned light coconut milk
1 teaspoon fresh lime juice
Pinch of cayenne pepper
1 teaspoon honey
1/4 teaspoon soy sauce
1/4 cup water
1 garlic clove, peeled
10 medium uncooked shrimp, peeled and deveined

Snow Pea Ingredients
1 cup fresh snow peas
1 garlic clove, minced
1 teaspoon sesame seeds
1 teaspoon olive oil
1/2 teaspoon toasted sesame oil

Prepare grill. Place all ingredients for peanut sauce except shrimp in blender or food processor; puree. Pour mixture over shrimp; let stand 15 minutes. Thread shrimp onto skewers; discard any excess marinade not clinging to shrimp. Grill 2 to 3 minutes per side, or until shrimp are opaque. Meanwhile, blanch snow peas in boiling water 2 minutes; drain and rinse with cold water. Cook garlic and sesame seeds in olive and sesame oils 2 minutes. Add drained snow peas; heat through, tossing well. Serve with shrimp.

What's in it for you?	
Total fat	10.5 g
Saturated fat	2.9 g
Healthy fats	7 g
Fiber	1.9 g
Carbohydrates	8.8 g
Sugar	5.1 g
Protein	9.5 g
Sodium	128 mg
Calcium	51.5 mg
Magnesium	40.6 mg
Selenium	13.1 mcg
Potassium	220 mg

Vegetable Tofu Stir-fry

2 servings ■ 602 calories per serving

1 tablespoon olive oil
1/2 teaspoon toasted sesame oil
1/4 teaspoon crushed red pepper flakes
1/2 onion, sliced
2 garlic cloves, sliced
1 cup broccoli florets
1/2 red bell pepper, sliced
6 large button mushrooms, halved
1 teaspoon soy sauce
4 small 2-ounce blocks baked tofu, cubed
2 green onions, chopped
1 small bunch cilantro, chopped
1 teaspoon sesame seeds

In wok or large skillet, heat olive and sesame oils and pepper flakes over medium-high heat. Add onion and garlic; stir-fry 2 minutes. Add broccoli, bell pepper, mushrooms, and soy sauce; stir-fry until vegetables are crisp-tender, 2 to 3 minutes. Add tofu, green onions, cilantro, and sesame seeds; stir-fry until heated through.

What's in it for you?	
Total fat	23 g
Saturated fat	3.3 g
Healthy fats	18.9 g
Fiber	11.1 g
Carbohydrates	43 g
Sugar	16.4 g
Protein	62.2 g
Sodium	873 mg
Calcium	400 mg
Magnesium	273 mg
Selenium	13.5 mcg
Potassium	2,403 mg

Tofu or Turkey Dogs with Sauerkraut

2 Servings ■ 298 calories per serving

4 tofu (meatless) or turkey hot dogs
1 cup sauerkraut
Whole wheat buns (optional)
2 tablespoons favorite mustard, such as spicy brown
   or coarse-grained

Simmer hot dogs in water with sauer-kraut until heated through, about 5 minutes. Drain; serve with mustard (with or without buns).

What's in it for you?	
Total fat	26 g
Saturated fat	9 g
Healthy fats	15.4 g
Fiber	0.7 g
Carbohydrates	3.8 g
Sugar	2.1 g
Protein	11.2 g
Sodium	1,219 mg
Calcium	158 mg
Magnesium	27 mg
Selenium	1.9 mcg
Potassium	160 mg

YOU Sides

Rock Asparagus
4 servings ■ 38 calories per serving

1 pound asparagus spears, rinsed, dried, and trimmed
1 teaspoon extra-virgin olive oil
Kosher salt, to taste (optional)
1/4 teaspoon *each:* dried thyme, oregano, basil, and black pepper
Optional garnish: diced tomato

Heat oven to 350°F. Toss the asparagus in a 13 x 9-inch baking dish or a shallow 3-quart casserole pan with the olive oil, kosher salt if desired, thyme, oregano, basil, and black pepper. Arrange asparagus in a single layer in the dish. Bake uncovered 12 to 13 minutes for thin asparagus or 15 to 18 minutes for thick asparagus, or until crisp-tender. Garnish with tomato if desired.

What's in it for you?	
Total fat	1.5 g
Saturated fat	0.2 g
Healthy fats	1.1 g
Fiber	1.4 g
Carbohydrates	5 g
Sugar	1.8 g
Protein	2.9 g
Sodium	5 mg
Calcium	27 mg
Magnesium	22 mg
Selenium	4 mcg
Potassium	352 mg

Tomato-Avocado Salsamole

2 servings ■ 90 calories per serving

1/4 cup finely chopped red onion
1 teaspoon minced jalapeño, or more to taste
1 tablespoon lime juice
1 tablespoon cider vinegar
1 teaspoon minced garlic
1/4 teaspoon salt
1 ripe avocado (preferably Hass), peeled, pitted, and coarsely
 mashed
1 medium tomato, chopped
1/4 chopped cilantro

Combine onion, jalapeño, lime juice, vinegar, garlic, and salt in bowl. Add avocado, tomato, and cilantro; stir well. Serve immediately or, to store, reserve avocado pit, add to mixture to prevent browning, cover tightly with plastic wrap, and refrigerate. Serve with lightly toasted whole wheat pita cut into triangles.

What's in it for you?	
Total fat	8 g
Saturated fat	2.1 g
Healthy fats	5.3 g
Fiber	3.1 g
Carbohydrates	8 g
Sugar	2 g
Protein	2 g
Sodium	25 mg
Calcium	20 mg
Magnesium	54 mg
Selenium	0 mcg
Potassium	805 mg

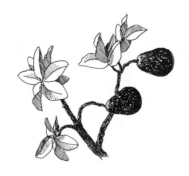

Cinnamon Baked Apples with Tangerines and Cranberries
4 servings ■ 146 calories per serving

2 large baking apples, such as McIntosh or Rome Beauty
   (or substitute pears)
1 1/4 cups unsweetened apple juice, preferably unfiltered organic
1/2 cup (2 ounces) dried cranberries (or substitute cherries)
1/4 teaspoon ground cinnamon
1/4 teaspoon ground cloves
2 seedless clementines or tangerines, peeled, separated into segments

Heat oven to 400°F. Cut apples in half lengthwise; cut out and discard cores, seeds, and stems. Place 1/4 cup of the apple juice in an 8-inch baking dish or casserole pan. Place apples cut side down on juice. Bake 15 to 18 minutes or until apples are tender. Meanwhile, simmer remaining 1 cup apple juice in a small saucepan over medium-high heat 5 minutes. Add cranberries, cinnamon, and cloves; reduce heat and simmer uncovered 10 minutes, or until cranberries are plumped, stirring occasionally. Remove from heat; stir in clementine sections. Arrange apple halves cut side up on serving dishes. Pour any remaining liquid from dish into cranberry mixture; spoon over apples.

What's in it for you?	
Total fat	0.6 g
Saturated fat	0.1 g
Healthy fats	0.3 g
Fiber	4.1 g
Carbohydrates	37.7 g
Sugar	30.4 g
Protein	0.7 g
Sodium	15 mg
Calcium	30 mg
Magnesium	13 mg
Zinc	0.1 mg
Selenium	0.2 mg
Potassium	281 mg

Cinnamon Apple Sauté à la Mode

2 servings ■ 220 calories per serving

2 small apples, such as Jonagold or Ambrosia
1 tablespoon apple butter
1 tablespoon unsweetened apple juice or cider, preferably organic
1/2 teaspoon ground cinnamon
6 walnut halves, toasted, coarsely chopped
1/2 cup nonfat or low-fat vanilla frozen yogurt

Cut apples into quarters; discard stems, cores, and seeds. Cut apple quarters into thin slices. Heat a large nonstick skillet over medium-high heat until hot. Add apples; cook until apples begin to brown, about 4 minutes, tossing occasionally. Stir in apple butter, apple juice, and cinnamon; continue to cook 5 to 8 minutes, or until apples are tender and sauce thickens, tossing frequently. Transfer to serving plates; top with nuts. Serve with frozen yogurt.

What's in it for you?	
Total fat	8.4 g
Saturated fat	0.8 g
Healthy fats	7.0 g
Fiber	6.7 g
Carbohydrates	38 g
Sugar	27.6 g
Protein	3.6 g
Sodium	23 mg
Calcium	83 mg
Magnesium	35 mg
Selenium	2 mcg
Potassium	346 mg

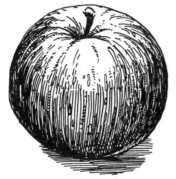

PROOF AGAINST M.D.s

369

Roasted Pear with Raspberry Coulis, Chocolate, and Pistachios
2 servings ■ 184 calories per serving

1 large red pear
1/2 cup white wine (high-quality)
6 ounces frozen unsweetened raspberries, thawed, or
   1 cup fresh raspberries
1 tablespoon mini semisweet chocolate chips
1 1/2 tablespoons coarsely chopped pistachios, toasted

Heat oven to 400°F. Cut pear in half; remove core with a melon baller or metal measuring teaspoon. Arrange pear halves, cut side down, in a shallow baking dish. Pour wine over pears. Bake 18 to 20 minutes, or until pears are tender when pierced with the tip of a sharp knife. Meanwhile, puree raspberries in food processor; strain and discard seeds. Transfer roasted pears to serving plates, cut side up; sprinkle chocolate chips over the pears (the heat of the pears will melt the chips). Combine pureed raspberries and liquid remaining in baking dish in a small saucepan. Cook over high heat until sauce is slightly thickened. Spoon sauce over and around pears; sprinkle with pistachios. Serve warm or at room temperature.

What's in it for you?	
Total fat	5.2 g
Saturated fat	1.4 g
Healthy fats	3.3 g
Fiber	4.9 g
Carbohydrates	31.8 g
Sugar	24 g
Protein	2.7 g
Sodium	7 mg
Calcium	45 mg
Magnesium	32 mg
Selenium	2 mcg
Potassium	344 mg

Sliced Peaches with Raspberries, Blueberries, and Chocolate Chips

2 servings ■ 46 calories per serving

2 small ripe peaches, sliced
1/2 teaspoon ground cinnamon
Pinch of nutmeg
1/4 cup (1 ounce) fresh raspberries
1/4 cup (1 ounce) fresh blueberries
1 1/2 tablespoons mini semisweet chocolate chips

Combine sliced peaches with cinnamon and nutmeg; transfer to two serving plates. Top peaches with raspberries, blueberries, and chocolate chips.

What's in it for you?	
Total fat	0.4 g
Saturated fat	0.1 g
Healthy fats	0.28 g
Fiber	2.6 g
Carbohydrates	11.5 g
Sugar	8.9 g
Protein	1 g
Sodium	0.5 mg
Calcium	22 mg
Magnesium	11.5 mg
Selenium	0.1 mcg
Potassium	202 mg

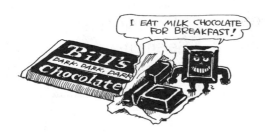

I EAT MILK CHOCOLATE FOR BREAKFAST!

Bill's DARK, DARK, DARK Chocolate

YOU Snack

Simon's Popcorn
4 servings ■ 61 calories per serving, 10 percent from fat

1/2 cup popcorn kernels
Flavored cooking spray (butter, olive oil, or garlic)
Garlic salt or cinnamon

Place popcorn in a 2 1/2-quart microwave-safe container; cover and cook at high power 4 to 5 minutes, or until popcorn is popped but not scorched. If the microwave oven does not have a rotating turntable, use oven mitts to grasp and shake the covered container after 3 minutes of cooking. Immediately pour the popcorn onto a baking sheet and coat with cooking spray. To further flavor the popcorn, immediately sprinkle on your favorite seasoning blend such as garlic salt or cinnamon.

What's in it for you?
Total fat	0.8 g
Saturated fat	0.1 g
Healthy fats	0.7 g
Fiber	0.4 g
Carbohydrates	5 g
Sugar	0 g
Protein	1 g
Sodium	0 mg
Calcium	1 mg
Magnesium	0 mg
Selenium	1 mcg
Potassium	0 mg

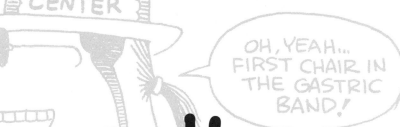

Appendices
The Medical Options

Solutions If You Plateau
or If Your Fat and Health Have
Spun Out of Control

About the Appendices

We know exactly what you think. When someone mentions that he's using a medical "aid" for weight loss — be it a drug or even surgery — you view the options as cop-outs. But for some people, these so-called cop-outs are real answers. If you've hit the wall, or if you have a mental block about losing the last thirty pounds, or if you've completely lost control, there are medical solutions that can help — or even reverse — obesity problems. They range from the relatively tame (like temporary prescription drugs) to the massively major (like gastric bypass surgery). And, depending on the situation, they can work for the person who has a handful of pounds to lose or a few hundred to lose. If you had prostate or breast cancer, you'd seek medical help. Being forty to one hundred pounds overweight at age 50 poses as much risk to you as breast or prostate cancer. That's right: It doubles your odds of dying or disability in the next seven years. While we believe that the majority of weight issues can be handled with the YOU Diet and YOU Activity Plan, we also want to make you aware that there are people who can benefit from medical interventions. And those procedures, which we'll briefly outline in these appendices, fall into three categories:

■ Prescription Drugs: used as a jump start, or to help people when they've reached a weight-loss plateau.

- Plastic Surgery: bodily fine-tuning that's used *after* someone has lost weight.
- Bariatric Surgery: major procedures for people who are massively overweight and have repeatedly bombed out at diet and exercise, and whose lives are in danger.

Even if you need to lose only a little weight, you may know someone who can benefit from one or more of these treatments. We offer these explanations not as across-the-line endorsements for everyone, but as a base of knowledge that can help you understand the physiology of medical solutions and give you a basis for exploring whether these options will work for you or a family member.

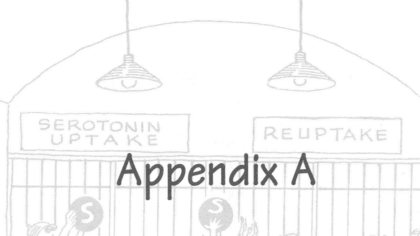

Appendix A

This Is Your Fat on Drugs

The Medical Jump Start to Waist Management

Diet Myths

- Using weight-control drugs is a sign of failure.

- OTC weight-loss drugs are safe.

- Caffeine makes you hungry.

In sports, drugs are viewed as cheating. In school, drugs are viewed as a quick ticket to suspension. In music, drugs may be viewed as another member of the band. But in weight-loss circles,

drugs have the reputation for being extreme or even being the dirty way to lose weight. Used the right way, under the right supervision, however, pharmaceuticals that influence weight can help change your brain chemistry to help you reach your goals.

Why? Because they're kick starts for times when you may reach a plateau after you've started to succeed with diet and exercise with the YOU Plan.

They're what can help you get over the hump.

YOU-reka! Weight-control drugs — in the form of doctor-supervised drugs, not OTC weight-loss fads — help you regulate your brain chemicals, so you think less about "dieting" if you need help to break plateaus. It's like a coach helping an athlete through a slump. Whatever their use, you do need to know that they're not miracle weight-loss methods, at least not at this point. They won't microwave fat from your belly in thirty seconds. But they can help you achieve about a 5 percent to 10 percent weight loss while you're taking them. That's significant, especially when you're stalling. But the only way to maintain the change is to simultaneously incorporate and supplement with the lifestyle and behavioral changes that we discuss in your overall waist management plan. Here are some hard numbers for the average person: Lifestyle change alone will usually get you 7 per-

378

cent loss of your total weight without major difficulty. Drugs alone will get you the same benefit, on average. But if you combine efforts, you can double the benefits to 14 percent.

Because these drugs have side effects, prescription weight-loss medications should be used only by patients whose complications from obesity are more serious than the possible side effects. They're

A Good Side to Bad Drugs?

Very soon, more and more classes of drugs will be developed to help control appetite, and some of them have their biochemical roots in the mechanisms of illegal drugs. One of the newest classes of weight-loss drugs — cannabinoid blockers, one of which is called rimonabant — are used to prevent cannabinoid receptors from making you hungry. Those receptors in your brain are the ones

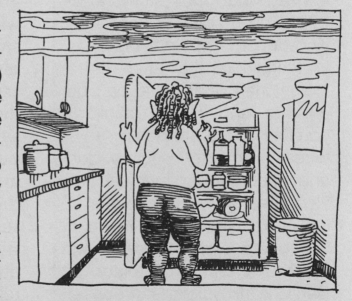

that are activated when someone smokes marijuana (cannabis is the scientific name for marijuana) and goes on to devour the top two shelves in the pantry (hence the marijuana munchies). How do they make you hungry? By blocking CCK and leptin, which encourages hedonistic eating. Drugs that block cannabinoid receptors are suspected to work because those blockers help reduce cravings. The cannabinoid receptors are also found in your liver, muscle, and belly fat and they affect how your body uses and stores food. Blocking these receptors results in less fat in the blood (triglycerides), less risk of diabetes, amd more of the healthy HDL cholesterol, dude.

not to be used for cosmetic weight loss. They're approved for people with a body mass index of 30 or above (see Figure A.1 on page 382), or 27 or above with obesity-related conditions like high blood pressure and diabetes. For many people, though, obesity causes an altered body image that also has medical consequences. We are comfortable prescribing them for women with a waist greater than 36 inches or men with a waist greater than 39, or for people who have diabetes, depression, sleep apnea, arthritis, high blood pressure, low self-esteem, or significant arterial disease. But the one prerequisite is that the patient has earnestly attempted changes in eating and activity. None of these drugs has been shown to sustain effectiveness once it is stopped, but the weight losses obtained while the drugs are taken have an added effect: In our and our colleagues' experience, they've helped patients gain confidence, get off the plateau, and lose the sense of guilt and shame associated with obesity.

Here's how these kick starts work: They help control the balance

YOU WHO Barbie

It turns out that your waist divided by your height is as valuable as the BMI in predicting the risks of obesity to your health. Your waist height odds (WHO) should be less than 50 percent, but keep in mind that Barbie is 25 percent and Ken is 36 percent. The average for men is 58 percent and for women is 54 percent.

of chemical reactions in your brain, so that your appetite is never in a monsterlike free-for-all for food. (The downside is that you may revert to old habits when you come off them.)

Generally, drugs that influence weight are classified by the mechanism through which they work. Many, like the ones listed below, work by controlling pathways in the brain (specifically through the brain chemicals that we discussed in Part 3), while others, which we'll explain later in this appendix, have an effect on the digestive process.

Drugs That Influence Norepinephrine: Some antidepressants work to control eating by easing anxiety, so that you don't experience the mood shifts associated with overeating. While some antidepressants actually increase weight, at least one — called bupropion (Wellbutrin) — has been shown to be effective for weight loss by influencing levels of norepinephrine (the fight-or-flight neurochemical), as well as increasing the pleasure-seeking dopamine. It creates a synthetic saber-toothed tiger: The norepinephrine increase that suppresses hunger causes your heart rate to increase and your blood pressure to increase, also speeding your metabolism. One study showed that people who took Wellbutrin maintained a seven- to twenty-pound weight loss for a year. (The downside is that the study was done with a dose of Wellbutrin that is associated with an increased risk of seizures — 300 to 400 milligrams.) Wellbutrin is often used in conjunction with a class of drugs called SSRIs (selec-

Figure A.1 **Tale of the Scale** This Body Mass Index (BMI) table lets you easily see what category you fall into. Just find your weight across the bottom and your height in the left column to see where the lines cross. The most common way governments and doctors keep track of our fat is through tables like this BMI table.

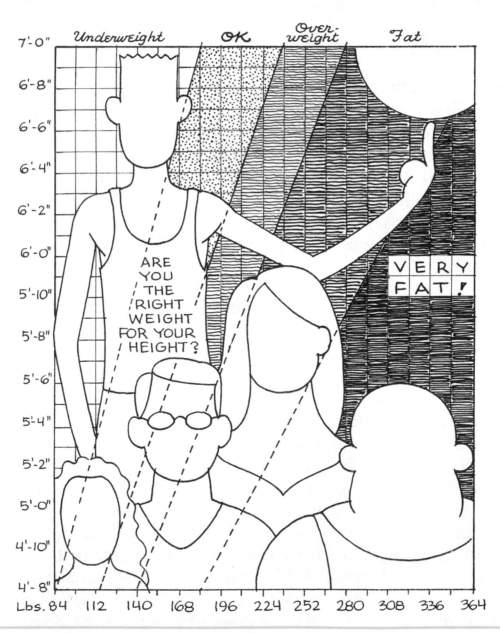

tive serotonin reuptake inhibitors) to reverse the weight gain and sexual side effects (decreased libido and delayed orgasm) that are sometimes associated with some SSRIs like Zoloft. (Some SSRIs like Celexa and Lexapro are shown to decrease appetite by increasing CCK and oxytocin.)

Caffeine and nicotine also work as appetite suppressants the same way — by increasing norepinephrine, suppressing appetite, and speeding metabolism (and heart rate). These drugs can be an effective part of a waist management plan (just not in the form of actual cigarettes). The herb ephedra, which is found in many "miracle" weight-loss solutions, has the same mechanism of action but can cause heart attacks. Just because something is natural doesn't mean it's good for you; tornadoes and bubonic plague are natural, too.

Drug Thugs

You think you're doing something right: You're overweight, which causes high blood pressure, so you go on medication to bring your BP down. Or maybe you're depressed about being overweight, and you take an antidepressant to help deal with self-esteem issues. The irony of it all? Many of the drugs used to treat those issues have been shown to make you *gain* weight. Beta-blockers, one of the drugs most commonly used for hypertension, for instance, have been shown to cause weight gain and decrease metabolic rate by 10 percent. Several classes of antidepressants have also been shown to increase body weight, as has insulin (used to help control diabetes, which can be caused by obesity). The lesson: Don't automatically assume that medications — even ones designed to help a specific problem — will help your weight-loss efforts. We recommend that you ask your doctor about weight side effects of drugs and try addressing weight issues with nutrition and activity levels first, before starting a prescription regimen that may leave you with an increase in the very thing you're trying to decrease.

Figure A.2 **Get the Message?** Neurons communicate with each other by sending and catching chemical signals. Serotonin, for instance, makes you feel good when your synapses are catching it. When there aren't enough for your neurons to catch, that's when you feel depressed. Drugs that stimulate the feel-good aspect may help promote weight loss.

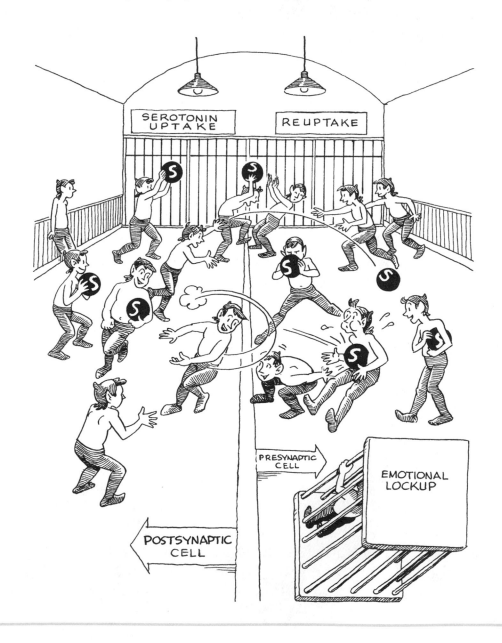

Drugs That Influence Serotonin: The drug sibutramine (Meridia) has been shown to suppress appetite by acting like the feel-good brain chemical serotonin, so you don't experience the dramatic increases and decreases in brain chemicals that lead to hedonistic eating. Most folks can lose roughly 7 percent of their weight but not much more with this drug alone. By the way, the popular weight-loss drug phen-fen had the same physiological action too, but it was taken off the market because of its link to pulmonary hypertension (that's high blood pressure in arteries that supply the lungs). An interesting side note: Increasing serotonin has been shown to reduce carbohydrate intake, so it becomes a physiological chicken-egg discussion: Do comfort foods work to help curb depression? Or do we eat because we're depressed?

Drugs That Influence Dopamine: Currently, no weight-loss drugs work by changing your reward-seeking dopamine levels, but dopamine may hold the key to why you crave the foods that make you feel good. Sugar's been shown to increase dopamine levels — and that spins you into a cycle of addiction.

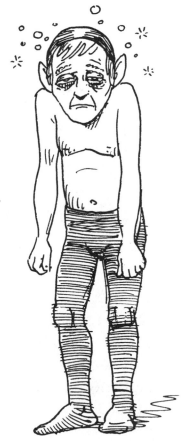

You eat sugar, which makes you feel cloud-high. When that feeling diminishes, you crave sugar to feel good, and so on. Of course, another radical direction is to address the psychological pain directly instead of using food as an emotional bandage.

Drugs That Influence GABA: Drugs that affect gamma-aminobutyric acid (GABA) levels are used for anesthesia and anti-seizure medications, because GABA acts to slow you down, calm you down, and put you to sleep. We don't recommend a lifetime of general anesthesia for weight control, but two antiseizure medications — topiramate (Topamax) and zonisamide (Zonegran) — have been shown to cause weight loss. They work because the drugs calm the nerve activity in your brain that signals you to eat (plus, you can't very well snort down a dozen glazed doughnuts when you're snoozing head-over-chest on the recliner). Topiramate, in fact, is a drug of choice for some weight-loss docs, but its class of drugs does have potential side effects; these drugs can make you feel disoriented, as if you're in a zombielike state.

Drugs That Influence Your Gut: While a number of weight-loss drugs can help change the circuitry in your brain to help you control your weight, other drugs influence the functions of your gut. The drug orlistat (also known as Xenical) works by inhibiting the diges-

The Future of Gut Drugs

One of the most promising drug therapies involves the injection of CCK or things that have a chemical structure similar to the Crucial Cravings-Killer peptide. (Remember, CCK causes your stomach to hold on to food for a long time and sends messages to the brain through the vagus nerve to say you're full.) The body produces specific enzymes in the small intestine to degrade CCK, but new developments show that you can stop that action. Ingesting or inhaling CCK that can access the bloodstream may help increase satiety levels.

tion of fat — specifically by blocking the enzyme lipase, which is responsible for breaking down dietary fats to prepare them for bile and absorption. When fat isn't broken down, the body can't absorb it, so you'll take in fewer calories. Orlistat seems to be safer than other weight-loss drugs and effective at helping you lose about 10 percent of your body weight. And it also seems to help with cholesterol, because it inhibits the absorption of fat. One disadvantage of orlistat is that you absorb less of the fat-soluble vitamins A, D, and E from your food, so you need to take a multivitamin at night. Another side effect is that you experience a toilet trifecta: more frequent stools, more gas, and caca that's oilier than a mechanic's garage. Luckily, you can counteract the effects with natural fiber in the form of psyllium husks, which seem to reduce the symptoms by bulking up your stools. You can also reduce the side effects by having a little fat (and less fat, in total) with each meal instead of all of your daily fat at dinner alone. Too much fat, and you'll know it with a full-time appointment with

FACTOID

The supplement called Hoodia — originally used by African tribal leaders so they could go on long hikes without going hungry — seems to show some effectiveness by stimulating the hypothalamus to increase the energy source of the body (called ATP). One early study showed that people taking Hoodia ate 1,000 fewer calories per day than those not taking it. But there's one catch: There's been more hoodia sold in the last year than has actually been produced in all of African history — meaning there are many companies claiming to have it in the bottles they're selling, when there's none in there. The herb Garcinia (at 300 milligrams) seems to work by the same mechanism, through changing ATP levels. One study showed that Garcinia decreased body weight by 5 percent in eight weeks.

your bathroom if you want to avoid soiling your undergarments.

The drug works by not allowing your body to absorb fat, effectively teaching people what foods have fat. It's like a candle for many patients — it teaches them how close you can get to the fire without getting burned. Just because a package says the food is cholesterol-free (or the like) doesn't mean it's free of fat. (You know by the fact that fat will go right through you.) Many docs say this drug is useful as it teaches you which foods have hidden bad fats in them so you avoid the aging that hidden saturated and trans-fats cause in addition to losing weight. Many specialists find orlistat a very useful addition to a successfully started waist-loss program that has stalled. Other gut-related drugs are also worth exploring.

- Because the drug glucophage (Metformin) increases insulin sensitivity, it seems to reduce inflammation in the liver, so the hormonal cross talk that is so important to prevent metabolic syndrome or polycystic ovary disease is preserved. Sugar levels return to normal as insulin is able to perform its role in pushing these tasty molecules into cells for consumption (blocking the production of new sugars that are made every half hour as energy stores are used up). Side effects include gas and nausea, not a bad combo to force less calorie intake. If you become dehydrated, this drug can cause severe problems — so it is not for those who like to exercise for two hours or more at a time.
- Acarbose (Precose) works in a similar way to the drug orlistat, but on sugars. While orlistat inhibits the absorption of fat, acarbose inhibits an enzyme in the metabolism of carbohydrates — meaning that it blocks carbohydrates from breaking down in the gut and being absorbed by your body. (The side effect is that sugars can cause diarrhea and also can be fermented, resulting in more gas.) Think of this as a subtle reminder to eat the right foods.
- A new drug called Zelnorm (tegaserod) works by stimulating serotonin receptors in your gut (remember, your intestines are

your second brain), and it also works by triggering other neuro-transmitters that decrease intestinal sensitivity and make you feel good, so you eat less. (People with more sensitive intestines have more pain with gas.) By working differently from fiber and laxatives, Zelnorm can be an alternative for those with irritable bowel syndrome.

YOU TIPS!

Drugs: Just Say Maybe. Any of the drugs we discussed earlier in this appendix are practical jump starts to use when you've reached a plateau or need help getting over a hump. So when you start your diet, schedule an appointment with your doc when you're likely to hit the hump — about day thirty. If you fit the BMI or waist profile from earlier in the appendix, we suggest you and your doc think about Wellbutrin. The drug is thought to work by helping emotional eaters decrease cravings. The reason why it works: It helps us not think and obsess over food. It can program our bodies to get back into our natural position — that is, not substituting a six-pack of Hershey bars for a spouse who doesn't listen, a boss who doesn't understand, or a child who feels like rolling soup cans down aisle four. Very soon, more and more new classes of drugs will be developed to help curb cravings and appetites, and they're worth exploring with your doctor. But these are short-term boosters to help you along your path.

> **FACTOID**
>
> One of the newer weight-loss interventions involves OTC Zantac (an acid-relieving drug). It may work by activating CCK, so that you feel full. Some studies have shown that cimetidine, the prescription acid-relief form of Zantac (vanitidine), in a dose of 400 milligrams three times a day, may yield a 5 percent decrease in waist size.

Try a Waist Management Cocktail. When many people quit smoking, one of the first things they'll do is complain about the weight they've gained after quitting. There's something to that. While cigarettes are bullets to your lungs, they do

Myth Buster seem to help people control weight — possibly, in part, through the destruction of taste buds. But they also seem to help by increasing metabolic rate by up to 10 percent as well as helping to reduce appetite.

Well, the chances of our offering up cigarettes as a waist-control method are roughly the same as the eight-track tape making a comeback. We don't want to rule out nicotine as one of those early-program jump starts you can use to jump over a hurdle to increase your metabolism and reduce your appetite. Studies have shown that nicotine — in the form of patches and gum, *not* in the form of cigarettes — when combined with a modest dose of caffeine (as in two cups of coffee) can help reduce weight for those who use it. It's not a long-term solution but one that can help you adjust and automate. We've prescribed a 7-milligram nicotine patch to help some over a hurdle, combined with two cups of coffee (average cups, not the high-test espresso type — it would be only two-thirds of one of those babies). Of course we ensure that the patient doesn't have side effects triggered by the caffeine, such as migraine headaches, GERD, increased heartbeats, or anxiety. Caffeine will raise your metabolic rate just a tad to burn more calories. Combine the two if your weight-loss program stalls. They can act as that crutch to help you over the hump. This is one tip, like all others in this appendix, that you should share with your doctor, to play it safe. Plus you need a prescription.

Appendix B

Skinny Skin Skin

When Plastic Surgery Is an Option

Diet Myths

- If done well, plastic surgery pretty much guarantees bodily happiness.

- Liposuction can help you lose a lot of fat fast.

- Some procedures can eliminate cellulite.

One of the reasons many of us want to lose weight is to look better, but sometimes — even after losing weight — that doesn't happen. That's because all that fat you were carrying around has stretched your skin to the size of a hot-air balloon and made it droopier than a basset hound's ears. But unlike some side effects, there are ways around this one. If you've gone through the rebooting process and then experience the effects of saggy, stretchy skin, you might be considering adding another player to your waist management team: the plastic surgeon.

Like a relief pitcher in baseball, the plastic surgeon can come in to complete your new image by sculpting, shaping, and rebuilding your body. Before we start, let's make two things clear: Plastic surgery isn't about perfection, and it has its risks. In reality, plastic surgery can very well be about trading in one deformity (saggy skin) for another (scars that can run longer than the Amazon), but for some people the trade-off is worth it.

Myth Buster

We know the knock: Only egocentric people use plastic surgery in a quest for exterior perfection. (Say that to someone who's lost a lot of weight and has stomach skin hanging down to the knees.) But you don't have to be desperately seeking saline implants to benefit from plastic surgery. For many who undergo plastic

FACTOID

Anyone who claims they can remove fat cells without surgery is more fraudulent than a credit-card thief. Ads for "mesotherapy" appear in the yellow pages, on telephone poles, and in your in-box — but stay away. They purport to do it by injecting a drug into your skin over the course of ten to twenty sessions; the drugs in these treatments haven't been shown to be effective. Of course, some chemicals — like sulfuric acid — might actually work, but we'd prefer you save these chemicals for clogged sinks.

surgery after weight loss or as a supplement to weight loss, some procedures can improve health as much as they improve appearance. Of course, plastic surgery isn't for everybody, and it's not something we endorse if the idea makes you squirm. Having plastic surgery doesn't turn you into a Barbie, doesn't make you more vain than a mirror-hogging gym-goer, and doesn't make you a cheat. If you're comfortable with it, you can view it as the polish on the washed car, the foam on the tall latte, the kiss after the first date. It helps make your weight loss feel complete — so you can be comfortable with your newly reprogrammed body.

Stretching the Truth

Anyone who's gained or lost weight knows what it can do to your skin: Pack on too much fat, and you'll create stretch marks that look like a

family of earthworms. Lose a lot of fat, and your skin will pour off your body like vats of pancake batter. Of course, we all know that skin is elastic and has a rubber band's ability to expand and snap back; one look at a woman who gives birth and regains a flat tummy

393

Figure B.1 **Thick Skin** Stretching tears the skin at the level of the dermis — that's the lower level of your skin that makes new cells, not the outer level of skin called the epidermis. (Unfortunately, the stretch marks associated with weight gain that happens in this deeper level do appear on the outer level.)

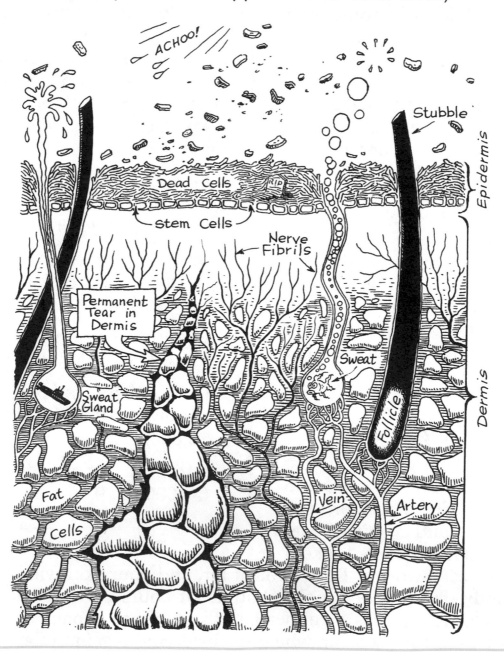

a few months later is evidence of that. So the question for those of us who lose a lot of weight is this: Why doesn't our skin snap back to normal after our weight does?

Think of your skin as one of those large Hefty plastic garbage bags. When it comes out of the box, it's folded up nice and tight. Fill it up with trash, and it expands, stretches, and bulges. Durable yet flexible, most bags can withstand the typical dumping of cans, papers, turkey carcasses, anything you throw into it. Your skin works the same way — it's durable, it stretches, and it can withstand most of the junk you toss into it. But what happens when you put on too much weight? When you fill your human Hefty bag with pies, nachos, and turkey carcasses? It'll keep stretching and stretching and stretching, but at some point, just like a bag, the skin will tear (see Figure B.1). It will tear at the level of the dermis — that's the lower level of your skin that makes new cells, not the outer level of skin called the epidermis,

FACTOID

It's about as easy to remove cellulite as it is to remove a suspect-looking mole with a plastic spoon. It can't be done.

Myth Buster

About 90 percent of women have some of the cottage-cheese-looking fat in their thighs or butts, and that's natural. Human skin is tethered to the underlying muscle by connective strands of collagen — and that prevents excessive motion. Dogs lack these; that's why their skin can move so easily. No creams (which mostly use caffeine as the active ingredient), medicine, lasers, or massage will work to remove cellulite marks. One technique vigorously marketed out of France is called Endermologie. It may temporarily reduce the appearance of cellulite. But it's only temporary and not worth the big bucks (or even little ones), in our opinion.

though the stretch marks associated with weight gain do appear on the outer level.

Just in the way that the bag becomes stretched to the point of tearing, your skin does too — and at that point, it's too late for it to snap back in place. So even if you take the trash out of the bag (by losing fat), you won't be able to restore the bag to its original state (of nice, tight skin). So it's very likely that you'll keep the skin of your 250-pound body, even if you now weigh 150.

The Plastic Possibilities

Whether you've lost a lot of weight or a little, you can fine-tune your skin with some small-scale procedures once you've lost the weight. These are the most common and — as long as you use them for the right purpose — reasonable solutions for very specific problems.

Tummy Tucks: Given the number of plastic-surgery shows on TV these days, flat stomachs are everywhere. Now, tummy tucks aren't for people with massive weight loss but primarily for people who develop a football-size pouch under their belly button (they're mostly done for women who develop a pouch after childbirth). Here's how they work: The excess skin is pinched, and the flap of skin is removed. On top of the rectus abdominis muscle (that's the six-pack muscle), you have a cellophanelike casing. It's a thick, leathery sac that wraps your innards together, a little like a denser sausage casing. When you gain weight, not only does your skin stretch, but that casing stretches as well. In the tummy tuck, besides cutting and reconnecting the skin, doctors will also pull that casing back together so it's tight and flat. Women who have had large babies can have muscles on their stomach that have weakened and separated during the process, and no number of crunches will fix that appearance, but plastic surgery will. Another bonus: Because the rectus is attached to the external obliques (the muscles on the sides of your torso), the tightening will improve the overall tone of all your abdominal muscles — potentially decreasing back pain and improving posture and lower-body strength.

Face and Neck Lifts: The genetic reality is that some people have more chins than Elvis has platinum records. If, thanks to your ancestors, you store fat in your neck even when the rest of your body is as sleek as a jaguar, then you can have the walrus rings removed from your neck. To tighten the skin on your face, the surgeon will make cuts that run inside your hairline at the sides of your forehead, run parallel with your hairline down your temples, emerge from your hair just above your ears, then go in front of your ears, under your lobes, and up into the hair behind your ears. The surgeon can also make a cut under the chin to work on your neck. Next, your skin is separated from the tissue and muscle below it (in most cases, those

FACTOID

It seems that using lotion on skin before it stretches (as in the case of a pregnant belly) may help reduce the chance of developing stretch marks, because the moisture may help maintain the dermis. However, once the dermis tears apart, there's nothing you can do. A lot of people may recommend lotions with alpha tocopherol (vitamin E) or aloe in them to help. No research has shown that vitamin E or its derivatives or aloe will make stretch marks fade. Once that layer underneath the skin is ripped, in theory you can only prevent it from getting worse. But some of our medical friends swear from patient and personal experience that aloe and/or vitamin E will reduce the size and improve the look of stretch marks. Things that make stretch marks worse: getting fatter and lack of exercise. Steroids and sun damage also weaken the skin's collagen. By the way, one thing that does facilitate skin healing (though not the total disappearance of stretch marks): walking. In one study, identical wounds healed in twenty-nine days for walkers and thirty-nine days for nonwalkers.

Figure B.2 **Get Tucked In** In tummy tucks, not only is the excess skin removed, but the underlying muscle (rectus fascia) is tightened to give patients a buff belly.

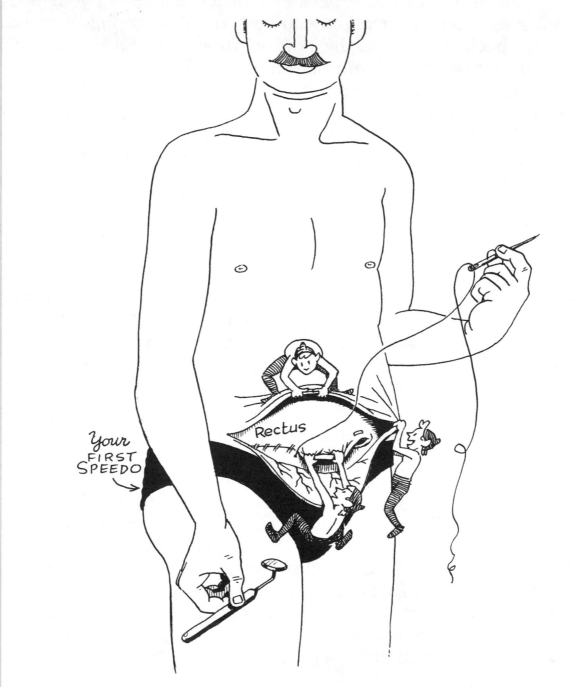

get tightened too). Then the surgeon can remove excess fat in your face with liposuction (see below), pull your facial skin up and back, trim off the excess, and stitch it back to the line where the cut was initially made. If your hair is nice and full, and you have a good surgeon, it will be hard to see the scar on this one (unlike the tummy tuck).

Liposuction: Straws may suck the cola out of cups, and vacuums may suck the crumbs out of the carpet fibers, but when it comes to the fat-removal process, liposuction sucks big-time. A fairly safe procedure (with three to five days of recovery time), liposuction has a place in a waist management plan. **YOU-reka!** But know this: Liposuction is no better as a weight-loss technique than a leg amputation. Liposuction is a sculpting technique; it'll help remove fat from problem areas, but it won't help you lose a significant number of pounds. So the question you need to ask yourself before considering liposuction is this: Is there an intolerable element to your body that, if changed, would make you happy? For example, are you disproportioned (a size 4 upper body and size 10 lower body)? Or do you carry your weight in one particular area only (like love handles on men)?

Liposuction has little effect on weight because fat is light. Remember that loving barb,

Myth Buster

> **FACTOID**
>
> It's best to keep a new surgical incision moist with a gentle moisturizer, but don't overtreat it. Our general rule: You shouldn't put any medicine or anything else on your skin that you wouldn't put in your eye. But get this: One study showed that covering a scar with porous paper (like Steri-Strips) for six months reduced the likelihood of an ugly scar — probably because the tape helps keep the healing scar moist.

"fat floats." A liter of fat weighs about two pounds (and the lipo max is five liters of fat removed). The ideal patient is about 10 percent above the ideal body weight, with isolated fat in one area (and that one area is often genetically driven; in other words, all the members of a family are shaped with excess fat in the same place). People who undergo massive weight loss can still use liposuction, but it should be in combination with other procedures to get their bodies in the proportion they want.

Here's how it works: About fifteen minutes before the actual sucking procedure, but while you're anesthetized, you're pumped full of fluid in the area of focus. The fluid contains saline (a salt solution), epinephrine (to control bleeding by making the arteries in the fat

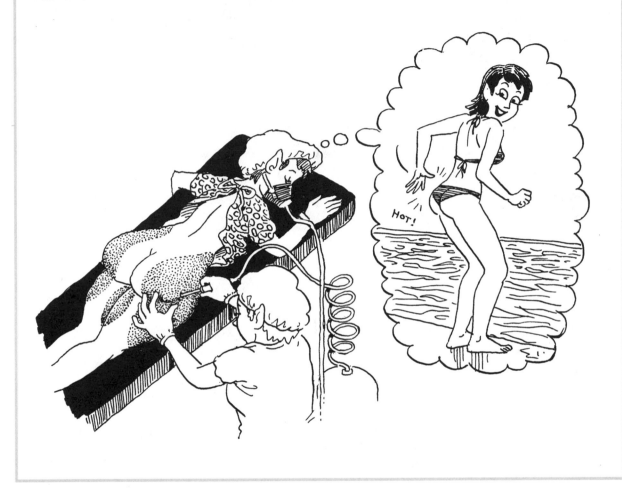

Figure B.3 **Vacuum Cleaners** With liposuction, the body can be sculpted with a straight instrument that serially churns and sucks out fat from selected areas.

constrict, or spasm), and lidocaine (to numb the pain). If you're having the procedure done with general anesthesia, you'll get different amounts of these drugs, which is important, because getting too much lidocaine causes many of the most serious complications associated with liposuction. When the fluid is pumped in, you'll swell up like the Michelin Man because you'll be given an amount of fluids equal to the amount of fat that's going to be sucked out (about one liter of fluid in for one liter of fat removed, depending upon the technique being used).

Then doctors suck out the fluid and the fat in one of two ways. In the first procedure, doctors take a tube of straw-shaped metal, shove it under the skin, and push it where it needs to go. They shove it in and out, in and out, cutting little tunnels of fat that are removed. In the second procedure, doctors use a power tool that looks like a coffee stirrer. Vibrating about 4,000 times a minute, the tool breaks apart fat cells and sucks them up

and out. Both are acceptable procedures in the right hands and allow for precise contouring. The key phrase? "The right hands." See "Do Your Own Checkup" for finding a plastic surgeon.

YOU TIPS!

Maintain Your Holding Pattern. Before you have any kind of plastic surgery for your skin, your doctor should insist upon a healthy nutritional status — primarily so you can heal properly after surgery (that is, maintaining a diet with healthful ingredients). You will also have much better outcomes if you actually train for surgery like you would for a road race, by exercising. You will need to be sedentary after surgery, so being strong beforehand just makes you bounce back better. Your doctor will also use diet and exercise to assess your ability to stay at your current level of weight. The doctor will want to know if your weight's been stable over the last six to twelve months. If you've been fluctuating either up or down, there's no point in having the surgery. If you're prone to gaining weight again, you'll simply stretch it out and defeat the purpose of the surgery. And if you're still losing weight, the surgery may be a bigger waste of money than the psychic hotline, because you run the risk of sagging again after the surgery.

Take a Reality Check. It all sounds more blissful than an oceanside piña colada: no more fat; no more loose skin; ah, the ideal body. But many people have a tough time adjusting to life in the plastic era. Why? There are psychological reasons: Weight gain occurs slowly — and most times, with the exception of some surgical procedures, weight loss happens slowly as well. You have time to psychologically adjust to your new body, whether it's getting bigger or smaller. But when you have plastic surgery (especially with removal of your skin), the changes are fast, drastic, and, in some cases, emotionally heartstopping. It took ten years to get fat and mentally adjust to your sense of "you," but when somebody whacks off twenty pounds of excess fat and skin and stitches you up like grandma's needlepoint, it takes a whole different mind-set to deal with the effects.

Yes, losing weight and losing excess skin are what you've always wanted, but you need to be prepared for the scars, for the body adjustments, for the attention you'll be given. While some people bask in the compliments they receive on their new bodies, others are embarrassed or shamed by positive feedback, because it reminds them of how noticeably overweight they once were. Lots of obese people never look in the mirror, so your new body may take some getting used to. There are also physical reasons that people are disappointed after plastic surgery. It's not like blowing your nose. Some of these surgeries are quite invasive, and there are drains, swelling, some pain, immobilization, and other discomforts that come with them. Some patients expect to look twenty-five years old when they're done. That just isn't real. The best you can hope for is a fitter, well-rested, ten-years-younger you.

Do Your Own Checkup. With some skin-altering procedures, it seems as if everybody and his mother's gardener thinks he can do them. But for any of these procedures, you need a board-certified

403

plastic surgeon. Liposuction docs should perform more than 100 procedures a year, and those doing surgeries for massive skin reduction should be doing a minimum of one and hopefully more a month. The board-certified plastic surgeon will be equipped to handle complications (remember, in liposuction procedures, the fat gets stabbed, and one potential risk is the stabbing of vital things and things that bleed a lot residing under or in the fat).

It doesn't matter whether you sign up to have surgery done in a hospital or an in-office doctor's OR; there's only one way to determine if the facility meets standards of high quality for service and cleanliness. That is, it needs to be accredited by the country's health-care do-gooder group called the Joint Commission, the patient's safety champion. You can search for facilities at www.jcaho.org. It's the backup and reassurance you need when someone's about to slice a few bricks' worth of skin off your belly.

Just because the corner guy is offering the "latest" or "newest" or "most cutting-edge" procedure doesn't mean you should be first in line. The plastic-surgery field is full of fraud, and you don't want to be a lab rat in someone else's experiment. Make sure the tool, technique, or procedure has scientific backing. One good place to start: Check the surgeon's website to see his results or ask for the "brag book" of sample cases like yours. Some plastic surgeons specialize in extreme weight-loss patients and can show pictures with disappearing bat wings and shots with and without skin aprons. But remember that no one shows off images of complications or poor results, so ask to see at least a dozen pictures. It helps if the surgeon is a diplomate in a plastic surgical society such as the American Society of Plastic Surgeons (ASPS), the American Society for Aesthetic Plastic Surgery, the International Society of Aesthetic Plastic Surgery (ISAPS), or the American Association of Plastic Surgeons (AAPS) — which means having to keep up with the latest and greatest. And ask for references. After all, just because the corner plastic surgeon buys a quarter-million-dollar device doesn't mean that you need to bankroll the financing.

Now Stop. We've all seen pictures of them; they're people who treat cosmetic operations like massages. The more they have, the better they feel. But the truth is that these people have more plastic than an in-debt college student. Yes, it's tempting to have additional procedures, but plastic surgery can be as addictive as any drug. The sign that you're in a constant quest for — *watch our fingers making quotation marks in the air* — "perfection" is that you're planning your next surgery as soon as you're finished with the one before it. So, yes, find your trouble spots and decide what will make you happy. Then pick an end point where you want your body to be and deal with the reality of what you're going to look like when you get there. Look in the mirror, tell yourself what changes would give you satisfaction, and then stop. If you can't stop — if you're constantly considering lipo-ing this or tucking that — then it's not your skin you need checked; it's your head. Bottom line: Before deciding on a procedure, you have to accept the fact that you're not seeking perfection; you're seeking improvements in your body and your happiness.

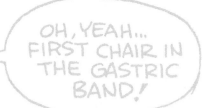

Appendix C

The Extreme Team

What to Do If Your Weight Is Out of Control

Diet Myths

- Weight-loss surgery is the easy way out.

- If you have gastric bypass surgery, you never have to worry about dieting again.

- Once you have the surgery and recover from it, the hard part is over.

For basketball players, desperation is the full-court shot at the buzzer. For accountants, desperation is 11:59 p.m. on April 15. For parents of an antsy kindergartner, it's a malfunctioning SpongeBob DVD. But for people struggling with weight issues, desperation is the feeling that comes when you've morphed from being overweight to going overboard. But here's the difference between most desperate situations and this one: While basketball players rarely make full-length heaves and 1040s can't be completed in sixty seconds, people with extreme weight situations do have a life raft that can change desperation to salvation: weight-loss surgery.

Most people view weight-loss surgery the way they view steroids in sports — that it's cheating, it's unnatural, it's an unfair advantage, it's cutting corners. But there are plenty of people — way too many, in fact — who have coffin-enticing obesity in the form of a body mass index of 35 or higher, with consequences like diabetes and high blood pressure. And for this segment of the population, especially if they have repeatedly tried and failed at a diet and exercise regime, weight-loss surgery may be an effective solution.

Myth Buster Some people simply can't lose weight like everyone else and often beat themselves up about being undisciplined or out of control. Many are very disciplined, successful, and in control in other aspects of their lives but are just wired differently in the weight department. Finally, there's a real alternative for people who are incapable of succeeding without help: weight-loss surgery.

In nearly every other medical situation in our lives, we experience a symptom, we try to treat it ourselves, and then we seek professional help if we can't. We need to start thinking about obesity as if it's any other health problem that prompts you to see a doctor — be it a bullet wound, a lump in your breast, or cholesterol numbers that need commas.

The truth is that many people have tried every over-the-counter antiobesity option; they have a library of diet books, a garage full of exercise equipment, and neurons full of frustration. But no matter what they try to do to lose weight, they either can't take it off or can't keep it off. For these people, the answer isn't always the over-the-counter way, because a life of obesity requires more than a commitment to a three-day all-juice fast or some ab machine that claims to banish your belly using electrodes. Heavy-duty bodies require heavy-duty help.

And that's OK. If you — or someone you love — falls into this category, then you have a serious condition that should make you feel you'd do whatever you could to try to reverse it. Technically, it's defined as 100 pounds above the ideal weight for men and 80 pounds above ideal weight for women, or men with 48-inch waists or larger and women with 41-inch waists or larger.

Think for a second: If you had prostate or breast cancer (which both have about the same risk of death per year for people over fifty as does a waist size of 38 for women and 45 for men with risks like high blood pressure, sleep apnea, diabetes, and cholesterol problems), you'd take action. You'd talk to doctors, you'd schedule surgery to remove the tumor, and you'd make lifestyle changes that would help lower the chance that you'd ever contract the disease again. You wouldn't pop a cough drop, then throw up your hands in defeat if menthol weren't the magic tumor killer. You'd get professional — even drastic — help. You would even let someone cut you open if the therapy was effective.

It's a mistake to think you're a weakling or a fool if you consider the operation option. Morbid obesity (morbid!) is as concrete a health problem as a sprained ankle, a heart problem, or cancer. In fact, at least 5 percent of morbidly obese people have a specific genetic problem that renders their brains unable to receive the leptin signals that they're full. So no matter what the cause of your weight problem, there's no shame in seeking one of the most effective cures for obesity that modern medicine has developed. Weight-loss surgery works. And it works more effectively — and faster — than any traditional dieting method for people with morbid obesity. Surgery can reduce your excess weight by half, whereas weight-loss drugs get you only 5 percent to 7 percent while you're on them, and lifestyle changes buy you *on average* another 7 percent of total weight if you're on your best behavior.

The success of weight-loss surgery is defined by the loss of excess weight — that is, not how much total weight you lose, but rather the difference between your current weight and your ideal weight. (For women, the ideal weight is 105 pounds for five feet of height, and 5 pounds for every inch after. For men, it's 106 pounds at five feet and 6 pounds for every inch taller. Those are for medium-framed people. Some adjustments are made if you're larger or smaller framed.)

FACTOID

For Medicare reimbursement, surgical centers need to be certified by either the ASBS or the American College of Surgeons (ACS). Medicare has recently agreed to pay for bariatric procedures even if no other comorbidity was found. This could change the reimbursement landscape for growing procedures, like banding — which are sometimes offered to less heavy patients (those with a BMI of 30 and at least one comorbidity).

Surgical options aren't for people who are just a little overweight. They're not for people worried about losing their runway-model job or their clothes not fitting. They're for people whose health is at extreme risk, who are four fries away from putting the grave-digger on speed-dial, because the effects of excess fat increase your risk of developing such day ruiners as coronary artery disease, hypertension, sleep apnea, infertility, chronic back pain, hernias, infections, gallstones, and depression.

Still, these options are the foundations for tomorrow's cutting-edge (and cutting-weight) procedures — the operations that may help people who don't have extreme weight problems. Of course, we still want you to adopt lifestyle changes, like regular walking and pushing away from the corn dogs (to be successful with surgery, you have to adopt more lifestyle changes than ever). But you should also know there is help that can save you and improve your quality of life if you are completely out of control.

Alternative Routes: Have You Got the Guts?

If you were driving along and came upon an urgent flashing sign that warned you of a twenty-mile backup a few miles ahead, you'd peel off at the next exit, hop onto back roads, stop at gas stations, and find your way around the mess. You'd do anything to avoid staying stuck in the same spot for hours. You wouldn't want to feel like you were going nowhere. And you'd probably take your chances that the country roads would turn out to be more effective than the parking lot of a freeway.

Well, if you're in an extreme waist situation, you're in the parking lot. You're stuck. You've stalled. You might even be running out of gas. And you haven't found that magic car-carrying helicopter that can take you from the desperation of feeling like a refrigerator to the healthy, happy feeling that doesn't always revolve around the refrigerator. But some nice alternative routes can get you out of this disastrous jam of yo-yo dieting and morbid obesity. Even better, they're the foundations for future waist management procedures that can change the way we all live.

Most important, these solutions are real options with life-changing results. Consider these statistics:

1. A twenty-five-year-old obese man (with a waist size of 40 inches or greater) has a 22 percent reduction in his longevity (that is, he will lose twelve years of his life).
2. A twenty-pound weight loss corresponds to a 53 percent reduction in obesity-related deaths — and most of these procedures are designed to help people lose five times that much weight.
3. Weight-loss surgery reduces diabetes-related deaths by 80 percent — and some procedures can even *cure* diabetes in over 90 percent of the cases.

What's most amazing is that changes in your risk factors like hypertension and cholesterol, but especially diabetes, start before the significant weight loss even starts in the first few days after surgery. (We know, it sounds like a tabloid headline: "Drop Your Cholesterol in Half! By 3 p.m.!") Your body, the smart little devil that it is, senses that the trend of weight and waist gain or loss is more important than your actual body weight or waist size; for these risk factors, it's not necessarily your waist size or how much you weigh that influences the risks, but which direction your body is heading in. Again and again, patients are off their insulin and hypertension drugs at one month or less after surgery. After surgery, your body starts behaving the way a normal body might behave, regulating the ghrelin and leptin cycle and other ways that your gastrointestinal tract may signal satiety and appetite. One patient told her surgeon that she was sure that he had operated on her brain, not her stomach, because the voice that continually told her she was hungry was turned off for the very first time. Weight-loss surgery may also work by decreasing markers of inflammation in your blood (like C-reactive protein) almost immediately. No matter the mechanisms, the effect is clear — and fast.

So, if obesity has forced one foot in the grave (and ten fingers in the pie), there's no reason to ignore surgery like a two-toothed hitchhiker. It isn't magic and won't create permanent success without lifestyle changes, but it will absolutely make a huge change in almost everyone who does it. Our understanding of how the stomach works has allowed us to develop procedures that manipulate the physiology of the stomach and the digestion process, to help people better control their weight. While a bunch of different surgical procedures exist, they all fall into two categories. They're either restrictive — meaning the procedures limit the room in your stomach and thus the amount of food you can eat. (This is sort of like saying you can't cram any more people into a phone booth; there's only so much it can hold.) Or they're malabsorptive — meaning that they change your body so you can't absorb all the excess calories. Nearly all of them can now be done through a thin, flexible scope, or laparoscopically, without cutting your muscle wall. Some procedures combine the best of both tactics. Below, we'll outline how they work. For more logistics and specifics about weight-loss surgery options and preparation, see www.realage.com.

Myth Buster

But let's be clear: These are major surgeries that, like skydiving and bumper cars, have as many risks as they have rewards. Most of all, you have to know going in that you have to commit to preparing for the procedures and changing your postoperative lifestyle with an appropriate diet and behaviors. Do that, and they'll turn out to be effective procedures that aren't just about improving your looks or sparing your desk chair — they're all about improving your health. Dramatically.

And you also have to be prepared to define what success is. Success isn't defined by how happy you are or how thin you are. It's defined by continuous weight loss of 50 percent of your excess weight. In those terms, surgeries have a success rate of more than 90 percent at one year, with an average over five years between 55 percent and 70 percent.

Myth Buster

You also need to understand that two of these procedures are permanent and irreversible, and you will need to commit to certain routines (like taking a multivitamin and B_{12} daily; drinking lots of water; taking it easy on alcohol, caffeine, sodas, and acidic foods; and not drinking during meals) to stay healthy for the rest of your life. You also need to know that every patient reacts a little differently, so while some patients breeze through, others have a lot of adjusting to do to regain their vitality.

Gastric Banding: Restrictive

In this procedure, the surgeon places a belt-like band around the stomach — up high on the stomach. When the belt is tightened, it constricts the stomach to form an hourglass shape (see Figure C.1) — leaving a very small pouch at the top of the stomach for food to get stored as it enters from the esophagus. The band creates a one-

413

Figure C.1 **Band Aid** Gastric banding limits the amount of food that can enter the stomach, with an inflatable inner tube placed around the stomach.

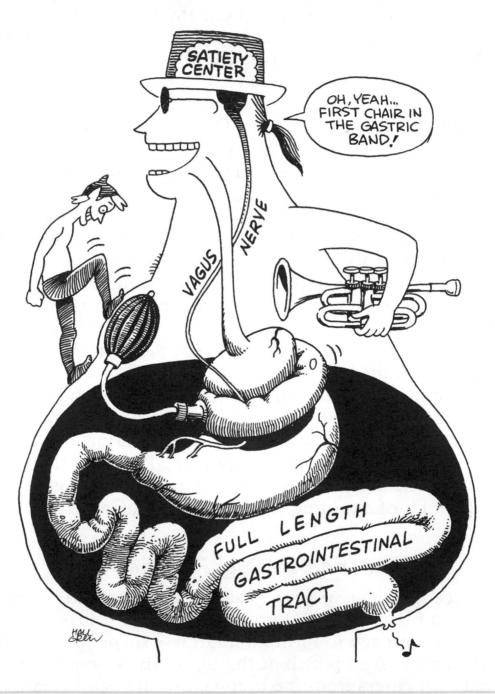

lane road that needs to accommodate dozens of lanes of traffic, a bottleneck that slows the movement of food through your GI system, so there's no way you can physically get more traffic into the bottom half of your stomach. When your food has to travel through that belt-tightened hourglass to the intestine, it means that you stay full for a long time, and you literally can eat only a small meal (this also forces you to eat slowly and chew thoroughly).

The big-band effect is that it simply limits your food intake so you can't eat (and store) excess calories. Doctors can also tighten or loosen the band depending on how much you're able to get down, so this is a procedure that has some flexibility to it. (Think of it as when Popeye squeezes Bluto's neck. When he squeezes, Bluto's head gets bigger. When the band gets tightened, it creates more of a bulge in the stomach and a tighter hole in the middle of the hourglass.) The pluses: Like an intramural-team T-shirt, it's reversible, and it has the lowest risk of all surgical options. The downside is that because your stomach shrinks, you have to cut food down to the size of the nail on your pinkie, which means you may be more likely to feast on junkier foods than bulky foods like spinach.

Duodenal Switch: Malabsorptive

Take a driving trip of any distance, and you know the difference between Route 1 and Alternate Route 1. Route 1 may take you right through the city's downtown so you can stop at the shops, see the houses on the historical register, and putter through the thirty-five traffic lights within a half-mile drag. Fine, in some cases. But if you're just trying to get to the other side of town, then you'll take Alternate 1 — the loop that goes around the town, avoids the lights, and gets you from the post office to the pet salon without having to worm along in traffic that's slower than a sedated slug. A malabsorptive procedure is Alternate Route 1: It cuts out the gastrointestinal main street so that food can go toll booth to exit ramp without having to stop at fat-storing traffic lights along the way.

In the duodenal switch (see Figure C.2), the intestines are cut and

Figure C.2 **Change Paths** Malabsorption is created by dividing the intestines immediately after the stomach and by-passing most of the small bowel. That way, only a short common channel remains for food to be absorbed. The high amount of nonabsorbed food can overburden the colon and cause loose poop.

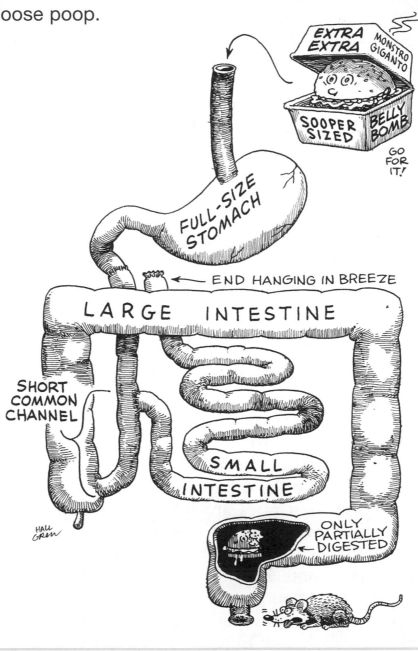

reattached, to quicken the time it takes food to go through the system so that not all the nutrients can get fully absorbed. (It cuts out about 80 percent of the distance food travels in the intestines, from 600 centimeters to 100 centimeters — from more than nineteen feet to about three feet.) The switch allows the intestines to separate the flow of food from the flow of digestive juices like bile, and that's what helps you avoid absorbing all of the calories. Farther down the intestinal line, the two paths get reconnected where the food and fat juices get mixed together like a margarita before you launch it into your municipal sewer system. During the time the two paths are separated, less fat will be absorbed into the bloodstream and eventually stored on your belly. It's a simple physiological statement: If you can't absorb excess calories, you can't store them.

In a way, restrictive procedures like banding are a little bit like having a smaller gas tank. If you cut the size of your fuel tank to one-tenth its original size, your car simply won't be able to hold as much gas. But malabsorptive procedures are like having a leak in your tank. With a leak, your engine wouldn't even be able to get the gas, no matter how much you put in there. In malabsorptive procedures, your body doesn't get the excess calories to store as fat — and in a way it leaks them out of your body (out your back alley).

The switch is typically the most effective procedure and allows people to eat normal-size portions. But you'll probably need to take supplements for the rest of your life (see www.realage.com for specifics), because your body won't digest the nutrients you do eat. Plus the draconian nature of this operation leads to the highest complications rates of any bariatric procedure.

Gastric Bypass: Restrictive and Malabsorptive

Like a good doubles team, a healthy marriage, or oatmeal topped with fruit, gastric bypass has the strength of two parts molded into one. Traditional bypass surgery combines the best of both restrictive and malabsorptive methods — and that makes it the right answer for lots of people who desire surgery. In gastric bypass, surgeons staple

Figure C.3 **Take the Bypass** The compromise procedure of gastric bypass makes the stomach smaller and removes some intestine, but it leaves much more "common channel" small bowel than the duodenal switch, which is a purer malabsorption operation.

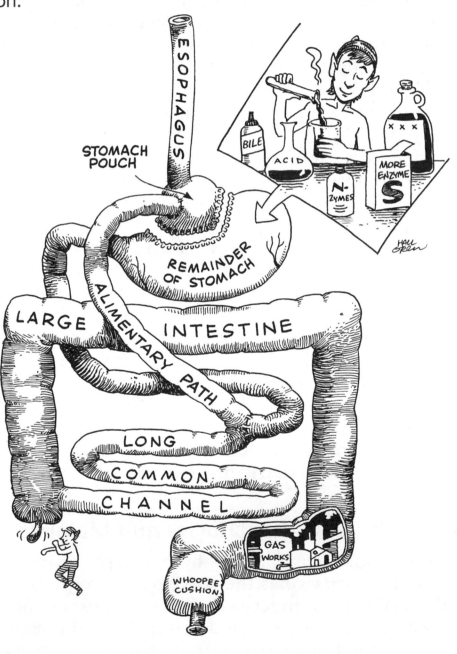

off a little pouch of the stomach (about the size of an egg) to accept the food you eat (see Figure C.3). That's the restrictive element, since you can't eat too much food at once without getting sick. The remainder of the stomach drains into the first section of the small intestine, but no food passes into this section of the intestine, so no absorption can take place. To allow some absorption, a downstream limb of the intestine is sewn to the top of the stomach. So the food goes into the little stomach pouch and then passes into the midpoint of the small intestine, where it continues along the normal pathway for 200 centimeters (about six feet) before it hits the large intestine. In the end, about one-third of the small intestine is bypassed, but not as much as with a duodenal switch. That's the malabsorptive element. In addition to keeping you from absorbing large amounts of excess calories because key components of food digestion are cut out of the process, there is a change in hormonal response to foods that leads to satiety.

How did surgeons ever figure out this crazy idea for losing weight? They latched onto the fundamental ideas for this procedure when removing stomachs in people with ulcer disease (before antacids, H2 blockers, or proton pump inhibitors). Surgeons went in there like special-ops forces and just took out what was causing the problem. But they found that patients developed symptoms and couldn't eat when food bypassed the stomach and got dumped right into the intestines; in that scenario, nutrients entered the bloodstream too quickly, as they got mainlined directly into the sensitive absorptive areas of our bowels. This ailment earned the title dumping syndrome, and suffering patients would feel nauseated, clammy, and sweaty. That all sounds about as appealing as a piping hot cup of Budweiser — unless you're trying to change your size from a redwood to a twig. The surgeons found that those patients who were not experiencing digestion problems were eating smaller portions — and eating healthy foods, since high sugar content really got the dumping syndrome cooking. So that made researchers believe they could curb appetites surgically by bypassing the stomach during the digestion process.

Forcing food to skip some of your small bowel will fix your metabolic problem almost immediately by triggering chemical changes that reverse high blood sugar and hypertension. While weight reduction is fast (about four to seven pounds a week at first), the procedure also has a higher complication rate than the more popular gastric banding.

Gastric Pacing: The Procedure of the Future for All of Us?

Throughout the day, we receive lots of signals that make us want to eat: come-hither burger commercials, coupons for $2.99 buffet specials, unopened bags of sugar wafers flirting with us every time we pass the pantry. But the future of waist-control surgical procedures could come in the form of a message-delivery system that sends signals that help keep us full or feeling full. This system was developed just like bypass procedures — by surgeons working on ulcer disease. They found that when they cut the vagus nerve, the brain no longer stimulated the stomach to make acid, and intestinal contractions slowed down. In effect, disrupting the vagus nerve sent a message that put the intestines to sleep, and the doctors realized that if you could control the message, then you could control the feelings of satiety.

To do that, scientists developed a gastric pacemaker that can be placed on the stomach near the vagus nerve. That pacemaker sends signals to the brain that you're always full by mimicking the actions of CCK (remember, Crucial Cravings-Killer). So that means it will take a lot less pumpkin pie to get you full — and you won't eat as many calories because the pacemaker will send the signal that it feels like Thanksgiving dinner even if you've had only a pretzel stick. Clinical trials are now being done, and the really exciting part about gastric pacemakers is that they could become the option for those in the middleman's zone — those with a large enough waist to be frustrated by dietary stalling but not wide enough to risk gastric banding or bypass surgery. Even better, the pacemaker could be adjusted for voltage to adjust the signals depending on your needs. How well does it work? We don't know yet, but the early reports are that it doesn't work as well as restrictive procedures; however, it's less invasive because no organs are being manipulated, and eventually it could even be placed endoscopically, with no cuts at all. And most likely, its descendants will serve as the basis for hybrids and new technologies that will be developed for people with any kind of waist issues.

YOU TIPS!

Interrogate Yourself. We have nothing against using crutches when we break an ankle, tear a knee ligament, or need to trip a purse-snatcher, so there's no reason not to consider weight-loss surgeries if you qualify for them. They're effective, they're fast, and they have the potential to turn a blimp of a body into a dragster. But they don't come without risks and potential complications, and they necessitate long-term behavioral changes.

Weight-loss surgery will do more than give you the confidence to reintroduce tank tops into your wardrobe. It can also save your life. Still, you have to know that it's not for everyone — and it can be challenging. So when you investigate options, be aware of the ways to lower your risks and increase your odds of success. Your first order of business is asking yourself these two questions:

Are You a Candidate?
You're eligible for surgery if you fit one of these three categories:

- If you're 100 pounds or more over your ideal weight.
- If you have a BMI over 40.
- If you have a BMI over 35 with hypertension, diabetes, arthritis, sleep apnea, serious lipid abnormalities, or altered body image.

For all of them, you need to be willing to make the life changes — exercise and diet — that will make these procedures work. Without them, these procedures won't be successful. After an initial "bounce" downward, you could be back at marathon munching before you know it. You will also need to be realistic about the potential side effects, like hair loss, dumping, diarrhea, and vomiting.

Whom Do I Trust to Switch My Duodenum or Band My Stomach or Bypass My Gastric?

You wouldn't want an orthodontist removing a tumor, an orthopedic surgeon doing a heart transplant, or a urologist doing a nose job. So the same rules apply here: Find a specialist. Ideally, you'll use a facility and team that will do the procedure laparoscopically, as opposed to open. Laparoscopy means that the surgeons will make small incisions and do the procedure through tubes (it'll appear as if they're working with chopsticks). Laparoscopic surgery means you'll heal faster with less pain, but sometimes the surgeon has to resort to the old-fashioned way.

You'll want to find a hospital that does at least 150 procedures a year — such hospitals have much lower complication rates than those that don't. Whoever your surgeon is, be sure there's an entire team of support both pre-op (to minimize complications) and post-op (to give you the best chance for success), including a nutritionist and psychiatrist. You can eat your way through — and thus destroy — any of these procedures. A support team can help you prevent post-op pudding backfires and give you resources to call upon as you're adjusting to your new eating habits — and new body. You should choose a hospital certified by the American Society for Bariatric Surgery (ASBS) (www.asbs.org).

Acknowledgments

Ted, Ted, Ted, Ted. We cannot say his name enough. Ted Spiker brought the multiple complex pieces together in an accessible and humorous fashion that is edgy but never condescending. Gary Hallgren continues to amaze us with his wit and raw artistic talent. He takes challenging concepts and contorts them into engaging cartoons packed with critically important content. View his illustrations with great care to observe every nuance. Craig Wynett is a seer and had the vision to bring us together. He always busts through the clutter with the big ideas that change the way we (and you) should think. These massive ideas are woven through the text and constitute many of our YOU-reka moments. Dr. Ellen Rome's brilliant intellect and dedicated desire to contribute information that would benefit the younger readership made her a crucial ally. Jeff Roizen's remarkable ability to gather raw data and interpret the sometimes disparate results helped us teach America about the hard science of obesity research. We thank Joel Harper for his tireless efforts to make the YOU Workout the perfect tool for us to get procrastinators to exercise. Dr. Keith Roach's clinical insights kept our aim on target. While the hours of conference calls, research, and writing were sometimes exhausting, this powerful team always pulled in the same direction to resolve content and style conflicts. Steve Phillips helped us with his very sophisticated understanding of emotional eating. Finally, our agent Candice Fuhrman's superb insights and honest commentary allowed this book to grow into the manuscript America deserves, and Linda Kahn's priceless reviews of the manuscript helped us tune up the final document.

We also want to thank the group at Free Press (Simon & Schuster) who so enthusiastically supported this material and dedicated themselves to bringing our ideas to the world. Thanks especially to our insightful editor, Dominick Anfuso, and his assistant, Wylie O'-Sullivan. We appreciate the courageous leadership of Martha Levin, and the tireless support of Jill Siegel, Carisa Hays, Linda Dingler, and Suzanne Donahue.

We are indebted to our wonderful collaborators at RealAge.com, including Charlie Silver, Shelly Bowen, Jennifer Perciballi, and especially Val Weaver for coming on strong at the end (and for the two *Vegetarian Times* recipes), and Discovery Health, including Eileen O'Neil, Donald Thoms, John Grassie, and of course Billy Campbell.

In a book of this scope based in science, no one human commands all the needed knowledge, so we sought advice from many world experts who selflessly shared their insights in the true academic tradition. We list them all here without details of their contributions in order to save space for the actual book, but we deeply appreciate their dedication to their specialties and willingness to sacrifice their time in helping craft the most scientifically accurate book on obesity possible. We thank Dr. Linda Bartoshuk, Dr. Mark Bessler, John Campodonico, Jason Conviser, Kathy Chambers, Irwin Davis, Ruth Davis, Dr. Lisa DeRosimo, Mark Eldaief, Dr. Kevin Fickenscher, Michael Gershon, Donoyan Green, Tracy Hafens, Dr. Byron Hoogwerf, Dr. William Inabnet, Gail Jolly, Evan Johnson, Paul Katz, Judith Korner, Ivan Kronenfeld, Dr. Jon Lapook, Karen Levin, Dr. Ben Lewis, Chris Malcom, Dr. Beth Mintzer, Dr. Michael O'Donnell, Dr. Arthur Perry, Susan Petre, Dr. S. Sethu Reddy, Dr. Paul Rosenberg, Sean Shilinsky, Nancy Unobskey, Sidney Unobskey, Meredith Uran-Skuro, Dr. Bernard Walsh, Jim Wharton, and Dr. Jim Zins.

— Michael F. Roizen and Mehmet C. Oz

Most diets and diet books fail you because you regain more than you lost — and that is an epic tragedy of wasted effort. I need to thank the many special people who helped us make this book one that leads to your ideal waist size. So I am grateful to the many other people who did much more than discard the emails when we asked them (sometimes desperately) to help us explain what hadn't been known even five years ago about hunger and satiety. John La Puma, a doctor who doubled as a chef at Rick Bayless's Chicago restaurants, taught me more than I now know about food and cooking. And Donna Szymanski had the patience to correct me and make the recipes more times than can be counted on all fingers and toes.

I need to thank the twenty or so fourth-year medical students each year who took the ten-day, ten-hour-a-day course that Dan Zakri and I taught — you taught me more than I taught you. I'd like to also thank the numerous tasters who visited our home to participate in the yearlong quest for perfect recipes that were great-tasting, were easy to make, and contained only foods that made you healthier. And the Wattels of Lettuce Entertain You indulged and encouraged even when their own patrons shunned the food with hearts next to them in the late 1990s ("times will change"). Our family was fully engaged — with Jeff as our MD, PhD, student research assistant; and Jennifer and Nancy as critical tasters and readers; joined at times by the "enlarged family" of the Unobskeys and Campodonicos, and Dr. Axel Goetz, Ruth Klein, and Irwin Davis. Ruth especially made the diet chapter easier to follow and helped create the shopping lists. I also need to thank Tracy Hafen, who taught me a magnificent amount about exercise; Sukie Miller and Anita Shreve, for saying the early chapters were just what she wanted to read; the many gerontologists and internists who read sections of the book for accuracy; others on the RealAge team who validated and verified the content, and contributed their expertise to the book; and Shivani Chadha and Kate Poneta, the research associates who worked tirelessly to analyze the nutrients of all the recipes we tested.

I also want to acknowledge the passion and tough love from the staff of the Center for Partnership Medicine at Northwestern

Memorial Hospital in Chicago, especially Dr. Dan Dermann, Drew Palumbo, and Dean Harrison. And my partners who allowed me the time to complete the work: Dr. Aaron Gerber and Mike Kessel.

My administrative assistant Beth Grubb made this work possible: she made sure the weekends (and most nights) were free of CAVs games to work on *YOU, YOU-Turns,* and *YOU-reka Moments.* I could not have done this were The Division of Anesthesiology, Critical Care Medicine, and Pain Management at the Cleveland Clinic and its staff not the best in the world. But it is and they are. It's no accident that the Cleveland Clinic has been ranked by *U.S. News & World Report* number one for twelve years in a row in cardiac care: Toby Cosgrove, Joe Hahn, Mike O'Boyle, Roberto Llamas, and Jim Blazer are the best at their positions and insist on innovation and simple excellence — they understand the need to prevent illness and promote wellness. And thanks to all the outstanding colleagues at the Clinic who answered our many questions. And my prior and current other associates: Anne-Marie Ruthrauff, Michelle Lewis, and Candy Lawrence each deserve special thanks, as do some RealAge partners: Martin Rom and Charlie Silver; and Diane Reverand, who told me not to worry about offending medical colleagues — as long as the science was solid, they would understand we were trying to motivate YOU to understand that you can control your genes and jean size.

Nancy, and our children, Jeffrey and Jennifer: I want to thank you for more than your critical reviews and scientific expertise. Your encouragement and patience, constant love and support really are saint-like. Thanks, Saint Nancy.

I hope and believe this book will help YOU to take control of your waist. That would be the best reward any physician could want.

— Michael F. Roizen

I thank my colleagues in Cardiothoracic Surgery for supporting the belief that surgeons can heal with our pens as well as with the cold steel of a scalpel edge. They freed me to write and brainstorm, especially Dr. Eric Rose, Dr. Craig Smith, Dr. Yoshifuma Naka, Dr.

Mike Argenziano, Dr. Henry Spotnitz, Dr. Allan Stewart, Dr. Barry Esrig, and the other superb surgeons on our team. The physician assistants, especially Laura Baer, and the nurses in the OR, ICU, and floor cared so meticulously for my patients that in my free time I could turn my mind totally to this book without the need to "pick up the pieces" from my clinical work. My clinical office manager, Lidia Nieves, has a razor-sharp mind (and memory) that prevented any patient's care from being compromised. My administrative coordinator, Michelle Washburn, not only made sure that all the tasks surrounding the book were done on time, but also read countless drafts of the text and provided incredibly insightful commentary. Finally, our divisional administrator, Diane Amato, shared her precious intellect with me without concern for her time and provided critically important edits and broad opinions about the direction of our work. We would have had an inferior book without their advice and support.

Thanks to all my colleagues in other specialties who provided quality control by offering thoughtful feedback on our writing. We list them in our joint acknowledgment by name, but their tireless responses to my sometimes tedious questions will always be appreciated. Thanks to the wonderfully talented (and busy) public affairs group at New York-Presbyterian, including Bryan Dotson, Alicia Park, and Myrna Manners, who have taught me to communicate complex messages in an accessible fashion. Thank you Ivan Kronenfeld for all your guidance.

My parents, Mustafa and Suna Oz, taught me to work hard for my life goals and never let go, even when success appears a fading hope. My parents-in-law, Gerald and Emily Jane Lemole, shared their strong value system and desire to look for the more profound answers in seeking truth. Thanks to my wife and coauthor, Lisa, who all our friends unanimously agree is the "brains" of the family. It is fun to marry and work with one's soul mate. Our siblings — Seval, Nazlim, Laura, Emily, Michael, Samantha, and Christopher — selflessly offered honest commentary on our work. Our four children — Daphne, who inherited the bug and has written her first book; Arabella; Zoe; and Oliver — bring joy to our lives with their every breath. Thanks for sacrificing numerous weekends in the name of "Waist Management."

— Mehmet C. Oz

Index

abdominal muscles, 252, 256, 258, 264–72, 282–84, 306, 396
Acarbose (Precose), 388
Activity Plan, YOU
   and add-ons, 277–78
   benefits of, 256
   and bonus moves, 279–84
   and cardiovascular exercises, 256, 258, 262, 278, 279
   cheat sheet strategies for, 252
   and choosing a trainer, 264
   every day, 257
   preparation for, 262
   as step on YOU path, 17, 19
   three times a week, 257–73
   and waist size, 256
   and YOU-Turns, 248
   See also exercise(s); physical activity; Twenty-minute Workout;
      specific exercise
addictions, 29, 201, 211, 228, 385, 405
adiponectin, 136, 172–73
adrenal glands, 170, 169, 171, 203
age, 49, 161, 169, 182, 195
alcohol, 71, 74, 86, 159, 301, 413

allergies, 100, 98, 99, 107, 112, 328
American Association of Plastic Surgeons (AAPS), 405
American College of Sports Medicine (ACSM), 264
American College of Surgeons (ACS), 410
American Council on Exercise (ACE), 264
American Society for Aesthetic Plastic Surgery, 405
American Society of Bariatric Physicians (ASBP), 380
American Society for Bariatric Surgery (ASBS), 410, 422
American Society of Plastic Surgeons (ASPS), 393, 405
amino acids, 75, 83, 84, 82
amphetamines, 61, 385. See also CART
anorexia, 61
antidepressants, 381, 383
antioxidants, 121, 126, 129
antiseizure medications, 386
appetite
    anatomy of, 58–63
    and body temperature, 167
    and emotions, 56, 204–7
    and failed diets, 227, 231
    forms of, 56
    and hormones, 170–74
    and inflammation, 126
    myths about, 55
    and physical activity, 185
    physiology of, 17, 56–71
    and protein, 180, 294
    and steps on YOU path, 17
    and weight-loss drugs, 379–89
    and YOU Diet, 295
    and YOU-Turn, 243
Apricot Chicken and Green Beans with Almond Slivers (recipe), 356
arteries
    function of, 138–40
    and health risks of fat, 134–40, 143–47, 151, 152–53, 156, 159

430

and hormones, 165, 171
inflammation of, 102, 152–53, 253, 402
and weight-loss drugs, 379–80
and YOU Diet, 294
arthritis, 61, 103, 380
artificial colors, 129
Arugula, Watermelon, and Feta Salad (recipe), 341
Asian Salmon with Brown Rice Pilaf (recipe), 350
aspirin, 159, 253
Atkins diet, 44
ATP, 181, 186, 387
audit, of physical activity, 192
automatic eating, 22–25, 47, 249–51, 286–87, 290–92, 296, 311
avoiders
    and Activity Plan, 256
    and failed diets, 212–14, 227, 238

back, 256, 265–70, 282, 396, 401
bariatric surgery. *See* weight-loss surgery
bariatricians, 380
behavior change, 310, 378, 421
belly fat. *See* omentum
Bent-over Back Rows (exercise), 282
beta-blockers, 383
Bicycle (exercise), 283
bile, 81, 88, 111
birth-control pills, 173–74
bitter orange, 110
blame, 27, 165, 210–12, 218–19
blood pressure
    and failed diets, 229
    and genetics, 44–45
    and health risks of fat, 44, 136, 137, 143, 145, 145–48, 150–51,
        155, 169–70
    and herbs/supplements, 110

blood pressure (*continued*)
  and hormones, 170
  ideal, 133, 164
  and inflammation, 103
  myths about, 133, 161
  and physical activity, 186, 189
  testing of, 308
  and weight-loss drugs, 379, 381, 385
  and weight-loss surgery, 407
  and YOU Strategies, 253
  See also hypertension
blood sugar
  and digestion, 88, 89, 93
  fasting, 162
  and health risks of fat, 136–37, 141, 147–48, 149–51, 155, 162, 163
  and hormones, 170
  and inflammation, 118, 130
  testing of, 161, 253
  and weight-loss surgery, 418
  and YOU Diet, 294–96
  and YOU Strategies, 252
  blood tests, 143, 161, 164, 171, 175, 308. *See also specific test*
  blue tongue test, 95
body
  as ally, 16
  biology of, 17–18, 25
  design of, 17
  as gym, 256
  and how your body thinks, 20
  ideal, 41–51
  individuality of, 25
  knowledge about, 250
  listening to, 260
  reprogramming of, 16, 42, 47, 57, 66, 250, 286–87, 310

See also body image; body mass index; *specific body part*
body image, mirror, 50
body mass index (BMI), 380, 382, 389, 408, 421
brain
   and appetite, 58–63, 67
   and depression, 115
   and digestion, 77, 84–89, 90, 92
   and emotions, 106, 200, 206
   and failed diets, 210–11, 212, 217–18
   and inflammation, 100–101, 106, 114, 124
   myths about, 97
   and physical activity, 180, 185
   and portion control, 287
   stress on, 124
   and weight-loss drugs, 378–80
   and weight-loss surgery, 420–21
   and YOU Diet, 294
   and YOU Strategies, 252–54
   See also specific part of brain
breakfast, 168, 297, 301, 321, 330
Broiled Trout, Orata, or Branzini with Rosemary and Lemon
     (recipe), 358
bupropion (Wellbutrin), 381, 389

C-reactive protein (CRP), 121, 153, 162, 164, 253, 412
caffeine, 377, 382, 390, 413
calcium, 75, 110, 118, 145, 175, 289
calories
   calculating daily, 293–94
   counting of, 16
   and digestion, 80–82, 92
   and fast food, 321–22
   and food journals, 306
   and health risks of fat, 147–48, 152
   and hormones, 168, 169, 174

calories (*continued*)
  and inflammation, 107
  myths about, 80–81, 97
  and physical activity/exercise, 184, 188–89, 267, 283–84, 293
  and preparation for YOU Diet, 292–95
  and resting metabolic rate, 293
  slowing of intake of, 287
  and weight-loss drugs, 386
  and weight-loss surgery, 412, 420
  and YOU Diet, 310
canabinoid blockers, 379
cancer, 86, 103, 153, 160
capsaicin, 94–95
carbohydrates
  and appetite, 71
  and automating eating, 47
  as bad food, 288
  complex, 82–83
  and digestion, 73, 82–86
  and emotions, 201, 205–6
  as good food, 288
  and health risks of fat, 160
  and hormones, 171–72
  and ideal body, 44
  and inflammation, 118, 129
  myths about, 73, 81
  and physical activity, 188–89
  simple, 288
  and weight-loss drugs, 383, 388–89
  and whole grains/wheat, 319
  and YOU Strategies, 252
  and YOU-Turn, 246
cardiovascular training
  and audit of activity, 192
  benefits of, 185–87

and calories, 293

equipment for, 277, 278

and exercising the right way, 258–59

myths about, 177

overview of, 278

as part of Activity Plan, 256, 279

preparation for, 262

too much, 188

and YOU Diet, 307

and YOU fitness test, 194–95

Carrot, Raisin, and Yogurt Slaw (recipe), 348

CART (cocaine-amphetamine-regulatory transcript), 60, 61, 64, 66–68, 212

CCK (cholecystokinin)

and appetite, 68

and digestion, 86–88, 92–94

gastric pacemaker as mimicking, 420–21

and inflammation, 128

and psychology of failed diet, 229–30

and weight-loss drugs, 379, 382, 386, 389

Celexa, 382

cellulite, 391, 395

cheat/crib sheet

for Activity Plan, 252

for YOU Diet, 251–52, 288–89

for YOU Strategies, 250–52

chemistry

of emotions, 199–206

and weight-loss drugs, 378–86

and weight-loss surgery, 420

and YOU Diet, 294–96

and YOU Strategies, 253

and YOU-Turn in thinking, 243

See also specific agent

The Chest Cross (exercise), 260–61

chest/shoulders exercises, 256–65, 281
Chicken Kabobs with Tabbouleh (recipe), 360
chocolate, 86, 300
cholesterol
  and age, 161
  drugs for, 143
  and emotions, 206
  HDL, 143, 146–47, 156, 157, 159, 161, 164, 172, 294–95, 308, 379
  and health risks of fat, 135–36, 143–45, 146–48, 150, 152, 155–61, 411
  and hormones, 172
  ideal, 164
  and inflammation, 100, 102–3, 120–21, 128
  LDL, 136, 137, 141, 143, 146–47, 153, 156, 161, 164, 295, 308
  and physical activity, 187
  testing of, 253, 308
  and weight-loss drugs, 379, 388
  and YOU Diet, 294–96
chromium, 162–63, 253–54
cimetidine, 389
cinnamon, 163, 252, 289
Cinnamon Apple Sauté à la Mode (recipe), 369
Cinnamon Baked Apples with Tangerines and Cranberries (recipe), 368
The Clapper (exercise), 263
cocaine, 61. *See also* CART
coenzyme Q10, 186, 253–54
coffee, 86, 129, 138. *See also* caffeine
collagen, 395, 397
colon, 74–75, 108
comfort food, 385
comfort level, 242–44
contingency plans, 28, 247–48
coping patterns, 235–36

cortisol, 116, 169, 170, 175
Cranberries, Walnuts, and Crumbled Cheese over Greens (recipe), 340
cravings
  and emotions, 199–207
  and failed diets, 212–13, 221, 227
  and fiber, 295
  and weight-loss drugs, 379, 383, 389
  and YOU Diet, 303, 310
  and YOU Strategies, 252
  See also CCK
CRH (corticotrophin-releasing hormone), 170
Crunch (exercise), 282
Curried Split Pea Soup (recipe), 335

dairy products, 129. *See also specific product*
depression, 186, 200, 201, 206, 211, 218, 224, 380, 381–84
deprivation, food, 20, 21, 23, 66, 167, 287. *See also* starvation
desserts, 300, 324, 368–72
diabetes
  and genetics, 44, 148–49
  and health risks of fat, 44–45, 61, 134, 148–49, 162, 381, 411
  and hormones, 170
  and inflammation, 102
  and lifestyle, 148–49
  and weight-loss drugs, 380, 383
  and weight-loss surgery, 407, 421
Diet, YOU
  basic principles of, 286–88
  and calories, 292–95
  cheat/crib sheet for, 250–52, 288–89
  choices in, 294–301
  and defining the problem, 291
  Fourteen-day, 290, 303–18
  journal for, 288

Diet, YOU (*continued*)
  mantra, 245–46
  meals for, 294–320
  and medications, 308
  overview about, 286–88
  partnering up for, 305
  and physical activity, 310
  preparations for, 289–95
  as step on YOU path, 18–19
  Troubleshooting Guide for, 327–28
  and Twenty-minute Workout, 306–8, 310–11
  and YOU-Turns, 289–88, 307–8, 310, 327
  See also specific recipe
diets/dieting
  and comfort level, 242–43
  effects of, 28
  elimination, 128–29, 328
  has to be hard, 41
  and hormones, 166
  mistakes during, 209, 220, 245–49, 251
  myths about, 209, 211, 217, 220
  and planning to fail, 247–49
  promises of, 15, 22
  psychology of failed, 209–38
  reasons for failure of, 21
  thinking about, 57, 210, 221
  and weight-loss surgery, 412, 421
  yo-yo, 20, 216, 411
  YOU as challenging beliefs about, 21–22
  YOU-Turn in thinking about, 241–54
  See also specific diet
digestion
  and breaking down nutrients, 80–82
  and inflammation, 82
  main areas of, 82–89

myths about, 73, 80–82, 87–88
overview about, 76–80
preparation for, 76–77
and satiety, 90
tips about, 92–95
and weight-loss drugs, 381, 387
and weight-loss surgery, 412, 419
YOU Test about, 95
See also metabolism
dinner, recipes for, 350–65
DNA, 103, 121
doctors, 27, 308, 380, 390, 400, 402, 402–5
domino effects, 147
dopamine, 201, 205, 207, 381, 385
Downward Dog Pose (exercise), 248
drinks, 182, 301, 329. *See also* alcohol; soft drinks
drugs
    cholesterol, 143
    and emotions, 205, 206
    exercise as, 178
    food as, 67, 221, 224
    and genetics versus environment, 44–45
    illegal, 205–6, 379
    that slow weight loss, 328
    See also weight-loss drugs; *specific drug*
dumping syndrome, 419
duodenal switch, 415–19
duodenum, 75, 88

eating
    environment for, 321
    frequency of, 48, 251–52
    hedonistic, 200, 379, 385
    patterns of, 232–33
    preparation for, 327–28

eating (*continued*)

  and sample eating schedule, 311–13

  YOU Strategies for, 251–52

  See also automatic eating; meals

eating disorders, 51

elimination diet, 129–30, 328

emergency food, 252, 288, 295

emotions

  and brain, 106

  chemistry of, 199–207

  and failed diets, 220, 226

  and hormones, 204–6

  and inflammation, 106, 107, 114

  myths about, 97, 199, 206

  role in weight issues of, 17

  as signals of appetite, 56

  and steps on YOU path, 17

  tips about, 206–7

  and YOU-Turn, 243

endocrine system, 168–71

energy

  and digestion, 73, 76, 81–82, 84, 82, 89, 90, 91

  and health risks of fat, 136, 138, 140, 155

  and hormones, 168, 170–73

  importance of, 90

  and inflammation, 109, 117

  myths about, 73

  and physical activity, 181, 182, 183, 184, 185, 186, 187

  and weight-loss drugs, 387

environment

  for eating, 321

  and ideal body, 44–45

ephedra, 110, 383

esophagus, 78, 86, 129

estrogen, 64, 153, 169, 171, 172, 173–74

evolution, 42–44, 114
excuses, 192–94, 224–25, 232–34, 256, 284
Exercise Ball Moves (exercise), 283
exercise(s)
  add-ons, 257, 277–78
  and bonus moves, 279–84
  breathing during, 259–62
  and calories, 267, 284
  and cooldowns, 262–63
  counting during, 258–59
  and digestion, 84, 86, 91
  and excuses, 256, 284
  and exercising the right way, 258–59
  and failed diets, 232–37
  and fat, 20, 163
  forms of, 180–83
  and heart rate, 259, 262, 278, 306
  and inflammation, 116
  intensity of, 188
  as medication, 178
  and metabolism, 284
  outward signs of, 188
  and pain, 263
  and plastic surgery, 402
  preparation for, 262–63
  role in weight loss of, 20
  sex as, 278
  shoes for, 263
  spot-reduction, 184
  and steps on YOU path, 17–19
  and stress, 256
  too much, 188
  variation in, 257
  and waist size, 24
  and weight-loss drugs, 388

exercise(s) (*continued*)
  and weight-loss surgery, 421
  weight-training, 177, 185
  See also Activity Plan, YOU; physical activity; *type of exercise*
eyelid surgery, 393

face/neck-lifts, 393, 395
fast food, 41, 126, 210, 297–98, 321–22
fasting, 90, 110
fat
  absorption of, 387–89
  as bad, 133, 288
  brown, 57
  burning of, 17, 46, 91, 165–75, 177–95, 256, 306
  classic psychology of, 27
  domino effect of, 147–48
  fighting, 17
  as good, 57, 288, 295
  health risks of, 133–64
  importance of, 172
  myths about, 21, 41, 73, 104–5, 133, 161
  saturated/unsaturated, 70, 88, 100, 127, 129, 148, 152, 156–59, 250–51, 288, 303–4, 326, 388
  storing of, 17, 21, 42, 43, 46, 48–49, 57, 58, 74, 135, 250
  subcutaneous, 136–38
  trans, 83, 100, 118, 127, 129, 148, 152, 157, 251, 288, 302, 304, 326, 388
  types of, 136–37, 156–57
  as way of avoiding failure, 225
  weight of, 399
  words for, 303
  See also specific topic
fat cells, size of, 43
Fat Facts Test, 31–36
fat-free food, 119, 302

fatty acids, 48. *See also* omega-3 fatty acids
fiber
  and automating eating, 47
  and cravings, 295
  and digestion, 80, 89, 92
  as good, 288
  and inflammation, 103
  and weight-loss drugs, 388–89
  and whole grains/wheat, 319
  and YOU Diet, 296
  and YOU Strategies, 253–54
5–HTP, 252, 253
flexibility, 191, 191, 195. *See also* stretching/flexibility exercises
food
  absorption of, 107
  allergies, 99–101, 108, 112, 328
  anti-inflammatory, 251
  and automating eating, 47
  bad, 126, 212, 214, 216, 288, 290, 294
  comfort, 385
  as drugs, 67, 221, 224
  dumping, 304–5
  elimination of, 129–30, 328
  emergency, 252, 288, 295
  fat-free, 303
  good, 288
  journals, 252, 288–89, 306
  labels for, 69, 251–52, 302–3, 326
  mood, 203
  natural, 302
  premade, 295
  shopping for, 305, 307, 309
  substitution, 227, 288
  variety of, 227
  YOU-th-full, 291

food (*continued*)
  your turn to, 248
  See also meals; portion size; recipes
Food and Drug Administration (FDA), U.S., 112
food memory, 200, 212–13
Fourteen-day YOU Diet, 290, 303–18
fructose, 67–68. *See also* high-fructose corn syrup
fruits, 42–45, 48, 302
fullness
  gauge of, 226, 287
  See also satiety

GABA (gamma-aminobutyric acid), 201, 386
Garcinia, 254, 387
Garden Harvest Soup (recipe), 381
gas, 102, 104, 106, 109–10
gastric banding, 410, 413, 415
gastric bypass surgery, 81, 407, 417–19
gastric pacemaker, 420–21
genetics
  and blame, 27
  and diabetes, 149
  and health risks of fat, 148
  and hormones, 168, 171–72
  and ideal body, 44, 49
  and inflammation, 98, 102, 114, 117, 120
  and obesity, 123, 409
  and plastic surgery, 396, 400
  and steps on YOU path, 19
  and YOU Tips, 19
GERD (gastroesophageal reflux disease), 86, 87, 389
ghrelin, 59, 65–68, 71, 200, 287, 412
glucophage, 176, 388
glucose
  and digestion, 74, 82, 90

and health risks of fat, 148–52, 162
and hormones, 170–71
and ideal body, 44–45
and inflammation, 100–101, 120–21
and physical activity, 186
See also sugar
gluten, 98. See also wheat
glycogen, 91, 246–47
grapefruit oil, 118, 253–54
Greek Feta Salad with Peppers and Olives (recipe), 342
green tea, 127, 251
Grilled Peanut Shrimp with Sesame Snow Peas (recipe), 363
guilt, 27, 214, 215, 216, 217, 218, 380
gut
    inflammation in, 97–131
    weight-loss drugs that influence, 386–89
    See also specific part of gut
gyms, 256

Hafen, Tracy, 264
Harper, Joel, 264
health
    as purpose of losing weight, 311
    risks of fat, 28, 133–64
    and thinness, 133
heart attacks, 110, 134, 141, 143, 147–48, 159, 178, 187, 383
heart disease, 100, 153, 163, 166
heart rate, 194, 259, 262, 278, 306, 308, 381, 390
Hearts of Palm Salad with Tomato and Mushrooms (recipe), 347
height, 381
herbs, 110. See also specific herb
high-fructose corn syrup (HFCS), 67–68, 251, 288, 304, 319, 321–22
hip/hamstring exercises, 261, 266–70
The Hippie (exercise), 261
hippocampus, 213

Hoodia, 253–54, 387
hormones
  and appetite, 63, 71
  and digestion, 92
  and emotions, 204–6
  and failed diets, 212
  as fat burners, 165–76
  and health risks of fat, 137, 146–47, 153–55
  and inflammation, 118–22, 125
  myths about, 165–68, 173
  reprogramming of, 172
  sex, 173–74
  and YOU Strategies, 253
Hot Wild Salmon (recipe), 362
hunger
  and appetite, 58–71
  and digestion, 73, 87–88
  and emotions, 199, 203, 205–6
  and failed diets, 226
  and goal of YOU Strategies, 28–29
  and hormones, 170
  myths about, 55, 73
  test for, 226
hypertension
  causes of, 138
  and genetics, 44
  and inflammation, 100
  and weight-loss drugs, 383, 385
  and weight-loss surgery, 411–13, 420–22
  as weight-related illness, 61, 144, 380
hypnosis, 229–31
hypothalamus, 58–60, 90, 170, 200, 211, 387

ileocecal valve, 89–95
immune system, 101, 111, 121, 138, 147, 151, 160

446

impotence, 143, 148
inflammation
  of arteries, 152–53, 253, 402
  causes of, 100–104
  and digestion, 82
  fight against, 118–23
  and food-elimination test, 129–30
  gut, 97–130
  and health risks of fat, 136, 147, 148, 152–53, 156, 159, 162
  and hormones, 166, 173–76
  of liver, 388
  myths about, 97, 103–4, 106
  overview about, 99–104
  and smoking, 402
  and stress, 114–18, 124–26
  and weight-loss drugs, 387
  and weight-loss surgery, 412
  and YOU Diet, 294, 311
  and YOU Strategies, 252–54
insulin
  and appetite, 61
  and digestion, 90, 93
  and emotions, 205
  and health risks of fat, 135, 148–52, 163
  and hormones, 170, 176
  and inflammation, 100, 116, 120, 124, 130
  and obesity, 411
  and weight-loss drugs, 381, 387–89
  and whole grains/wheat, 319–20
International Society of Aesthetic Plastic Surgery (ISAPS), 405
Invisible Chair (exercise), 272

Japanese Ginger Salad with Pumpkin Seeds and Sprouts (recipe), 338
joint problems, 151, 155, 186

jojoba beans, 128, 254
Journal of the American Medical Association, 47
journals, food, 252, 288–89, 306

kidneys, 143, 145, 170
konjac root, 93
Kushner, Robert, 232

labels, 69, 251–52, 302–3, 319, 326
lactose, 74, 98, 103, 112. *See also* milk
laparoscopy, 412, 422
Leg Drop (exercise), 268–69
leg exercises, 266–73, 279–81
Lemon Caper Chicken with Sweet Potato Puree (recipe), 359
leptin
  and appetite, 59, 62, 63–65, 66–68, 70, 71
  and digestion, 87
  and emotions, 200
  and genetics, 45
  and inflammation, 128
  and weight-loss drugs, 379
  and weight-loss surgery, 412
  and YOU Diet, 289–90
Lexapro, 382
lifestyle, 45, 114–15, 140, 148–49, 378, 409, 410, 413, 421
Lip Lick, 308
lipid profile blood test, 161
liposuction, 391, 393, 398, 399–402, 405
Lisa's Great Gazpacho (recipe), 332
liver
  cirrhosis of, 105
  and digestion, 80, 81–82, 82, 90
  fatty, 105
  and health risks of fat, 135–38
  and hormones, 175

and inflammation, 100, 105, 106, 115–23, 126, 388
and weight-loss drugs, 379
and YOU Diet, 310
longevity, 172, 411
low-calorie diets, 48
low-carb diets, 246
low-fat diets, 55, 80–81
lunch, choices for, 298
Lunges (exercise), 279
luteinizing hormone/follicle-stimulating hormone test, 175
lycopene, 118

macrophages, 101, 111
Magical Breakfast Blaster (recipe), 330
magnesium, 74, 162, 289
mammillary body, 60, 212
mannitol, 303
mantra, YOU-Turn, 245–46, 248
marijuana, 62, 379
mast cells, 101, 111
mates, 123. *See also* support system
meals
  frequency of, 48, 251–52
  journal, 252, 306
  planning, 48–49
  preparation for, 287
  ready-made, 326
  sameness/variety in, 296
  strategies for, 288
  YOU Diet, 294–318
  YOUR choices for, 294–303
  See also eating; recipes
meat, 42–45, 43–44, 83
medical options, 18, 375–76. *See also* plastic surgery; weight-loss
    drugs; weight-loss surgery

Medicare, 410

medications. *See* drugs; weight-loss drugs

medicine cabinet, 253–54

meditation, 163, 229–30

Mediterranean Cauliflower Salad (recipe), 345

Mediterranean Chicken with Tomatoes, Olives, and Herbed White
    Beans (recipe), 354

Mediterranean diet, 47

melatonin, 207

men
  and BMI, 381
  and hormones, 172
  ideal weight for, 410
  waist size for, 24, 253, 380, 409

Meridia, 385

mesotherapy, 392

metabolism
  and appetite, 61
  and body temperature, 167
  and exercises, 284
  and hormones, 166–68
  myths about, 21
  phases of, 90
  and physical activity, 186
  and resting metabolic rate, 293
  "slow," 165
  and Twenty-minute Workout, 306
  and weight-loss drugs, 283, 388, 389
  See also digestion

Metformin, 176, 388

milk, 103, 111–12. *See also* lactose

mind
  and failed diets, 209–38
  reprogramming of, 220
  role in weight loss of, 17, 20

and YOU-Turns, 241–54
See also emotions; willpower
Minted Fresh Pea Soup (recipe), 337
mirror image test, 50–51
mistakes
  and preparation for YOU Diet, 291
  and restaurants, 324
  while dieting, 209, 220, 245–49, 252
  and YOU Diet, 310, 327
  and YOU Strategies, 250, 252
  and YOU-Turns, 29, 289–91, 310, 327
monosodium glutamate (MSG), 152
mood, 203–7, 211, 381
motivation, 244, 306, 380
mouth, 88, 212–13
muscle cells, size of, 43
muscle(s)
  adding more, 185
  and appetite, 65
  and digestion, 73, 81, 84, 82
  focusing on, 263
  foundation, 189–90, 256
  and health risks of fat, 152, 162
  and hormones, 171–74
  involuntary, 183
  mass, 181–86, 189–91, 260, 284
  myths about, 73, 80–82
  oblique, 265–66, 396
  peripheral, 191
  and physical activity, 177, 178–95
  quadricep, 271–72
  skeletal, 179
  and weight, 20
  weight of, 184
  and weight-loss drugs, 379

muscle(s) (*continued*)
  See also Activity Plan, YOU; exercise(s); *specific muscles*
myths, 21, 41. *See also specific myth*

National Strength and Conditioning Association (NCSA), 264
natural food, 302
nervous system, 151, 186–87
NF-kappa B, 119–24, 126
niacin, 159
Nice Thighs (exercise), 272–73
nicotine, 123, 140, 382, 390. *See also* smoking
nitric oxide, 203, 222
nonexercise activity thermogenesis (NEAT), 167
norepinephrine, 115, 203, 381, 382
NPY (neuropeptide Y), 60–61, 64–68, 71, 115, 204, 207, 212
nutritionists, 27–28, 289, 422

obesity
  as disease of inflammation, 103
  and genetics, 409
  and health problems, 28
  and lifestyle, 409
  and longevity, 411
  morbid, 409, 411
  and risk factors, 375, 412–13
  statistics about, 411
  and waist size, 409
  weird causes of, 123
  See also weight-loss surgery
  olestra, 116
omega-3 fatty acids, 48, 127, 157, 163, 174, 206, 251, 289, 295
omega-6 fatty acids, 157
omentum
  and health risks of fat, 135–38, 148, 153–55, 155
  and hormones, 172

and inflammation, 104, 105, 113–19, 126
and major principles for YOU Strategies, 250
and weight-loss drugs, 379
Orient Express Salad with Chopped Peanuts (recipe), 344
orlistat (Xenical), 386–87, 388
oxytocin, 222, 230–31, 382

partnering up, 305
PCOS (polycystic ovary syndrome), 173–76
Pecs Flex (exercise), 262–65
personality, 203, 232–37
phen-fen, 385
physical activity
    and appetite, 65
    audit of, 192
    benefits of, 185–89
    and burning fat faster, 177–95
    and calories, 293–94
    excuses about, 192–94
    and failed diets, 229
    fantastic four of, 189–94
    and health risks of fat, 145, 146–48, 152, 160
    and hormones, 166–68
    and ideal body, 44
    importance of, 185–87
    and inflammation, 130
    and metabolism, 186
    myths about, 165, 177, 180–81
    test about, 194–95
    and YOU Diet, 311–13
    See also Activity Plan, YOU; exercise(s)
physical examinations, 308–9
Pineapple-Banana Protein Blaster (recipe), 329
pizza crust, 306, 353

planning
    contingency, 29, 247–48
    to fail, 248–49
plastic surgery
    as addictive, 405
    additional, 405–6
    before-and-after photos of, 404
    disappointments about, 403
    and exercise, 402
    and face/neck-lifts, 393, 397–98
    and finding a surgeon, 403–4
    functions of, 375–76
    and insurance, 400
    and liposuction, 391, 393, 398, 399–402, 403–6
    myths about, 391–92, 395, 399
    reality check for, 403
    risks of, 392
    and saggy, stretchy skin, 392, 393–96
    and scars, 398, 399, 403
    training for, 403–4
    and tummy tucks, 396–97
plateaus, 18, 253, 309, 311, 327, 378, 380, 389
portion size, 47, 93, 287, 293
posture, 272, 306, 396–97
potassium, 74, 145, 175
PPARs (peroxisome proliferator-activated receptors), 120–21, 122–24, 126
Precose, 388
premade food, 294–95
protein
    and appetite, 180, 295
    and automating eating, 47
    and digestion, 73, 74–75, 80–81, 82–86
    and failed diets, 214
    as good, 288

and health risks of fat, 149, 151, 160
and ideal body, 44–45
and inflammation, 118–20
myths about, 73, 80–82
and physical activity, 144, 179–80, 182–86, 186
and rise of agriculture, 46
and whole grains/wheat, 319
and YOU Diet, 294–96
and YOU Strategies, 252
See also C-reactive protein
psychiatrists, 422
Push-ups (exercise), 261–62, 281–82

quercetin, 128
Quick Black Bean Soup (recipe), 336

ready-made meals, 326
rebounders, 278
recipes
    breakfast, 330
    dessert, 368–71
    dinner, 350–65
    drink, 329
    salad, 338–49
    for side dishes, 366–67
    snack, 372
    soup, 331–37
    and steps on YOU path for weight loss, 17–19
    and YOU diet and Activity Plan, 18
resistance training, 180–85, 189, 283–84
restaurants, 324–25
resting metabolic rate, 293
rhinoplasty (nose jobs), 393
The Rickety Table (exercise), 265–66
rimonabant, 379

Roasted Pear with Raspberry Coulis, Chocolate, and Pistachios
    (recipe), 370
Rock Asparagus (recipe), 366
Roll With It (exercise), 259–60
Royal Pasta Primavera Provençale (recipe), 355

saccharin test, 95
salads, 298, 338–49
salt, 45, 203
satiety
  and appetite, 58–63, 66–71
  and calories, 292
  and digestion, 81, 89, 92
  and emotions, 202
  and genetics vs. environment, 44–45
  myths about, 73, 81
  and portion control, 287
  and preparation for meals, 290
  and preparation for YOU Diet, 290–91
  signals for, 295
  and weight-loss drugs, 386
  and weight-loss surgery, 420
  and YOU Strategies, 252
  See also CART; leptin
schedule, sample eating, 311–13
Seated Drop Kick (exercise), 271
The Seated Pretzel (exercise), 266
self-assessment, 18
self-esteem, 221–25, 229, 380, 383
serotonin, 114, 115, 203–7, 242, 384–85, 388
serving size. *See* portion size
Sesame Cucumber Salad (recipe), 349
sex, 71, 173–74, 253, 278. *See also* impotence
shame, 215, 216–17, 218, 380
shoes, running, 263, 307

shopping, food, 305–7, 309, 314–18

shoulders. *See* chest/shoulders exercises

Simon's Popcorn, 300, 372

sleep/sleep apnea, 153–55, 207, 253, 379–80, 421

Sliced Peaches with Raspberries, Blueberries, and Chocolate Chips (recipe), 371

small intestine, 103–5, 106–13

smell, 77

smoking, 100, 102–3, 123, 390, 402. *See also* nicotine

snacks, 299–300, 327–28, 372

soft drinks, 70, 103, 138

sodium, *see* salt

soul, and failed diets, 221–25

soups, 295, 298, 326, 331–37

Spicy Chili (recipe), 351

Spicy Vegetable Lentil Soup (recipe), 333

Spinach-Walnut-Citrus Salad (recipe), 339

spot reduction, 184

Squats (exercise), 280

SSRIs (selective serotonin reuptake inhibitors), 382

stamina-based training, 180, 185–86, 192

starvation, 48, 61, 168, 201, 251. *See also* deprivation, food

Steady on the Plank (exercise), 264

Step Taps (exercise), 280–81

steroids, 124, 129–30, 171, 397

stomach
  and digestion, 75, 80, 87–89
  full, 73, 86
  growling, 93
  and inflammation, 97
  myths about, 97
  and physical activity, 189, 194
  See also omentum

strength exercises, 179–89, 191, 192, 252, 256–73, 283, 293, 306

stress
  and appetite, 64
  chronic, 114–15, 124, 126
  and emotions, 200, 203, 205–6
  and exercise, 256
  and failed diets, 211, 221, 226, 227–31
  and health risks of fat, 136, 140, 145
  and hormones, 169, 170
  and ideal body, 47
  and inflammation, 100, 103–4, 114–18, 124–26
  and physical activity, 188
  types of, 114–16
stretch marks, 393–95, 397
stretching/flexibility exercises, 256–57, 262–70, 272–73, 303–10
stroke, 134, 143, 148, 160
Stuffed Whole Wheat Pizza (recipe), 253
substitution food, 227–28, 288
sugar
  and appetite, 70
  as bad, 288
  and digestion, 73, 81–86, 88–89, 90–91
  dumping, 304
  and emotions, 203, 205–6
  and evolution, 42–43, 46
  and failed diets, 212–14
  and fast food, 321
  and health risks of fat, 138, 146–48, 152, 155
  and ideal body, 44
  and inflammation, 98, 102, 103, 114, 118, 130
  myths about, 73
  natural, 303
  and physical activity, 186
  simple, 45, 69, 81, 84, 88–89, 146–48, 152, 162, 187, 251–52, 304, 321
  and weight-loss drugs, 385–86, 388

and whole grains/wheat, 319

words for, 304

and YOU Strategies, 251–52

See also glucose; sweeteners

Sun Salutation (exercise), 268

Superman (exercise), 266

supplements, 110, 253–54, 417. *See also* vitamins; *specific supplement*

support system, 218–19, 249–50, 289, 327

surgery. See plastic surgery; weight-loss surgery

Sweet Beet and Gorgonzola Salad (recipe), 346

sweeteners, 130, 304

tai chi, 187

taste, 76, 88, 94–95, 199, 227, 389

teeth, 79–80

tegaserod (Zelnorm), 388–89

testosterone, 64, 169–76

test(s)

  avoider, 238

  and failed diets, 231–38

  Fat Facts, 31–39

  and hormones, 170, 175

  hunger, 225

  mirror image, 50–51

  overview about, 19

  personality, 232–37

  and physical activity, 194–95

  saccharin, 95

  and taste, 94

  why ask why, 230–31

  YOU, 95, 164, 230–31, 232–37, 238

  and YOU Strategies, 253–54

  See also test, YOU; *specific type of test*

thinness, 133, 134, 212, 224

thirst, 70, 252, 412. *See also* drinks
thyroid-stimulating hormone test, 175
Tight Pants Syndrome, 104
Tofu or Turkey Dogs with Sauerkraut (recipe), 365
Tomato-Avocado Salsamole (recipe), 367
tongue, 77–78, 95, 212–13
topiramate, 386
trainers, 27, 264, 289
triglycerides, 90, 120–21, 135, 136, 379
Troubleshooting Guide, YOU Diet, 327–28
tummy tucks, 394–98
Turkey Tortilla Wraps with Red Baked Potato (recipe), 357
Turkish Shepherd Salad (recipe), 343
Twenty-minute Workout, 256, 258–73, 306–10
Two-Onion Delight (recipe), 334

Up, Dog, Up (exercise), 264
urinary cortisol test, 175
urine test, 171

vanitidine, 389
Vegetable Tofu Stir-fry (recipe), 364
vegetables, 42–43, 48, 293
vitamins, 45, 74–75, 94, 159, 289, 318, 387, 397, 412–13. *See also*
    supplements
vomiting, 129

Waist Hang, 308
waist size
  and Activity Plan, 257
  and exercise, 24–25
  and failed diets, 214
  focusing on management of, 23–25
  and gender, 253, 409
  and health risks of fat, 134, 138, 148, 153, 155

ideal, 24, 138, 253, 409
importance of, 249
and major principles for YOU Strategies, 250
measurement of, 253
for men, 25, 253, 380, 410
and obesity, 409
and physical activity, 179, 188
and weight, 24
for women, 24, 253, 380, 409
and YOU Diet, 308–10
walking
and activity audit, 192
and failed diets, 218, 229
importance of, 189, 257
and pain, 327
as part of Activity Plan, 257
and stretch marks, 397
tips about, 189
and weight-loss surgery, 410
and YOU Diet, 303–10
and YOU Strategies, 252
weight
of fat, 400
fluctuation in, 246
goal for, 247
ideal/healthy, 50–51, 63, 409–11
and major principles for YOU Strategies, 250
and muscle, 20
reasons for losing, 310, 392
reasons for not losing, 42–47
side effects of excess, 44
and waist size, 24–25
and weight-loss surgery, 409–11
and YOU Diet, 309–10
YOU path for losing, 16–20

weight cycle, 214, 216, 224
weight-loss drugs
  and dopamine, 385–86
  functions of, 375
  future of, 386
  and GABA, 386
  myths about, 377–79, 390
  and norepinephrine, 381
  over-the-counter, 377
  and plateaus, 253, 309, 327
  popular image of, 378
  risks of, 385
  and serotonin, 381–88
  side effects of, 379, 382, 388
  that influence gut, 386–88
  weight-loss surgery compared with, 409
weight-loss surgery
  and brain, 420
  and calories, 420
  candidates for, 421
  common views about, 407
  duodenal switch, 415–17
  functions of, 375
  gastric banding, 413–15, 410, 417, 419
  gastric bypass, 417–20
  and gastric pacemaker, 420
  and ideal weight, 409–10
  malabsorptive, 412, 415–20
  myths about, 407, 412
  overview about, 408–11
  questions about, 421–22
  restrictive, 413–15, 412, 417–20
  risks/complications of, 413, 415, 419, 422
  routes for, 411–13
  side effects of, 422

success in, 410, 412

whom to trust to do, 422

weight-training exercise, 177, 185, 258–59, 277–78

Wellbutrin (bupropion), 381, 389

wheat, 98, 129, 304, 318–19, 352–53

"whole grains," 302, 319–20

Whose Side Are You On, Anyway? (exercise), 265

Why Ask Why test, 230–31

willpower

and appetite, 63, 65, 66

and emotions, 199

and failed diets, 209, 211, 213

and ideal body, 42–45

as insufficient force for losing weight, 15–16, 23

myths about, 55, 199, 209

and YOU Diet, 286, 295–96

and YOU-Turn in thinking, 242

women

and BMI, 381

and cholesterol, 308

and hormones, 169, 171–74

ideal weight for, 410

postmenopausal, 174

waist size for, 24–25, 253, 380, 409

www.choicescount.com, 288

www.jcaho.org, 404

www.mychoicescount.com, 219, 295, 306

www.oprah.com, 264

www.realage.com, 258, 264, 291, 305–6, 310, 327, 413, 417

X Crunch (exercise), 271

Xenical, 386–88

yo-yo dieting, 20, 216, 411

yoga, 257, 268–69

YOU Strategies
  cheat sheet for, 250–54
  for eating, 251–52
  flexibility of, 29–30
  focusing vs. relying on, 26–27
  major principles for, 250–51
  purpose of, 286
  See also specific strategy
YOU-reka Moments, 18–19
YOU-th-full food, 291
YOU-Turn
  and cheat sheet of YOU strategies, 249–51
  function of, 29
  mantra, 245–49
  and mistakes, 289, 292, 310, 327
  overview about, 241–44
  and principles of YOU Diet, 288–89
  tips about, 245–49
  and YOU Diet, 289–91, 311, 327

Z-trim, 119
Zantac, 389
Zelnorm (tegaserod), 388
Zoloft, 382

About the Authors

Michael F. Roizen, M.D., is a professor of anesthesiology and internal medicine and chair of the Division of Anesthesiology, Critical Care Medicine, and Comprehensive Pain Management at the Cleveland Clinic.

Mehmet C. Oz, M.D., is a professor and vice chairman of surgery as well as director of the Cardiovascular Institute and Integrated Medical Center, New York Presbyterian-Columbia University.